Shakespearean Maternities

Crises of Conception in Early Modern England

Chris Laoutaris

Edinburgh University Press

Edinburgh University Press Ltd
22 George Square, Edinburgh

Typeset in Sabon and Futura
by Servis Filmsetting Ltd, Stockport, Cheshire, and
printed and bound in Great Britain by
CPI Antony Rowe, Chippenham, Wilts

A CIP record for this book is available from the British Library

ISBN 978 0 7486 2436 2 (hardback)

Contents

Acknowledgements

This book has been a long time in the making. It began life as a doctoral project which was completed at University College London's Department of English Language and Literature. An interdisciplinary study of this nature would not have been possible without the help and support of a great many individuals who have contributed in tangible ways to its development at every stage. I owe so much to my family, whose encouragement and tireless devotion is – and will always be – the foundation of everything I do; in particular my mum, Thalia; my dad, John; and my brother, George to whose memory this book is dedicated. Although my brother did not live to see its publication, his wisdom, patience and courage have been silent shaping principles which have gently nurtured this study and which will continue to inform every other project I undertake in the future. He will always be, in some way, the mother of my invention.

Particular thanks are due to the academic and administrative staff at University College London. From the first day I enrolled at UCL's Department of English Language and Literature as an undergraduate student they have been a limitless source of inspiration and guidance. I am deeply indebted to Helen Hackett, who first ignited in me an interest in the field of early modern women's studies. Her influence on my work has been tremendous and I have benefited from her generosity and friendship in more ways than I have room to detail here. I am immensely grateful to René Weis, whose expertise has guided this project from its very earliest stages. His support, both professional and personal, is greatly appreciated. I must also express my gratitude for the inspirational tutoring of John Sutherland, Paul Davies and Bas Aarts, who have been decisive influences in the shaping of my writing over the years. Special thanks go to Kathryn Metzenthin and Anita Garfoot, the administrative team of the English department. I have benefited daily from their hard work and dedicated professionalism as well as their kindness.

UCL is continuing to provide a nurturing and stimulating culture for my ongoing research and I am incredibly grateful to the former Head of Department, now Dean of the Faculty of Arts and Humanities, Henry Woudhuysen (who also provided feedback on segments of the original thesis which has shaped the methodology of this book in significant ways) and to the current Head of Department Susan Irvine for their much-appreciated support.

I feel immensely privileged to have had the opportunity to work alongside Kate Moncrief of Washington College and Kate McPherson of Utah Valley State College. Sharing with them my passion for early modern maternity studies has been an enriching experience and one which has left an indelible impression on this book. An earlier draft of the fourth chapter appeared in their edited collection *Performing Maternity in Early Modern England*, published by Ashgate Press in 2007. I am similarly grateful to Caroline Bicks for her insightful comments on an early version of the same chapter and for our discussions on maternity and the Renaissance theatre. I must also extend my heartfelt gratitude to Kate Chedgzoy and Valerie Wayne for their sensitive and highly astute feedback on this project during its fledgling stages. This book would not have been published without their positive assessments. I owe a special debt to David Margolies for his much-valued support and wisdom. Our many conversations, both while I was teaching at Goldsmiths College (University of London) and after, have meant a great deal to me. I would also like to thank Katherine Duncan-Jones and Gordon McMullan for their observations on this study at the doctoral stage. Their judicious responses have made this a better book than it otherwise would have been.

Particular thanks go to Jackie Jones, who first commissioned the book, Máiréad McElligott, James Dale and Nicola Wood. Their professionalism, perfectionism and endless stores of patience are the bedrock upon which this project has been built. Dealing with them has, at every stage of the book's production, been a pleasant experience, and they have answered my, almost daily, questions on image layouts and manuscript presentation, dealt with copyright holders and picture archivists, and implemented editorial changes, with great grace and serene efficiency.

I would not have been able to complete this book, nor the long-term academic study which was its catalyst, had it not been for the vital financial aid of the Arts and Humanities Research Council who funded my graduate and doctoral research. I am also beholden in more ways than words can express to the British Academy for awarding me a post-doctoral fellowship for 2007–10. Their crucial support has seen me through the final stages of this book's completion and is the basis of my continuing research, teaching and writing. I am also grateful to the English department and Graduate School of UCL for funding my participation in international academic conferences during the course of my doctoral research. Without the invaluable assistance of these funding bodies so many of the academic projects I have been fortunate enough to be involved with would have remained unrealised.

Undertaking an interdisciplinary project of this kind meant that I often found myself having to journey into unfamiliar academic territory. I was, however, blessed with many willing guides who have helped me navigate these exciting, though daunting, landscapes of knowledge. I have had the privilege of working with people from many different fields – academics, historians, archivists, curators, librarians, researchers, archaeologists, scientists and chemists – who have generously given up their time to share their expert knowledge with me and, in some cases, even their own meticulous research. I am particularly indebted to Patricia Burstall, Bisham Church archivist, who is a gifted writer and enthusiastic local historian. I am also grateful to Alan Massey, honorary fellow of the Department of Chemistry, Loughborough University, for giving me exclusive access to his thrilling chemical analyses on early modern Witch-bottles. I have also been aided in my archaeological investigations by Brian Hoggard; Tim Pestell, Curator of Archaeology at the Norwich Castle Museum; Jacqui Pierce of the London Archaeological Archive Research Centre; Professor Ivor Noel Hume, formerly of the Guildhall Museum; and Hazel Forsyth, curator of the Tudor/Stuart galleries at the Museum of London. Special thanks go to Margaret Hannay, who kindly shared her own unpublished research with me; Robin Harcourt Williams, archivist at Hatfield House; Geoffrey Fisher of the Conway Library, Courtauld Institute of Art; Anthony Trowles of the Westminster Abbey Library; Chris Gravett and Ann Mitchell of Woburn Abbey; Sebastian Fattorini of Skipton Castle; Robert Yorke of the College of Arms; Jo Rowley of Pioneer Productions; the National Geographic Channel US; Ian Murray, archivist at the present Barber-Surgeons' Hall; John Fisher of the Guildhall Library; Rea Alexandratos, Dal Pozzo Project Coordinator for the Royal Collection, Windsor Castle, whose efficiency is a godsend; Lucie Strnadova at the Royal Collection, Windsor Castle; Nikki Braunton of the Museum of London; Jeremy Coote and Kathy Wright of the Pitt Rivers Museum, University of Oxford; Joanna Parker of Worcester College Library, University of Oxford; Colin Barber of Margate Shell Grotto; Matthew Bailey of the National Portrait Gallery, London; Rachael Cross of the Wellcome Trust, London; Heather Gordon and Liz Jenkins of the National Monuments Record, English Heritage; Ute Wenzel-Förster of the Städel Museum, Frankfurt; Ingrid Kastel of the Albertina Museum,

Vienna; Michele Visentin of the Centro Studi Antoniani, Padua; Marie Poulain and Raphaëlle Cartier of the Agence Photographique de la Réunion des Musées Nationaux, Paris; Florian Kugler of the Kunsthistorisches Museum, Vienna; Gunilla Dedesund, Permissions Editor for Lennart Nilsson; José Manuel Fernández at the Museo Nacional del Prado, Madrid; Nell Carrington of the Wallace Collection, London; Axelle Russo of the British Museum; Niki Pollock of the Special Collections Department, Glasgow University Library; Elizabeth Mcgrath of the Warburg Institute, London; Lesley Headdon of Penshurst Place; and all the staff at the British Library, Wellcome Library, Courtauld Institute of Art, Warburg Institute, Lambeth Palace Library, Guildhall Library, London Archaeological Archive Research Centre and Museum of London, who have assisted me in my research. I am also grateful to Viscount De L'Isle of Penshurst Place and His Grace the Duke of Bedford of Woburn Abbey for kindly allowing me to publish photographs of items in their collections.

Over the years my enthusiasm for academic research has been energised by the support of friends from whom I have drawn inspiration and encouragement. I owe particular thanks to Shona McNeill who first instilled in me a love of literature. Her knowledge, both literary and historical, continues to amaze me and her influence on my education and career are greater than she knows. I am also grateful to those with whom I have had many stimulating and fruitful discussions about my ongoing research, including Eleni Pilla; Maria Petrides; Jerri McIntosh; Yih Yee Wong; Yewande Okuleye; and Florentia Stavrou whose presence and support during the final stages of the manuscript's completion is much appreciated. I would also like to say a big thank you to Tasos Pelekanis for his technological expertise which has taken the strain out of the practicalities of digital imaging. I apologise to anyone who has in some way been part of this project but did not get a mention here.

Note on the Text

In transcriptions of manuscripts and early printed texts all i/j and u/v orthographical constructions have been modernised, unless otherwise stated. In the end notes of each chapter I have indicated the direct sources, including the accession numbers, of early printed texts referred to. The Short Title Catalogue (STC) numbers for early English texts have, where this information was available, been included in the bibliography. Where STC numbers were unavailable WING catalogue numbers, where possible, have been added.

List of Illustrations

This book is dedicated to the memory of my brother, George
(1975–2006)

Introduction: Constructing Maternal Knowledge

> I thinck the time best spent in tiring you with the idle conceits of my travelling minde . . . to convert my feare, dispaire, greefe, mistrust and other deepe rooted conceits which long time and wofull experience . . . bring forth . . . which hide the desired fruite of your labour from your knowledge till time have brought it to maturity . . .
>
> Lady Arabella Stuart to Sir Henry Brounker[1]

Between 2005 and 2007 Pioneer Productions launched its groundbreaking trilogy of documentaries, *In the Womb*, taking a global audience on a spellbinding journey into the very beginnings of life. State-of-the-art 4D technology and arresting computer-generated imagery met with live-action medical photography to open the world of the womb as never before. The foetus was shown developing in a nurturing yet perilous eco-system, interacting with its living environment and, in the case of multiple-births, with its siblings. This was bodied forth with touching immediacy in the documentary *In the Womb: Multiples* which revealed the womb to be a space in which early emotional ties could be formed and human boundaries tested. Twins and multiples were captured as they engaged in recognisable acts of social exchange, seeming to play, fight and even, in one particularly memorable instance, kiss (Fig. I.1).[2]

These documentaries mark an important historical phase in the biomedical epistemology of the womb which, in the twentieth century, was inaugurated by the pioneering photography of Lennart Nilsson. It was in *Life* magazine's edition of 30 April 1965 that Nilsson released his painstakingly assembled visual record of human life in its earliest stages of development. Introduced with the provocative caption 'Drama of Life before Birth', a veritable cabinet of foetuses, each locked in its diaphanous amniotic bubble, was showcased in finer detail than had ever been possible (Fig. I.2).[3] Since then the seemingly indissoluble marriage between the technologisation of the maternal body and the increasing

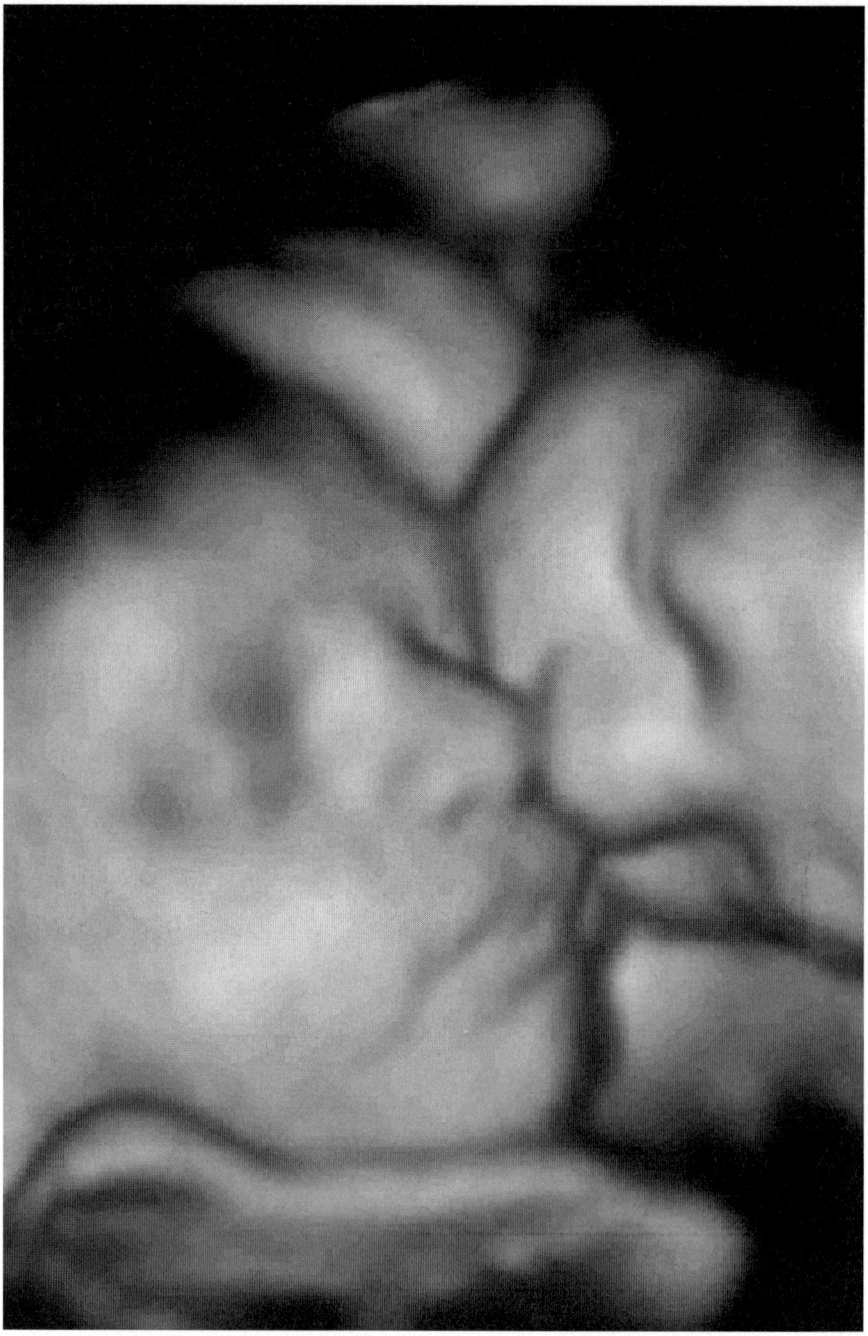

Figure I.1: Twins appearing to kiss in the womb. 4D reconstruction from the documentary *In the Womb: Multiples*, 2007. Pioneer Productions, National Geographic Channel US.

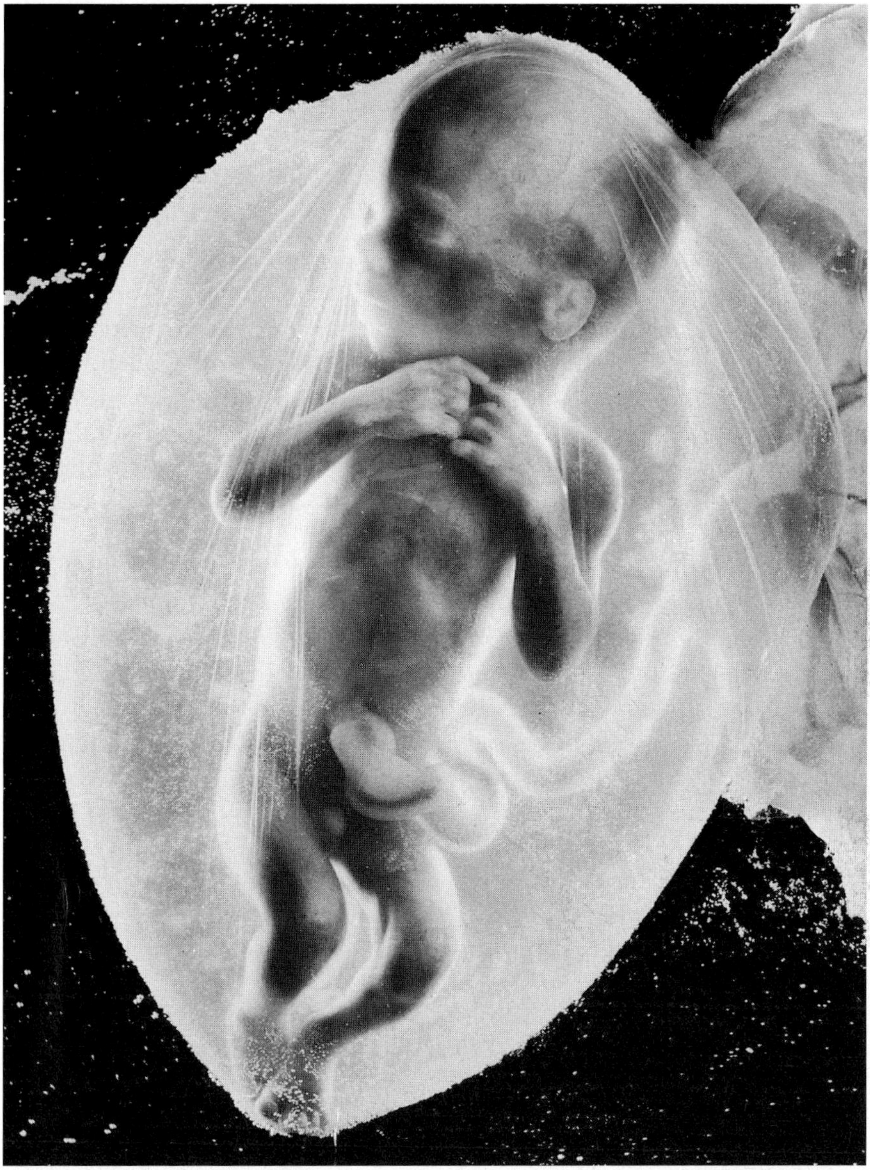

Figure I.2: Eighteen-week-old foetus from the pioneering photographic record of Lennart Nilsson, originally appearing on the cover of *Life* magazine on 30 April 1965. Lennart Nilsson/Albert Bonniers Förlag AB.

ability of medical science to *visualise* its interior reaches has been read back into histories of maternity, becoming a potent structuring narrative for researchers interested in the processes which have contributed to the womb's status as an empirically-regulated locus of certain knowledge.

In her *Reproducing the Womb: Images of Childbirth in Science, Feminist Theory, and Literature*, Alice E. Adams describes how the march of 'technologies that permit visual access to the fetus' threatens to occlude the subtle, mutually-shaping, dynamic between mother and child. In Nilsson's images, she maintains, 'the mother's body has disappeared' and hence 'they are based not on a model of cooperation or union between mother and fetus but on a model of maternal-fetal opposition . . . [since] the fetus is always alienated from its immediate (maternal) environment'. In such instances the articulation of anatomical 'truth' is coterminous with 'the clinical eye [which] brings about the erasure of the mother's body'.[4] Similarly Barbara Duden, in her *Disembodying Women: Perspectives on Pregnancy and the Unborn*, uncovers what she terms 'the new trend toward vision on command' which is 'concerned with the depiction of things that lie beyond the eye's horizon, which, to be "seen," must be explained by some authority'. The historian of childbirth and maternity must therefore 'question the certainties' which have led women to impart 'embodied reality to managed constructs . . . where pregnancy is defined in terms . . . of something called "life," for which we are all asked to take public responsibility'.[5] Such responses present the visualising technologies which have developed around conception, pregnancy and childbirth as the catalysts for debates about abortion and the rights of the unborn child which turn the self-contained ecology of the womb into the originary and pre-determining locus of personhood and acculturation. In her *Fetal Positions: Individualism, Science, Visuality*, Karen Newman defines the 'power of reproductive technologies to disperse maternity materially as well as socially' as both deriving from, and existing in perpetual tension with, a classical and early modern politics of vision:

> the constitution of fetology and obstetrics around the fetus as an individual in need of diagnosis and treatment . . . collapse[s] the mimetic and the simulated on behalf of a humanist hermeneutics enabling to "pro-life" rhetoric . . . On the other hand, the new visual apparatuses can potentially be harnessed to counter classical and Renaissance modes of representation, thus disrupting the cultural logic of individualism that relies on perspective – the rationalization of sight – and an observing subject interpellated to humanize such simulated images.[6]

What Duden, Adams, Newman and others have been working towards is a cultural awareness of the ways in which women have become historically complicit in their growing status as *knowable* subjects. This has taken place through a biomedical process which situates the accumulation of embryological and obstetric knowledge – and by implication the safeguarding of women's own health and safety during the birthing process – within a schema of gradual visual penetration in which the perspective of the mother recedes as the hidden world of the womb is drawn ever closer. In actual fact both Nilsson (in his published photographic collection, *A Child is Born*, which followed his *Life* debut) and the makers of *In the Womb* were careful to incorporate into their embryological studies visual references to pregnant mothers and their families, therefore engaging more sensitively in the varying social, emotional and domestic implications of childbirth than is apparent from the isolated foetal images which have commanded such media attention.[7] Yet as Adrienne Rich has described with reference to her personal experiences of pregnancy, in her inaugural study *Of Woman Born: Motherhood as Experience and Institution*, women are subject to precisely this sense of alienation as the wider social and medical productions of maternal knowledge begin to make demands on their conceptions of their own bodies:

> I realize that I was effectively alienated from my real body and my real spirit by the institution – not the fact – of motherhood. This institution – the foundation of human society as we know it – allowed me only certain views, certain expectations, whether embodied in the booklet in my obstetrician's waiting room, the novels I had read, my mother-in-law's approval, my memories of my own mother, the Sistine Madonna or she of the Michelangelo *Pietà*, the floating notion that a woman pregnant is a woman calm in her fulfillment . . .

Woman's 'physical knowledge of her pregnancy',[8] the distillation of centuries of obstetrical, biological and embryological teaching, acts upon other culturally-inscribed formations of maternity in ways which work to elide the heterogeneous, conflicting and contested nature of that knowledge. It is the obfuscation of these epistemological crises which has since led us to *visualise* the reproducing woman as the site of, in Rich's words, the 'calm' and certain expectation of the maternal process. Naturally, the physical dangers and traumas which attend pregnancy, labour and postpartum nurture have always placed an inescapable burden on women's understanding of the birthing process, no matter how historically conditioned that understanding may have been. What we must ask, however, is how it is that we have come to accept what we have been *made to see*, not by the 'institution' of motherhood, as Rich would have it, but by the many institutions which have, historically, laid claim to the wisdom locked in the darkened domicile of the maternal body.

Duden sums up the trajectory of many current histories of embryology from the Renaissance to the present in her concern with tracing how woman 'came to have a fetus that she "sees" ', a project requiring a close engagement with the development of 'optical devices' which have, throughout the evolution of maternal anatomy, 'enhance[d] the ability to see' into the maternal body. What, Duden reminds us, is being seen is not authentic *truth* but a 'managed image' mediated by the authoritative constructs of technology and medicine.[9] It is perhaps significant that Duden associates the earliest invention and application of these 'optical devices' with the work of the Renaissance embryologist Hieronymous Fabricius of Aquapendente (c. 1533–1619), a contemporary of William Shakespeare. Fabricius was the successor of the founding-father of anatomy at the University of Padua, the great Andreas Vesalius of Brussels (1514–64), and published his lavish images of foetal embryology in his *De Formato Foetu*, first issued in 1600 (Fig. I.3).[10]

Fabricius' floating embryos, snugly settled in pockets of truncated maternal flesh, are not a far cry from the anatomies of foetal development cultivated by Nilsson and the makers of *In the Womb*. With these homological examples before us it is clear how the age of Shakespeare could so easily become a determining point in a progressivist history which maps out the inexorable domination of the medical gaze. And it is partly in order to confirm this chronological narrative that in 1997 scientists descended upon a small corner of East London, bringing with them the latest in ground-penetrating radar technology.[11] Setting up their mobile laboratory in what is now little more than an unimposing garden adjoining the present Barber-Surgeons' Hall in Monkwell Square, they sought to determine the precise location of the seventeenth-century building whose elegantly curving wooden stools would have once been crowded with eager spectators jostling for a glimpse of the systematic unravelling of nature's greatest mystery. For until 1784 when it was torn down, it was on this site that England's first permanent anatomy theatre had stood. And it was under the auspices of this institution that the most cutting-edge advances in embryology would have been disseminated.

The barber-surgeons had been conducting anatomies as a single professional body since the Act of Incorporation, issued by Henry VIII in 1540, had united the Company of Barbers and the Guild of Surgeons, granting the new consolidated company the right to dissect the bodies of four executed criminals every year.[12] The driving force behind the union was Thomas Vicary (1495–1561), Master of the Company and Sergeant Surgeon to Henry VIII, who was responsible for importing many of the central tenets of Vesalian embryology into England, which he presented in his *Englishe Mans Treasure* in 1548. It was not, however, until February of 1636 that the barber-surgeons determined to commission 'a publique Theatre for Anatomycall exercises and

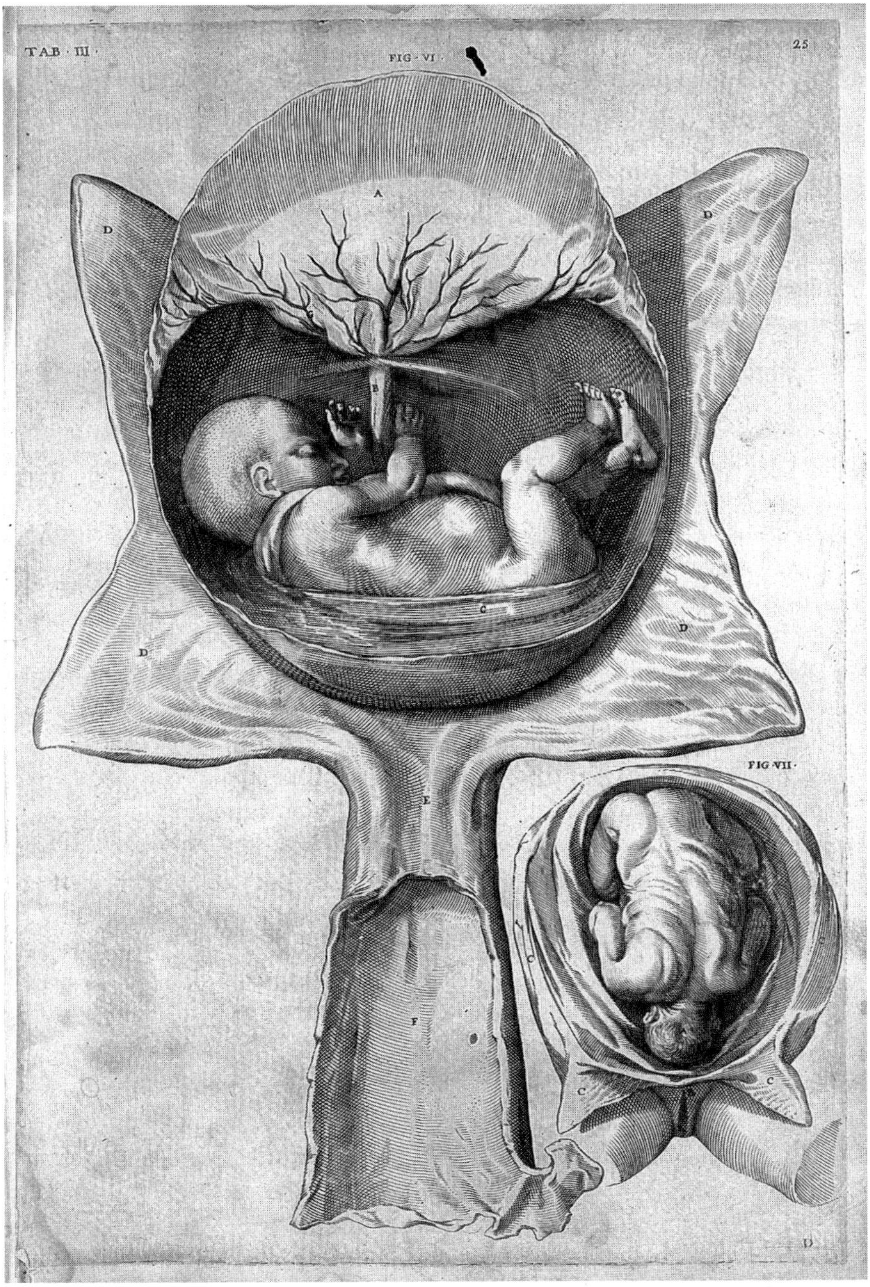

Figure I.3: Embryological dissections. Hieronymous Fabricius, *De Formato Foetu*, 1624. Wellcome Library, London.

Sceletons . . . ovally built for the Wor[shi]p and comoditie of this Companie', a project which would ensure that the unveiling of the body's interior spaces would take place in a purpose-built structure with optimal viewing conditions rather than in the makeshift surroundings of the barber-surgeons' kitchen.[13] The project was the culmination of what had been an ongoing effort on the part of the barber-surgeons to monopolise the prestige which accompanied the authoritative visual and tactile engagement with the bodily interior. A crucial field for the concentration of these efforts was the obstetrical branch of anatomy.[14] The archives of the present Barber-Surgeons' Hall bear witness to the company's attempts at redefining the process of childbirth as a necessarily surgically-mediated procedure. On 31 January 1610, for example, one James Blackborne was examined regarding 'his skill in the generatyve p[ar]tes of woman; and bringinge of women to bedd in their dangerous & difficult labors'. Though he was found 'fitt and allowed to Practize' as a male midwife, his licence to intervene in the biological processes of the female anatomy was distinctly defined as 'that Chirargicall p[ar]te of Surgery touching the generatyve p[ar]tes'.[15] In such instances the 'dangerous & difficult' nature of childbirth served as a validating pretext for the presence of the male physician in the birthing chamber.

How the projection of this authoritative knowledge penetrated the domestic setting of childbirth can be illustrated in the case of Barbara Gamage Sidney who, during her pregnancy in the winter of 1595, began to exhibit alarming signs as her confinement approached. Her symptoms, with which she 'took no rest, being . . . troubled with an extreme cough', were diagnosed as a case of the measles.[16] Because her husband, Robert Sidney, was away, his trusted agent Rowland Whyte kept him informed of her condition in a series of letters. Confessing that 'because she is with child it may prove dangerous', Whyte assured the concerned husband that 'she shall want no earthly help and attendance'.[17] To this end he enlisted the services of Dr Brown and one Jacob, possibly a male midwife, who remained at the house until her traumatic delivery was over, the former having slept there 'all that night'. Thankfully her 'safe deliverance of a goodly son' meant that their services were not required.[18] The account of the birth, which includes details of the precautions taken to promote the well-being of the new-born infant, is one of the most touching to have survived in any private correspondence from this era:

> her pains were sharp and natural, and God, according to his wonted goodness towards her, delivered her of the pain [b]y [*torn*] sending into this world a goodly fat boy, but as full of the measles in the face as can be. They gave

it some of the nurse's milk and saffron, which he sucked out of a spoon, and they keep it very warm. He sucks as well as any child doth, and cries as strongly. So that we hope in God he shall live long to both your comforts.[19]

The letters provide evidence that masculine presence in the birthing room was often an indicator of impending crisis. While making preparations for the attendance of the 'great ones' who would act as 'gossips' alongside the midwife, Whyte resolved that the male practitioner should reside 'in my chamber if my Lady should fall to travail though my Lady shall not know it'.[20] His insistence, at least initially, that the attendance of Jacob be kept secret from her suggests that he was solicitous in shielding the expectant mother from the anxiety that such knowledge would arouse. A portrait of Lady Sidney with her six children dated 1596, probably by Marcus Gheeraerts, hangs in Penshurst Place (Fig. I.4). She is visibly pregnant and the infant to whom she gave birth just one year before while travailing with the measles is seated beside her, clutching a coral-tipped silver rattle and a bunch of cherries, a traditional symbol of innocence. Like many pregnancy portraits of the time, the image occludes the crises which can beset a mother at birth, presenting the public face of motherhood as the wellspring of dynastic legitimation.[21] Serene in her self-assurance as the vessel of her husband's continuing

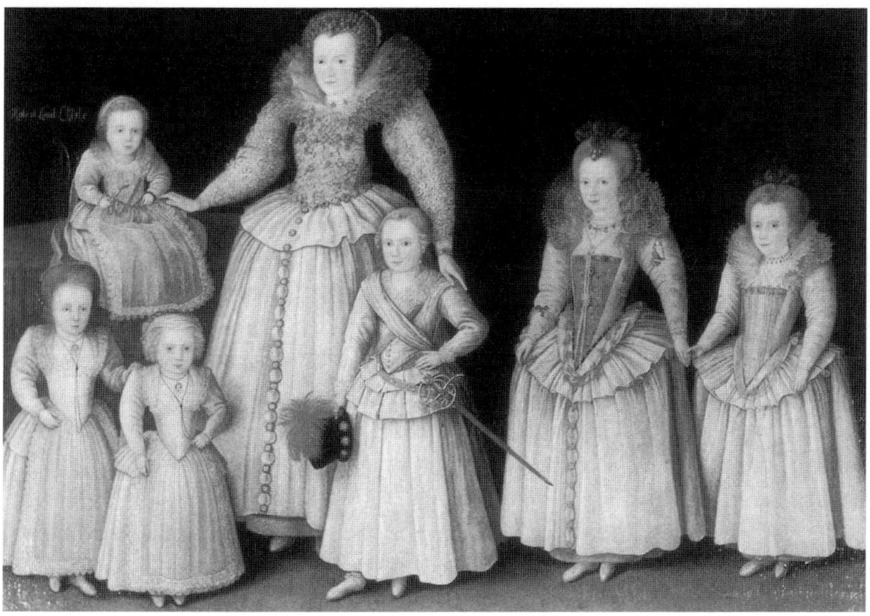

Figure I.4: Marcus Gheerarts II, Lady Barbara Gamage Sidney and six of her children, 1596, Penshurst Place. By kind permission of Viscount De L'Isle from his private collection.

lineage, she is the Renaissance counterpart of Rich's 'pregnant . . . woman calm in her fulfillment'.

The barber-surgeons' prescriptions for the medicalisation of childbirth, which find their practical corollary in the kind of childbed scenario recorded by Whyte, rely on their apparent access to accurate data about the secrets of conception, pregnancy and childbirth. The success of this endeavour has been recapitulated in subsequent historical accounts of the male midwife's gradual, though inexorable, penetration of the birthing room.[22] Such histories are problematised, however, by the competing accounts of contemporaries. In 1671 Jane Sharp challenged the omniscient vision of the anatomists in her *Midwives Book*. Writing about the difficulties of divining the structure of the developing embryo, she declared that precise knowledge of how 'each part is made . . . [and] fastned to the Mothers womb' is

> thought to be the hardest piece of *Anatomy*, because it is seldome to be observed, because if women dye in child-bed they first miscarry and dye afterward. Some follow *Galen* herein, who never saw a woman Anatomized; others *Columbus*, some *Vesalius*, but few or none know the truth. The stones of a woman for generation of seed, are white, thick and well concocted, for I have seen one, and but one and that is more by one than many Men have seen.[23]

In one stroke Sharp dismisses history's most lauded anatomical celebrities, the foundations upon which English embryological thought had been built: Galen, Vesalius and Realdus Columbus (1516–59), Vesalius' one-time student. The visual aetiology for the success of early modern embryology these medical men have propounded, Sharp avers, is founded upon a lie.[24] Rarely the object of actual dissections, the interior of the pregnant female anatomy is hardly ever *seen*. Sharp has targeted what will be the fulcrum around which this study will turn: if knowledge of the maternal body did not derive solely from the visual penetration of real bodies by the medical profession (though this did indeed contribute an important shaping influence), then just how was maternity – as body, principle, natural force, political instrument, locus of the sacred and the satanic – constituted in the age of Shakespeare? In other words, how did Shakespeare's contemporaries come to *know* the maternal body?

Sharp provides an important clue in her indication that the, albeit limited, visual access to embryological information all too often goes hand-in-hand with the tragic disruption of the proper course of conception, pregnancy or childbirth. It is difficult for us today, in the age of X-rays, Doppler sonography, magnetic resonance imaging and ultrasound scanning technology, to comprehend a time when the living body was not the primary vehicle for authoritative knowledge of the reproductive function. These technologies have made the penetration of animate tissue synonymous with the success of the institutions which are the transmitters and interpreters of what are deemed medical facts. In Shakespeare's day things were very different. Maternal knowledge came at a price: the physical health, spiritual sanctity, fertility, nurturing potential and even life of the body that was the source of that knowledge. Anatomists and male practitioners learned about the female reproductive biology by dissecting the dead female bodies that, although rare, sometimes came to their hands. They bribed midwives for aborted foetuses, stole bodies and body-parts illegally from tombs and graveyards, and intervened in crises in the birthing room. Natural historians examined instances of monstrous births and the anomalous productions of the natural world in order to understand better the mechanisms which underpinned vegetal, animal and ultimately human generation. Demonologists and legal authorities tested their theories of the preternatural properties of the maternal body when women, both as suspected witches and bewitched victims, found themselves in court over accusations of witchcraft. Heralds, genealogists and memorialisers explored the potential for the consolidation of social and political authority afforded by the emblematic associations attached to the dead mother. Maternal knowledge was fashioned at the liminal instant in which the body was most mutable, unstable, fragmented and equivocal, its ordinary biological processes always just beyond reach. The maternal body *known* was the maternal body in crisis.

The purpose of this study is to recuperate the ways in which such crises of conception provided the precondition through which the maternal body could be turned into bodies of knowledge. The reproductive anatomy was not a monolithic construct whose mysterious workings could simply be laid bare through invasive visual inspection. It existed rather as the site of a range of competing disciplines which sought to derive authoritative status through a mastery of its generative capabilities. In order to understand this we must resist reproducing the selectivity of authoritative histories. The triumph of the biomedicalised body – which has since been re-inscribed by historians of embryology as the epistemological goal towards which all intellectual and pedagogical branches of learning have been working – has obscured the significance of those other disciplines which fostered alternative ways of knowing the maternal. While this study will indeed pay due attention to those fields of endeavour which have since acquired the self-ratifying prestige of mainstream status, such as anatomy and natural history, it will also attempt to recover their dependence on the non-medical discourses which, incorporating myth, literary topoi, sexual analogy and archaeological and architectural motifs, served as potent ideological tools in the struggle for professionalised status. We will, however, also explore those bodies of knowledge which have been marginalised or entirely depleted of their intellectual and pedagogical currency as the biomedical and natural sciences have gained ground. Disciplines such as demonology and heraldry had a tremendous impact on the construction of maternity in early modern England, yet have not been recognised as contributors to the *material* foundations of reproductive knowledge in their own right. By restoring these disciplines to the wider intellectual and cultural landscape of which they were originally a part we will come to recognise that the maternal body was never the guarantor of humanity's unproblematic transition from intellectual darkness to the light of reasoned scientific discernment, but of an epistemological process in which disruption, uncertainty, contention and exchange were the constitutive and sometimes even deconstructive principles.

The barber-surgeons placed the commission for their new theatre in the hands of none other than Inigo Jones, Ben Jonson's collaborator and certainly the country's leading specialist in the architectonics of theatrical display. Surviving in copies penned by Isaac Ware, the plans for the anatomy theatre reveal its indebtedness to structural principles deriving from the work of one of the Renaissance's most influential architects, Sebastio Serlio, whose *Architettura*, published in 1545, Jones is known to have used (Fig. I.5).[25] Serlian amphitheatre models also provided the inspiration for some of England's finest playhouses, including Jones' Cockpit Theatre in Drury Lane, the schematics for which were executed between 1616 and 1618 (Figs I.6a and I.6b).[26] While the theatricalised setting of anatomy allowed the barber-surgeons to affirm the visual dynamic which provided the justificatory rationale for the professionalisation of their craft, the confident unitary perspective they hoped to monopolise was put under strain by the histrionic displays which infiltrated the teaching-space, opening up the spectacle of dissection to potentially dissident elements. The dissemination of anatomical knowledge was often accompanied by music and feasting and on the Continent, where anatomies were scheduled in the winter during the carnival period, students sometimes attended in full masquing regalia.[27] There is also evidence that similar practices occurred in England. Ordinances held at the current Barber-Surgeons' Hall indicate that 'dissolute' and boisterous behaviour was not uncommon among those practising the 'arte of barbery or surgery'. Indeed, offenders were reprimanded for committing 'odious & intoll[er]able inconveniences & abuses' and for their unruly behaviour while dressed in 'disguysed

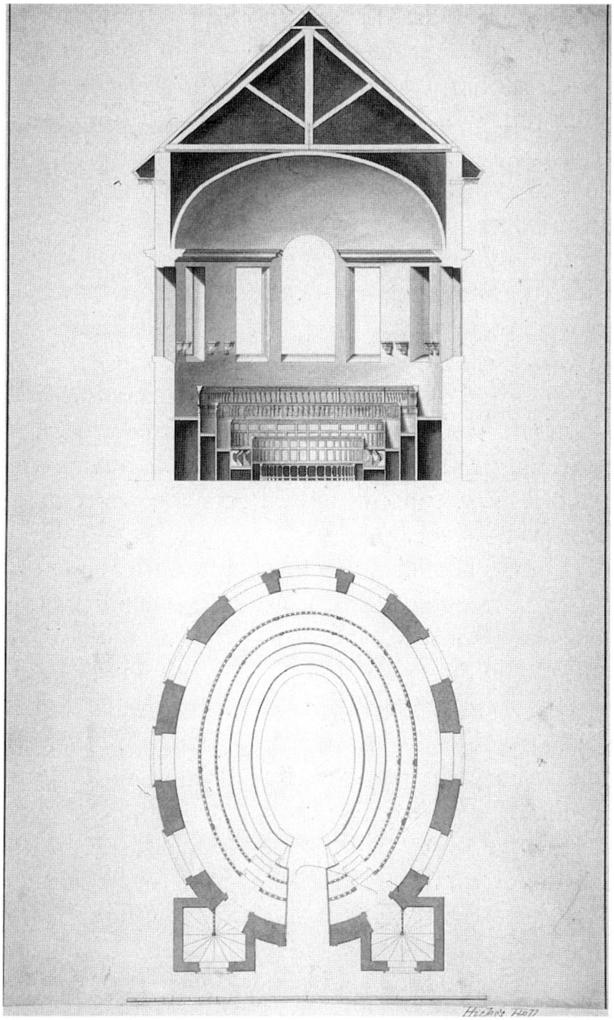

Figure I.5: Inigo Jones/Isaac Ware, interior of the Barber-Surgeons' Anatomy Theatre, Monkwell Street. Guildhall Library, City of London.

apparrell'.[28] In such instances the ideological and methodological principles which governed dissection were forced to give way to alternative ways of knowing.

The process which made the act of peeling back the body's layers susceptible to the satirical and politically disrupting rites of social inversion in the anatomy theatre – rendered readily transposable through the continuum of theatrical entertainments available to early modern subjects – would have found its mirror-image in the playhouse where the human body *in extremis* was similarly placed centre-stage. This makes the

6a

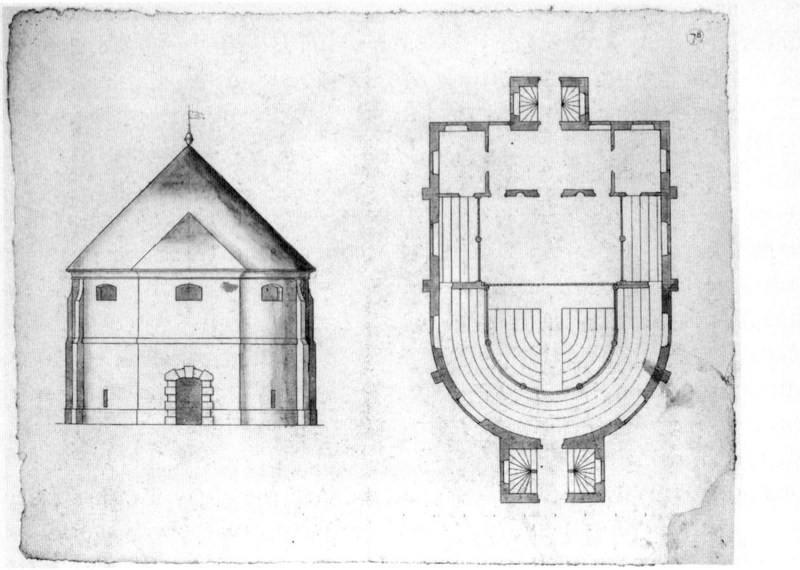

6b

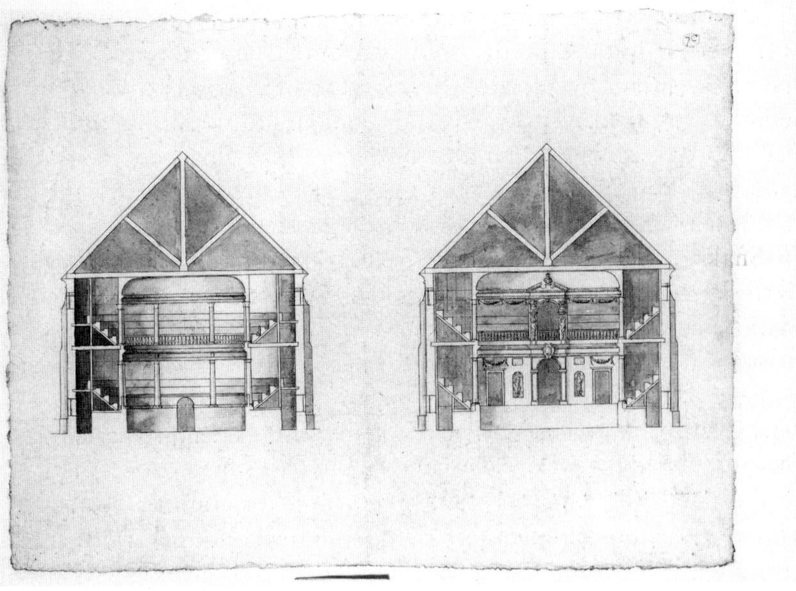

Figures I.6a and I.6b: Inigo Jones, designs for the Cockpit Theatre, Drury Lane. Worcester College Library, Oxford. By kind permission of the Provost and Fellows of Worcester College, Oxford.

Shakespearean theatre a crucial medium for exploring the dichotomous nature of the maternal crises which provided the basis for the authorisation of those branches of learning that sought to regulate and define the reproductive anatomy. As I hope to show, instances of tragic intervention in the ideal processes of conception, birth and nurture – such as disease, bewitchment, monstrosity and death – could also expose the potentially destabilising power of maternity, dismantling the epistemological certainties with which the maternal body had been invested in the interests of the nascent institutions which were being formed around the disciplines this study is subjecting to scrutiny. Above all it is the theatre's ability to allude to a range of managed spaces beyond audiences' immediate perspectival vision which is a guiding structural principle of the chapters which follow. As well as the anatomy theatre, the Renaissance grotto and garden, the courtroom in which women were brought to trial as suspected witches, and the early modern chapel or mausoleum, were all important testing-grounds for early modern figurations of maternity; spaces in which the reproductive body was rendered mobile, manipulable, resistant and affecting.

The process of visualising pregnancy and embryological development was indeed important to the Renaissance imagination,[29] and critics have responded by plotting Shakespeare's relation to what they have identified as the drive towards a gradual institutionalising of the demand for, appropriately echoing a phrase from *Othello*, 'ocular proof' of the maternal body's interior structures.[30] Studies extending the field of investigation beyond the ocular story of the reproductive anatomy in Shakespeare take their impetus from the seminal work of Mary Beth Rose.[31] Although Rose provided much-needed evidence that Shakespearean maternity did indeed merit closer scrutiny, she simultaneously delimited the range of 'options' through which this could be achieved: 'If, in comedy, the maternal role remains invisible, unrepresented, in tragedy it . . . is constructed almost entirely in terms of the private world of desire.' According to this assertion, maternity in Shakespeare is thus either wholly 'invisible' or confined to the enclosed spaces of the home, since,

> motherhood . . . remains most resolutely limited to the private realm, inscribed entirely in terms of early love and nurture. As a result, motherhood in this formulation can be dramatized only as dangerous or as peripheral to adult, public life.[32]

While Rose excludes the dramatic and representative reach of maternity from 'public life', her work has proved a crucial starting-point for those psychoanalytical studies which sought to restore the interplay of influences between mother and child. In her immensely important *Suffocating Mothers: Fantasies of Maternal Origin in Shakespeare's Plays* Janet Adelman examines the way in which Shakespearean constructions of maternity encode 'a primitive infantile terror derivative from the period when the mother or her surrogate was not seen as a whole and separate person, when she – or the body-parts through which she was imagined – had the power to make or unmake the world and the self for her child'.[33] This, largely Freudian, schema of a latent but poisonously ever-present childhood trauma, which animates fantasies of detachment and nostalgic re-attachment to an originary maternal presence, is countered by Theresa M. Krier in *Birth Passages: Maternity and Nostalgia, Antiquity to Shakespeare*. By drawing on alternative influences, particularly those of Luce Irigaray, Melanie Klein and D.W. Winnicot, Krier insists that a new understanding of the processes of childhood development and nurture can be attained, 'creat[ing] a field in which literary critics may speak also of praise, celebration, exultation, exaltation, gratitude, and transformation' as the positive outcomes of parturition.[34] Mounting a 'resistance to the pathos of nostalgia', she identifies the potentially creative interchange that can inform the mother-child bond following the transitional phase of birth, a process which can 'shape and sustain a space between them for fluencies of language, affect, thinking, and formal creation'.[35]

If such approaches to maternity recapitulate the idea of the womb as the transhistorical constitutive site of what Karen Newman calls 'fetal personhood',[36] largely focusing on the impact of the mother on the child's cognitive and behavioural development, contemporary anthropological studies have sought to centralise women's experiences of their own bodies at the specific cultural and temporal moment in which childbirth and maternal nurture occurs.[37] This objective has also underpinned the historicising work which has sought to restore the cultural specificity of maternity in early modern England.[38] While these critical perspectives have sounded a rallying-call for feminist scholars, providing the basis for a more sensitive approach to the study of motherhood, they are largely confined to those rituals which are most germane to the environs of the domestic sphere in which women, as communities, experienced childbirth and undertook the daily work of maternal nurture and care-giving. Going beyond the private realm to recover the far-reaching intellectual, cultural, epistemological, archaeological and spatial implications of maternity to the Renaissance imagination is the purpose of this present study.

Establishing a critical language with which to speak about the relevance of maternity to the public sphere and its constituent political discourses has been the subject of recent studies which have made important strides in this new area. In her *Midwiving Subjects in Shakespeare's England*, Caroline Bicks counters the 'persistent trend' which has 'read the midwife and other women of the birthroom as comprising a private and empowered female society – one distinct from the patriarchal world beyond its walls'. The birthing chamber, Bicks argues, was not 'formed in reaction to a public, central male sphere' but was the space 'that midwived subjects into being'.[39] Most recently, Kathryn M. Moncrief and Kathryn R. McPherson, in their edited collection *Performing Maternity in Early Modern England*, have revealed the ways in which an understanding of the maternal body as both active and *acting* is able to expose the mysogynistic faultlines which turn the maternal body into the locus of epistemological certainty, arguing 'that maternity – both public and private, physically embodied and enacted – must be considered performative and that the maternal body, as a result, functions as a potent space for cultural conflict, a site of imagination and contest'.[40]

Such approaches have provided vital groundwork for the opportunities afforded by the Shakespearean text as a means of uncovering the wider-ranging impact of maternity, which this study will, it is hoped, extend to the spaces – medical, natural historical, legal and sacred – which provided the 'theatres' in which the reproductive body and its functions accrued social, intellectual, aesthetic and pedagogical value. Recuperating this occluded history of maternity requires a particularly interdisciplinary methodology. A central principle of this study will therefore be its engagement with the material remains which mediated the reproduction, dissemination and practical application of maternal knowledge within the spatial contexts which formed the setting for its management and deployment.[41] What the following chapters will have in common is an interest in various forms of archaeological recovery, deploying their materials of evidence from a range of textual, iconographical and three-dimensional artefacts which constituted the alternative epistemologies of maternity from which early modern subjects could draw. Anatomical broadsides, pornographic plates, portraits, cabinets of curiosity and their contents, early natural historical specimens, fountains and artificial islands, earthenware and ceramics, mysterious magical artefacts, costume, funerary monuments and statuary, take their place in this study alongside archival manuscript material, early printed sources and, of course, the Shakespearean text. Such an approach, I believe, will bring us closer to understanding the fluid, less rigidly demarcated form of the disciplines under consideration. As we will see, the bodies of knowledge which we will be exploring are not by any means cohesive and self-sufficient constructs, but overlapping and mutually determining. As such they reflect the heterogeneous nature of the Shakespearean maternities whose legacy is our inheritance today.

In the first chapter I hope to overturn the assumption that the popular early modern genre of anatomical satire developed purely as a reaction against, and should therefore be understood antithetically to, the early modern discipline of human dissection. In actuality the proponents of the new anatomy, whose figurehead was the pioneering Vesalius, appropriated a satirical vocabulary which turned the wayward maternal body into a powerful vehicle for the professionalisation of their craft. Shakespeare's Hamlet takes his place among the English satirists whose anatomical probing of a diseased and corrupting reproductive female corporeality was in part shaped by the reforming rhetoric of the Wittenberg school of anatomy which arose from this radical culture of dissection. Hamlet's obsessive scrutiny of the 'matter' of maternity, however, works to dismantle the epistemological certainties which the luminaries of the Vesalian anatomical regime claimed to derive from their satirical postures of anatomy.

The Renaissance grotto and garden, as we will see in the second chapter, were politicised cabinets of wonders in which a maternalised, and potentially monstrous, nature was subjected to the regimen of natural historical investigation in the interests of colonial expansionism. These spaces encapsulated emergent theories which stressed that aberrations of creation were part of the inherent or *common* mechanisms which governed the production of all life-forms, requiring careful supervision, suppression and control. Shakespeare's *Tempest* puts these ideas to the test as Caliban engages in a struggle with Prospero over the reproductive knowledge afforded by the natural properties of the island's grotto-spaces. Prospero's attempts at defining Caliban as a threat to the procreative destiny of the island's wonder, Miranda, and hence to the social and political order itself, are unsettled as the play gradually erodes the difference between the monster and the natural historian upon which the colonial programme depends.

The material artefacts of witchcraft and superstition, which form the focus of the third chapter, will provide a pivotal medium through which to explore how the specifically maternal functions of the witch's body were believed to facilitate her demonic influence. Indeed, the *archaeologies* at our disposal offer new insights into the corporealised basis of the disruptive effects of magic on the maternal role; the processes of domestic production, fertility and nurture. Shakespeare's *Macbeth* is steeped in the accoutrements of witchcraft and it is in the maternal knowledge which serves as the necessary precondition for their deployment that the play locates its dramatic deconstruction of the rituals of power. Shakespeare deliberately equivocates the material adjuncts of kingship with those belonging to the satanic crafts, and in doing so reveals that both are founded on the invasive manipulation of the blood and bodily matter of those over whom the artful purveyors of these mysteries would have dominion.

As we will see in the final chapter, the age of Shakespeare gave rise to a poignant language of maternal memory. The inception of a *mother's legacy* tradition, changes in the religious and social functions of the death-ritual and stylistic innovations in the manipulation of stone and marble began to convey the spiritual, emotional and ideological contours of the maternal posture in new and dramatic ways. By the time Shakespeare completed *Antony and Cleopatra* the heraldic funeral was being gradually replaced by other ceremonial and commemorative acts which centralised the role of the family and provided women with the conceptual tools for the re-evaluation of their status as participants in, as well as subjects of, the memorialising practices which sought to define their place in the patriarchal economy. In her own maternal postures of death Cleopatra, Shakespeare's most monumental of heroines, commandeers an empowering, and even subversive, form of female self-commemoration which allows her to script her own posthumous history.

The disciplines which form the core of this study exploited, precipitated or asserted their authority through a growing conception of the maternal body as the corollary of an autonomously acting nature, a nature governed by its own inherent, immutable laws whose operations could be properly understood through the processes of probing, dissecting, classification, legal definition and historical containment. As this study will attempt to show, however, maternity proved stubbornly resistant to, and stimulated the interrogation and reconceptualisation of, the very bodies of knowledge which sought to lay claim to its unique and mysterious powers.

Notes

1. Arabella Stuart, *The Letters of Lady Arabella Stuart*, ed. Sara Jayne Steen (Oxford: Oxford University Press, 1994), pp. 168–70.
2. The three documentaries were *In the Womb*, *In the Womb: Animals*, and *In the Womb: Multiples*. These were first broadcast in the UK by Channel 4, with the first documentary appearing with the title *Life before Birth* in 2005. The series was broadcast in the United States by National Geographic Channel US. I would like to thank Jo Rowley and Pioneer Productions for kindly providing me with the image and with information about the series.

3. Nilsson's images are also reproduced in *Life Science Library: Growth*, eds. James M. Tanner, Gordon Rattray Taylor and the editors of Time-Life Books (London and Holland: Time-Life International, 1968), pp. 62–75.
4. Alice E. Adams, *Reproducing the Womb: Images of Childbirth in Science, Feminist Theory, and Literature* (Ithaca and London: Cornell University Press, 1994), pp. 143–4 and 137 respectively. In relation to the 'new fetal images' produced by Nilsson and subsequent pioneers of the visual culture of the womb, E. Ann Kaplan asks if 'the focus on the fetus [is] the latest form of the age-long male utopian urge to control reproduction, to control the [by implication maternal] body, perhaps to the extent of eliminating it altogether', 'Sex, Work, and Motherhood: Maternal Subjectivity in Recent Visual Culture', in *Representations of Motherhood*, eds Donna Bassin, Margaret Honey and Meryle Mahrer Kaplan (New Haven and London: Yale University Press, 1994), p. 269.
5. Barbara Duden, *Disembodying Women: Perspectives on Pregnancy and the Unborn*, trans. Lee Hoinacki (Cambridge: Harvard University Press, 1993), pp. 16 and 4 respectively.
6. Karen Newman, *Fetal Positions: Individualism, Science, Visuality* (Stanford: Stanford University Press, 1996), pp. 110–13.
7. See Nilsson's, *A Child Is Born* (London and New York: Doubleday, 1990) for representations of the family in various domestic, medical and social contexts. This text has appeared in numerous editions since 1965. When Channel 4 aired the *In the Womb* series it included an engaging voice-over from the poet Roger McGough, which used the narrative medium of verse to articulate these broader emotional and familial concerns even while the interior of the womb and foetus were being presented.
8. Adrienne Rich, *Of Woman Born: Motherhood as Experience and Institution* (New York and London: W. W. Norton and Company, 1986), p. 39.
9. Duden, *Disembodying Women*, pp. 4, 47 and 17 respectively.
10. The edition I have consulted is the *De Formato Foetu* (Francofurti: 1624), BL, 549.1.20.(1). For an edition which includes Fabricius' embryological research on birds see *Opera Anatomica . . . De Formato Foetu, Formatione Ovi et Pulli* (Patavii: 1625), BL, 781.1.1. English translations are provided in *The Embryological Treatises of Hieronymus Fabricius of Aquapendente: The Formation of the Egg and of the Chick; The Formed Fetus*, trans. Howard B. Adelmann (New York and London: Cornell University Press, 1942). Fabricius' teacher was Gabriel Fallopius (1523–62) who made important observations on the ovarian follicle. Fabricius would go on to tutor William Harvey (1578–1657) at the University of Padua. For more on the development of embryology as a discipline see Joseph Needham, *A History of Embryology* (Cambridge: Cambridge University Press, 1959); and *The Human Embryo: Aristotle and the Arabic and European Traditions*, ed. G.R. Dunstan (Exeter: University of Exeter Press, 1990), pp. 136–57.
11. These scientists were Bill McCann and Paul Mackie, from the Clark Laboratory of the Museum of London. The discovery of the anatomy theatre is reported in Nigel Hawkes, 'Grisly surgery site discovered', *The Times* (3 September 1997). I am grateful to Ian Murray, archivist at the present Barber-Surgeons' Hall, for discussing the hall's history with me,

and for allowing me complete access to the archival material located there. The full results of the geophysical survey carried out on the site of Inigo Jones' anatomy theatre (site code: BSG97), including those of the ground-penetrating radar completed in 1997, and the subsequent excavation which was carried out in 1998, are detailed in Robin Wroe-Brown, *Barber-Surgeons Hall Garden: An Archaeological Research Evaluation* (Museum of London Archaeology Service, May 1998), unpublished. For more on the archaeological history of the site see Nathalie Cohen, 'The Hall of the Barber Surgeons', *London Archaeologist* 8 (6) (Autumn 1997), pp. 162–7. For a general history of the barber-surgeons see Jessie Dobson and R. Milnes Walker, *Barbers and Barber-Surgeons of London* (Oxford: Alden Press, 1979). See also *The London Journal* (27 November 1875), p. 344, Guildhall Library, A.45/9.

12. Dobson and Walker, *Barbers and Barber-Surgeons of London*, pp. 31–4.
13. The barber-surgeons' records for 11 February 1636, Sidney Young, *Annals of the Barber-Surgeons of London* (London: East and Blades, 1890), vol. 1, p. 132.
14. Anatomy theatres also provided venues for the display of anatomical specimens, many of which demonstrated a particular interest in the reproductive aspects of the female body. The interior of the Leiden anatomy theatre was admired throughout Europe and even in England, where an English account of its curious contents was circulated as *A catalogue of all the cheifest rarities in the publick theater and anatomie-hall of the university of Leyden . . .* (Leyden: 1591), BL, 7421.b.19. The inventory included 'The Skin of a childe when first born', 'the Sceleton of a New-borne-childe', 'An Abortus embalmed', 'A Woman's Pudenda', 'The Sceleton of a childe but 4 moneths old in the Womb' and 'A curious Sceleton of a child born before his time', sigs A2v–A5.
15. *Court Minutes 1607–1621*, Barber-Surgeons' Hall, MS B/1/4, 31 January 1610, f. 133.
16. 1 December 1595, C12/34. I am grateful to Margaret Hannay for drawing my attention to the letters which are most germane to my research and for supplying me with her unpublished transcriptions of the correspondence which forms part of the private collection of Lord De L'Isle, taken from *The Correspondence of Rowland Whyte and Robert Sidney, first Earl of Leicester*, eds Michael G. Brennan, Noel J. Kinnamon and Margaret P. Hannay (unpublished version). The letters are now housed in the Centre for Kentish Studies, Maidstone, call number U1475.
17. Ibid., 30 November 1595, C12/33.
18. Ibid., 5 December 1595, C12/36.
19. Ibid., 2 December 1595, C12/35. The additions in square brackets are the work of Noel J. Kinnamon, who transcribed these particular letters.
20. Ibid., 29 November 1595, C12/32. For more on the anxieties surrounding childbirth seen through the eyes of the women in the seventeenth-century Verney family of Buckinghamshire, see Miriam Slater, *Family Life in the Seventeenth Century: The Verneys of Claydon House*, London: Routledge and Kegan Paul, pp. 124–5.
21. For more on pregnancy portraits see Pauline Croft and Karen Hearn ' "Only Matrimony Maketh Children to be Certain . . .": Two Elizabethan

Pregnancy Portraits', *The British Art Journal* 3 (3) (Autumn 2003), pp. 19–24; Karen Hearn, 'A Fatal Fertility? Elizabethan and Jacobean Pregnancy Portraits', *Costume: The Journal of the Costume Society* 34 (2000), pp. 39–43; and Hearn's overview of the Renaissance pregnancy portrait in *Marcus Gheeraerts II, Elizabethan Artist: In Focus* (London: Tate Publishing, 2002), pp. 40–51.

22. A survey of the rise of the male midwife appears in Jean Donnison, *Midwives and Medical Men: A History of the Struggle for the Control of Childbirth* (New Barnet: Historical Publications, 1988). Renate Blumenfeld-Kosinski's *Not of Woman Born: Representations of Caesarean Birth in Medieval and Renaissance Culture* (Ithaca and London: Cornell University Press, 1990), broadly follows this trajectory. For a contemporary account of the tensions which existed between female midwives and male practitioners see Percivall Willughby's diary, *Observations on Childbirth, with Descriptions of Cases in his Practice*, 1630–78, BL, Sloane MS 529.
23. Jane Sharp, *The Midwives Book, Or the Whole Art of Midwifry Discovered*, ed. Elaine Hobby (Oxford: Oxford University Press, 1999), p. 103.
24. Elaine Hobby points out that Sharp's critique of Galen echoes that of Nicholas Culpeper in his bestselling *Directory for Midwives* (1651), ibid., n. 2 to p. 103.
25. The plans for the anatomy theatre were kindly supplied by John Fisher of the Guildhall Library (ref. 8478). For designs which proved to be of most influence with regard to theatrical style see Serlio's *On Architecture*, an English rendering of Books I-V of *Tutte L'Opere D'Architettura et Prospetiva*, trans. Vaughan Hart and Peter Hicks (New Haven: Yale University Press, 1996), vol. 1, pp. 82–5 (for the semi-circular theatre) and pp. 99–103 (for the rotunda models derived from antiquity). See also ff. 2v–3, 29v–30, 33v–34, and 36, Book III and Book IV of the English translation made for Robert Peake in 1611, in Sebastio Serlio, *The Five Books of Architecture: An Unabridged Reprint of the English Edition of 1611* (New York: Dover Publications, 1982). A photographic reprint of the edition of Serlio's *Architettura* (Venice: 1619) which was known to have been owned by Inigo Jones, containing annotations by John Webb, is held in the British Library, X.423/159.
26. Worcester College, Oxford (Jones/Webb, I/7B and 7C). For other manuscript records of theatre designs see 'Inigo Jones's Original Ground Plots and Profiles of Scenes', BL, Lansdowne MS 1171; and Simon Basil, designs for the theatre at Christ Church, Oxford, BL, Additional MS 15505, f. 21. Anatomy theatres and playhouses, including Shakespeare's Globe, shared Zodiacal decorative motifs. Compare Edward Hatton's description of the barber-surgeons' theatre in *A New View of London* (London: 1708), BL, 577.d.1–2, with the interior of the Cockpit Theatre in John Orrell, *The Human Stage: English Theatre Design 1567–1640* (Cambridge: Cambridge University Press, 1988), pp. 54–5. On the use of the 'heavens' and Zodiac in other theatre interiors see Andrew Gurr, *The Shakespearean Stage 1574–1642* (Cambridge: Cambridge University Press, 1992), pp. 122–3. In her *Staging Anatomies: Dissection and Spectacle in Early Stuart Tragedy* (Aldershot: Ashgate, 2005), Hillary M. Nunn also

considers the connections between the anatomy theatre and the indoor playhouse, but focuses on the 'perspectivist habits of viewing' they both shared, pp. 111–15. See n. 3, p. 148 of ibid. for the uncertainty surrounding the attribution of the designs thought to be of the Cockpit Theatre.

27. Giovanna Ferrari, 'Public Anatomy Lessons and the Carnival: The Anatomy Theatre of Bologna', *Past and Present* 117 (1987), pp. 50–106. There is also some indication that in England criminals, whose bodies would end up on the dissecting table, found themselves in a carnival atmosphere as they were being led to execution at Tyburn's gallows. Surviving accounts record that executioners and even the condemned themselves were sometimes costumed in the lively garb of fair-time celebrations. Popular contemporary euphemisms for execution included 'Tyburn fair', 'hanging fair', 'Paddington fair', and 'to dance the Paddington frisk'. As such executions could be accompanied by 'elements of black humour' or 'burlesque' which may have spilled over into the anatomy theatre, see Alan Brooke and David Brandon, *Tyburn: London's Fatal Tree* (London: Sutton Publishing, 2004), pp. 14, 19 and 39–40.
28. *Charter Act and Ordinance Book 1461–1607*, Barber-Surgeons' Hall MS A/6/1, Ordinances, 1606, f. 30.
29. For this see Laura Gowing, *Common Bodies: Women, Touch and Power in Seventeenth-Century England* (New Haven and London: Yale University Press, 2003), pp. 122–38.
30. For studies which centralise the visual/anatomical disclosure of the female body and its reproductive spaces to the study of Shakespeare's plays see Howard Marchitello, 'Shakespeare's *Othello* and Vesalius's *Fabrica*: Anatomy, Gender, and the Narrative Production of Meaning', in *Narrative and Meaning in Early Modern England: Browne's Skull and Other Histories* (Cambridge: Cambridge University Press, 1997), pp. 10–38; Michael Neill, 'Opening the Moor: Death and Discovery in *Othello*', in *Issues of Death: Mortality and Identity in English Renaissance Tragedy* (Oxford: Clarendon Press, 1997), pp. 141–67; Patricia Parker, '*Othello* and *Hamlet*: Spying, Discovery, Secret Faults', in *Shakespeare from the Margins: Language, Culture, Context* (Chicago: University of Chicago Press, 1996); Elizabeth Sacks, *Shakespeare's Images of Pregnancy* (London: Macmillan, 1980); Michael C. Schoenfeldt, *Bodies and Selves in Early Modern England: Physiology and Inwardness in Spenser, Shakespeare, Herbert, and Milton* (Cambridge: Cambridge University Press, 1999); Gail Kern Paster, *The Body Embarrassed: Drama and the Disciplines of Shame in Early Modern England* (Ithaca and London: Cornell University Press, 1993); Maurizio Calbi, *Approximate Bodies: Gender and Power in Early Modern Drama and Anatomy* (New York and London: Routledge, 1995); and Nunn, *Staging Anatomies*. For a wide-ranging chronological study which also takes in Shakespeare see Jacqueline Rose, *Sexuality in the Field of Vision* (London and New York: Verso, 1986).
31. Mary Beth Rose, 'Where are the Mothers in Shakespeare? Options for Gender Representation in the English Renaissance', *Shakespeare Quarterly* 42 (Fall 1991), pp. 291–314.
32. Ibid., pp. 305 and 313.

33. Janet Adelman, *Suffocating Mothers: Fantasies of Maternal Origin in Shakespeare's Plays, Hamlet to The Tempest* (New York and London: Routledge, 1992), pp. 3–8. For another reading which uses psychoanalytical techniques of enquiry see Coppélia Kahn, 'The Absent Mother in *King Lear*', in *Rewriting the Renaissance: The Discourses of Sexual Difference in Early Modern Europe*, eds Margaret W. Ferguson, Maureen Quilligan and Nancy J. Vickers (Chicago: University of Chicago Press, 1986), pp. 33–49.
34. Theresa M. Krier, *Birth Passages: Maternity and Nostalgia, Antiquity to Shakespeare* (Ithaca and London: Cornell University Press, 2001), Preface, xiv.
35. Ibid., pp. 11–12.
36. Newman, *Fetal Positions*, p. 17.
37. The work of E. Davies-Floyd and Carolyn F. Sargent builds on the foundational efforts of Brigitte Jordan whose *Birth in Four Cultures* (Eden Press, 1978) inaugurated a new era of ethnographic research into birth. In their edited collection, *Childbirth and Authoritative Knowledge: Cross-Cultural Perspectives* (Berkeley, Los Angeles and London: University of California Press, 1997), Davies-Floyd and Sargent express a desire to 'speak in the language of the birthing body' by restoring 'the deep physiology of birth as well as its cultural overlay'. Instrumental to this endeavour is the recognition of the ways in which authoritative knowledge of maternal processes is 'contested by nurses, midwives, holistic physicians, and other dissenters inside its ranks', pp. 13–15. Anthropological studies have found it much harder to account for the social and epistemological significance of crises in their analyses of childbirth, though one exception to this is Karen Ericksen Paige and Jeffery M. Paige, *The Politics of Reproductive Ritual* (Berkeley, Los Angeles and London: University of California Press, 1981), which puts forward the theory that 'those events in the human reproductive life cycle marked by ritual observances – birth, puberty, and menstruation – pose potential crises for preindustrial societies . . . [T]he solution to each of these dilemmas is often a ritual because in preindustrial societies direct political or legal solutions are often not possible,' p. 43.
38. Sara Mendelson and Patricia Crawford, *Women in Early Modern England 1550–1720* (Oxford: Clarendon Press, 1998), esp. pp. 148–64; Antonia Fraser, *The Weaker Vessel: A Woman's Lot in Seventeenth-Century England* (London: Phoenix Press, 1984), esp. pp. 71–96 and 537–65; David Cressy, *Birth, Marriage and Death: Ritual, Religion, and the Life-Cycle in Tudor and Stuart England* (Oxford: Oxford University Press, 1999), esp. pp. 15–94; Heather Dubrow *Shakespeare and Domestic Loss: Forms of Deprivation, Mourning and Recuperation* (Cambridge: Cambridge University Press, 1999); Richard Wilson 'Observations on English Bodies: Licensing Maternity in Shakespeare's Late Plays', in *Enclosure Acts: Sexuality, Property and Culture in Early Modern England*, eds Richard Burt and John Michael Archer (Ithaca and London: Cornell University Press, 1994), pp. 121–50; Audrey Eccles, *Obstetrics and Gynaecology in Tudor and Stuart England* (London: Croom Helm, 1982); Adrian Wilson, 'The Ceremony of Childbirth and its Interpretation', *Women as Mothers in Pre-Industrial England: Essays in Memory of*

Dorothy McLaren, ed. Valerie Fildes (New York and London: Routledge, 1990), pp. 68–107 and 'Participant or Patient? Seventeenth-Century Childbirth from the Mother's Point of View', *Patients and Practitioners: Lay Perceptions of Medicine in Pre-Industrial Society*, ed. Roy Porter (Cambridge: Cambridge University Press, 1985), pp. 129–44; Angus McLaren, *Reproductive Rituals: The Perception of Fertility in England from the Sixteenth Century to the Nineteenth Century* (London: Methuen, 1984); Jacques Gelis, *History of Childbirth: Fertility, Pregnancy and Birth in Early Modern Europe* (Cambridge: Polity Press, 1991); and John Dewhurst, 'The Alleged Miscarriages of Catherine of Aragon and Anne Boleyn', *Medical History* 28 (1980), pp. 49–56.

39. Caroline Bicks, *Midwiving Subjects in Shakespeare's England* (Aldershot: Ashgate, 2003), pp. 8 and 12.
40. Kathryn M. Moncrief and Kathryn R. McPherson (eds), *Performing Maternity in Early Modern England* (Aldershot: Ashgate, 2007), p. 1. A version of Chapter 4 of this study appears as 'Speaking Stones: Memory and Maternity in Shakespeare's *Antony and Cleopatra*', in *Performing Maternity*, pp. 143–69. In the same volume Moncrief reveals that 'the early modern understanding of the indeterminate nature of pregnancy' is essential to Shakespeare's challenging of 'authoritative evidence' in *All's Well That Ends Well*. Helena's pregnant body does not 'represent a "rebirth" of the shattered marital relationship, as pregnancy might, but serves instead to highlight uncertainty', ' "Show me a child begotten of thy body that I am father to": Pregnancy, Paternity and the Problem of Evidence in *All's Well That Ends Well*', pp. 40–2. Laura Gowing also rehistoricises the 'uncertain knowledge' of the early modern maternal body in *Common Bodies*, pp. 17–51. See also the wide-ranging approaches to maternity in Naomi J. Miller and Naomi Yavneh (eds), *Maternal Measures: Figuring Caregiving in the Early Modern Period* (Aldershot: Ashgate, 2000); Valeria Finucci and Kevin Brownlee (eds), *Generation and Degeneration: Tropes of Reproduction in Literature and History from Antiquity to Early Modern Europe* (Durham and London: Duke University Press, 2001); and Susan C. Greenfield and Carol Barash (eds), *Inventing Maternity: Politics, Science, and Literature, 1650–1865* (Kentucky: The University Press of Kentucky, 1999). Another important work which discloses the political import of birthing and maternal analogies is Helen Hackett's *Virgin Mother, Maiden Queen: Elizabeth I and the Cult of the Virgin Mary* (London: Macmillan, 1995).
41. Studies of maternity have only recently begun attending to its *material* histories by using the evidence derived from physical and archaeological artefacts. These include Amanda Carson Banks, *Birth Chairs, Midwives and Medicine* (Jackson: University Press of Mississippi, 1999); Jacqueline Marie Mussachio, *The Art and Ritual of Childbirth in Renaissance Italy* (New Haven and London: Yale University Press, 1999); and Nancy Demand, *Birth, Death, and Motherhood in Classical Greece* (Baltimore and London: Johns Hopkins University Press, 1994). Approaches to Shakespeare using these methodological principles are rare. Three examples are Catherine Belsey, *Shakespeare and the Loss of Eden: The Construction of Family Values in Early Modern Culture* (Houndmills:

Palgrave, 2001); Margareta de Grazia, 'Imprints: Shakespeare, Gutenburg and Descartes', in *Alternative Shakespeares*, vol. 2, ed. Terence Hawkes (New York and London: Routledge, 1996), pp. 63–94, a fascinating account of the relationship between the female reproductive anatomy and the early modern printing press; and Helen Hackett ' "Gracious be the Issue": Maternity and Narrative in Shakespeare's Late Plays', in *Shakespeare's Late Plays: New Readings*, eds Jennifer Richards and James Knowles (Edinburgh: Edinburgh University Press, 1999), pp. 25–39. Hackett reveals the ways in which the 'archetypal feminine activities of spinning and weaving' constituted an alternative type of cultural 'text' which informed the production, dissemination and consumption of maternal narratives, p. 32.

Chapter 1

Flesh and Stone: Dissecting Maternity in the Theatre of Anatomy

Behold the Woman: The Renaissance Anatomist in the Satyr's Mask

> [T]he death of the womb, is an entrance . . . [T]he womb hath discharged us, yet we are bound to it by cords of flesh . . .
>
> John Donne, *Death's Duel*[1]

It was after dark in Louvain when Andreas Vesalius of Brussels allowed himself to be locked out of the city gates once more. Days before, while 'looking for bones where the executed criminals are usually placed along the country roads', he had chanced upon the remains of a dried cadaver 'which had been partially burned and roasted over a fire of straw and then bound to a stake'.[2] Making successive clandestine visits to the gruesome site he was able to smuggle parts of the decayed body back into the city. His return, on an autumnal evening in 1536, was prompted by his desire to 'obtain the thorax, which was held securely by a chain', fastened to the gibbet from which the remaining parts of the corpse still hung. This episode from his student days is described in what is perhaps the founding text of modern anatomy, the *De Humani Corporis Fabrica* (1543):

> So great was my desire to possess those bones that in the middle of the night, alone and in the midst of all those corpses, I climbed the stake with considerable effort and did not hesitate to snatch away that which I so desired.[3]

This fulsome, even sensual, account of illicit body-snatching is augmented by Vesalius' boast, in elegant Latin prose sparkling with humour, that he had contrived an ingenious ruse in order to evade the detection of the authorities, constructing a complete skeleton from stolen body-parts so skilled in its execution that his claim to have bought the specimen in Paris went unchallenged. Vesalius' refashioning of the corpse as locus of desire intersects with a range of literary tropes to which his autobiographical narratives allude. Shades of courtly romance and Fabliau, in which the aspiring lover must suffer trials and hardships, or in more comedic vein, dupe his gullible social superiors, in order to win the object of his affections, flicker at the edges of these digressive set pieces. In his *Letter on the China Root* (1546) Vesalius presents a melancholic self-portrait in which he becomes a martyr for his art, one who would 'willingly spend long hours in the Cemetery of the Innocents in Paris turning over bones', even risking life and limb to obtain precious body parts, as was the case during one of his bone-collecting escapades in Montfaucon where he 'was gravely imperilled by the many savage dogs'. He does not try to conceal, but actually advertises, his frequent attempts at night-time grave-robbing, for which he encouraged his students to forge keys 'for the beautiful cemetery of San Pisano so that they might investigate the many burial monuments'.[4] The confessional mode of the text is further amplified by the disquieting admission that Vesalius would often 'keep in my bedroom for several weeks bodies taken from graves or given me after public executions'.[5] Nowhere does this open enumeration of the illegal, anarchic and even necrophilic aspects of anatomy come to the fore as it does in Vesalius' investigations into the female reproductive system. The identities of the women he has dissected are not entirely obliterated by the anatomist's blade but suffer partial reparation as a result of his own unconcealed sexual curiosity and appetite for scandal. The description of the uterine anatomy is framed by an unflinchingly macabre tale:

> The handsome mistress of a certain monk of San Antonio here [in Padua] died suddenly as though from strangulation of the uterus or some quickly devastating ailment and was snatched from her tomb by the Paduan students and carried off for public dissection. By remarkable industry they flayed the whole skin from the cadaver lest it be recognized by the monk who, with the relatives of his mistress, had complained to the municipal judge that the body had been stolen from its tomb.[6]

The anatomists' illicit means of procuring bodies form part of a larger drama of transgression in which the shameless violation of both sexual and religious propriety centres on two figures who could easily have been lifted from the Fabliau tradition: the lascivious monk, a microcosm for the corruptions of the Catholic Church; and the sexually incontinent mistress whose diseased uterus seems to make her the subject of divine retribution. The *Fabrica* contains further references to such loose women, including a 'prostitute of fine figure and in the prime of life, who had been hanged'.[7] And in his *Letter on the China Root* Vesalius reveals that even the virginity of a nun cannot be taken on trust until she is opened to reveal her 'ovaries, [which] however, were shrunken as happens to organs that are not used'.[8] Vesalius' lively delineations of the characters who make cameo appearances in his anatomical manual operate beyond the purely functional paradigms of medical explication and form an integral part of what I am identifying as the largely unacknowledged *satiric* impulse of the early modern anatomy, the nature of which will be the subject of the first half of this chapter.

Perhaps the most influential record of an anatomised woman ever to appear in any medical treatise, and one which will form the epitome of this chapter's rereading of the satirical ethos of the early modern anatomical discipline, is the much-lauded title-page of the *Fabrica*, a landmark in the history of European printing (Fig. 1.1).[9] More than any other this image cemented the association between the authoritative knowledge of the anatomical discipline and the privileged disclosure of the maternal body's deepest secrets, yet it is hardly what we might expect a formal medical lesson to look like. Animals jostle for space among the curious spectators, some of whom seem to be dressed in anachronistic costumes which have a distinct *all'antica* flavour. What would have appeared most shocking to contemporary eyes, however, is the dramatic use of the body of a female executed criminal who, Vesalius informs us, 'in fear of being hanged had falsely declared herself pregnant'.[10] Given the rarity of anatomical demonstrations of female bodies in the early modern period, it seems all the more extraordinary that Vesalius should wish to place a woman centre-stage in this way.[11] Her nakedness and the orientation of her body, which emphasises her exposed genitalia, would have pushed the boundaries of propriety and amplified the subtly subversive connection between sexual inquisitiveness and prohibited forms of acquiring anatomical data which form a recurring theme of the narratological apparatus of the *Fabrica*. Vesalius' laying bare of the empty womb, proving the executed woman's testimony to be a lie, compresses the erotic overtones of the image with the anatomists' mastery over the wayward female body. A good deal more is going on here than what we are *seeing*.

Taken together with the anatomical project for which it serves as the visual preface,[12] the *Fabrica*'s title-page reflects the peculiar cult of personality with which Vesalius hoped to be associated. To modern scientific sensibilities this will seem alien. A thief, a trickster, a dissimulator, an adventurer, a melancholic, a connoisseur of erotic perversions; Vesalius appears to go out of his way to present himself as a rogue and daring flouter of the law. But why should he wish to do this and why was he so interested in the lurid personal histories of the women he dissected? The answer will bring us closer to understanding Vesalius' strategic insistence on equating the success of anatomy, as a distinct body of knowledge, with the explication of maternal mysteries. This will

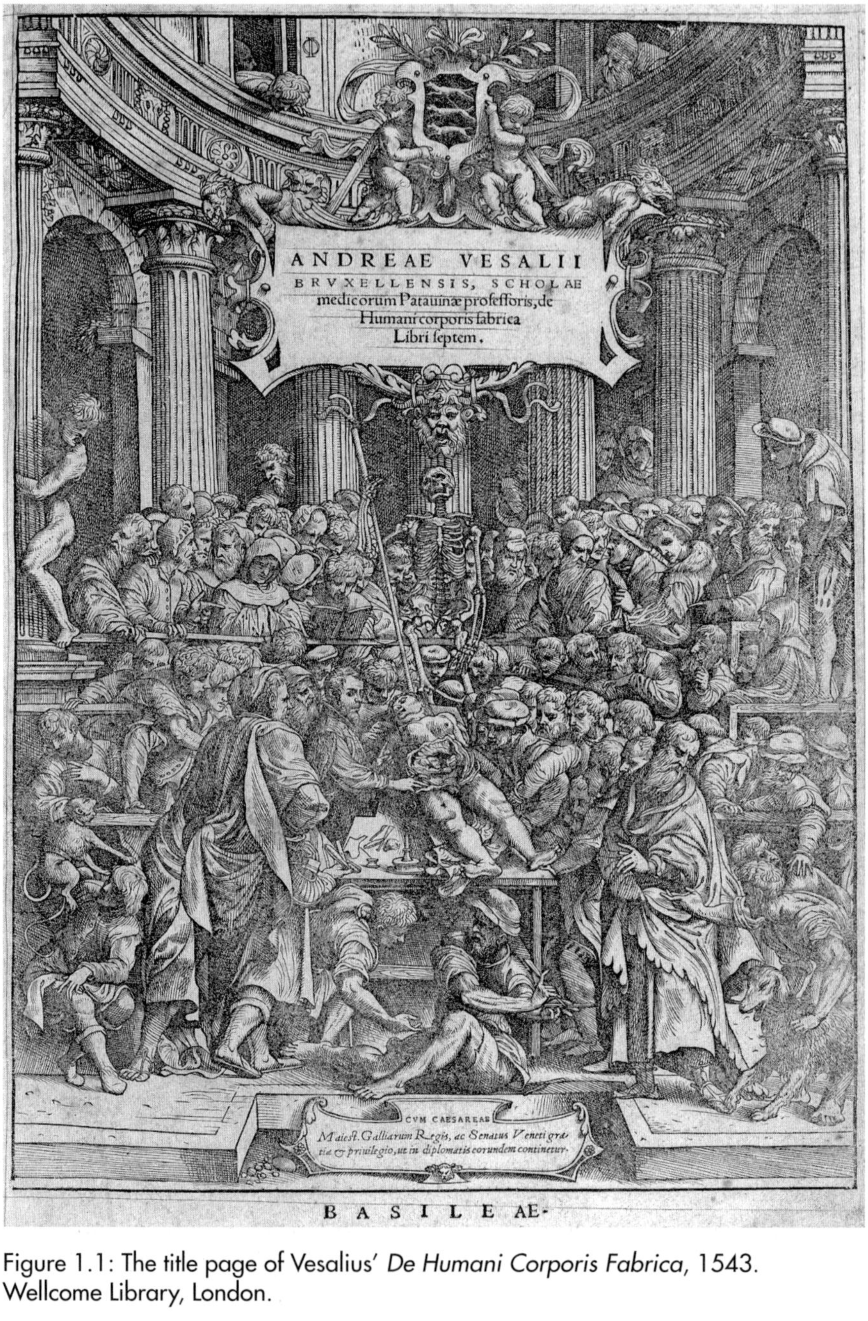

Figure 1.1: The title page of Vesalius' *De Humani Corporis Fabrica*, 1543. Wellcome Library, London.

enable us to go on, in the second part of this chapter, to reveal the ways in which Shakespeare's dissections of the maternal body in *Hamlet* both appropriated and interrogated a satirical tradition which, as I hope to show, supplied the anatomists with the propagandist machinery which proved so crucial to their pedagogical enterprise.

What better proof of Vesalius' refinement and good taste would his contemporaries have needed than his decision to place the commission for the revolutionary anatomical plates of the *Fabrica* in the hands of the renowned Titian workshop?[13] This may also have been a shrewd career move for the Paduan anatomist since Titian had by this time attracted the patronage of Charles V, whose favour Vesalius also hoped to win by lauding him as the *Fabrica*'s royal dedicatee. Instrumental to Titian's success was his friendship with the notorious Pietro Aretino, an association which had, according to his earliest biographer, Giorgio Vasari, 'brought Titian great honour and advantages, for the reason that Aretino made him known wherever his pen reached, and especially to important rulers'.[14] It was the cultural ethos of this privileged milieu, I would like to suggest, that Vesalius was accessing when he conceived the *Fabrica*'s iconographical and narratological apparatus, an endeavour which was to have a lasting, and wide-reaching impact on the study of the maternal body.

In 1543, the very year in which the *Fabrica* was published, Titian completed his monumental painting *Ecce Homo* ('Behold the Man'), which dramatises the moment when Pontius Pilate surrenders Christ and Barabbas to the judgement of the people, asking them to choose their sacrificial victim (Fig. 1.2). Among the portraits of contemporaries which are reproduced in the image, a mode of allusive presentation particularly favoured by Titian, the artist pays tribute to Aretino by depicting Pilate in the very likeness of his humanist friend.[15] This was the man who had, by the time of the *Fabrica*'s publication, already found his way into the public imagination after his involvement in a scandal which had sent shock-waves throughout Europe and which, as we will see, left its indelible mark on the history of anatomy. For it was in 1524 that Aretino's friend, Marcantonio Raimondi, was imprisoned in Rome for engraving a collection of highly explicit erotic images – the infamous *I modi*, or 'positions' – originally produced by Raphael's protégé, Giulio Romano. Undaunted by the fate of Raimondi, Aretino went on to produce a sequence of sonnets which he published in the more liberal city of Venice, the *Sonetti lussuriosi*, to accompany the sixteen pornographic plates (Fig. 1.3). The sonnets would be the beginning of Aretino's long battle with the censors over the right to circulate sexual

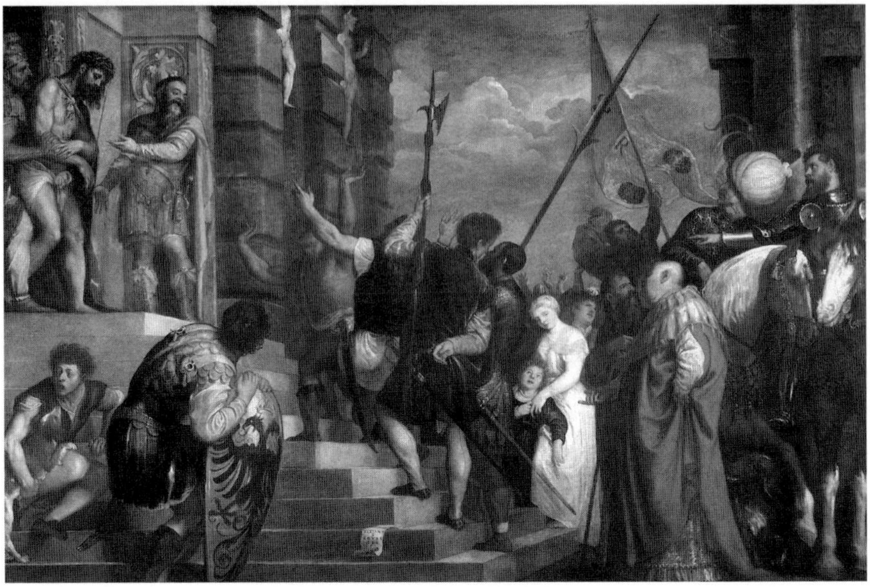

Figure 1.2: Titian, *Ecce Homo*, 1543. Kunsthistorisches Museum, Wien oder KHM, Wien (Vienna).

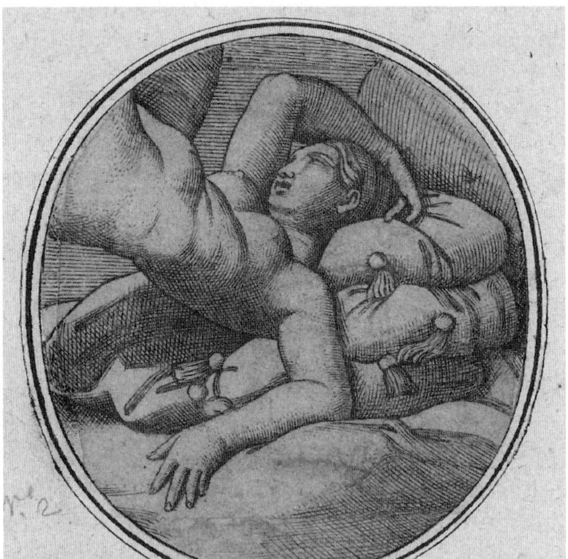

Figure 1.3: Marcantonio Raimondi or close followers, fragment from the *I Modi* series for which Pietro Aretino provided the textual accompaniments with his *Sonetti Lussuriosi*. British Museum, Department of Prints and Drawings. © The Trustees of the British Museum.

knowledge, and in a letter to the surgeon Battista Zatti of Brescia, possibly composed as a dedicatory epistle to the 1527 edition of the *Sonetti lussuriosi*, he condemned the authorities who, in order to 'forbid the eyes what delights them most', had 'cried out for this fine artist [Raimondi] to be crucified'. Comparing the contentious erotica to the Chigi Palace's 'marble satyr' – a mythological figure of brazen sexuality which would become his own personal *impressa* and the image with which he would be most readily identified[16] – he fashioned a paean to the unrestrained veneration of the male generative organs:

> It would seem to me that the tool Nature gave us to preserve the race should be worn as a pendant round one's neck or as a medal in one's hat, since it's the spring which feeds all the rivers of humankind and the ambrosia the world drinks on high-days and holidays . . . so we should allocate to it its own ferial-days and consecrate special vigils and feast-days in its honour . . .[17]

Aretino's encomium on the sexual organ, a satiric motif he helped to popularise, borrows from a tradition of pagan sacrifice, the worship of the phallic god deriving from classical accounts of Bacchic and Satyric festivals. It was at this time that Titian was popularising this very imagery in paintings such as *The Andrians* (c. 1523–4) which foregrounds, in a manner strongly reminiscent of Vesalius' title-page, the naked body of a woman reclining on folds of white cloth whose unflinchingly sexualised pose replicates a well-known classical statue of Ariadne (Fig. 1.4).[18] Over the years Aretino would develop and enrich this classicising iconography in order to forge a public persona as an interpreter of sexual mysteries, a charismatic libidinous rogue and a 'scourge' of folly's followers whose 'pen, armed with all its terrors, has succeeded in forcing them to reform themselves'.[19] Exploiting the fabled etymological connection between satire and the Satyr plays of ancient Greece,[20] Aretino combined the notion of satire as a sexually scurrilous tale reminiscent of the antics of the goatish Satyrs with the harsher, more reforming, function of Juvenalian satire.[21]

More than an entertaining diversion this satirical discourse, which centred round the sexualised body, became a vehicle for exposing the weaknesses of a pedagogical endeavour which relied greatly on the recovered fragments of the received wisdom – historical, linguistic and anatomical – newly available to scholars of the humanist curriculum. In the *Sonetti lussuriosi*[22] he insisted that carnal knowledge did not require the study of learned authorities but could be acquired 'without making the rounds of the schools to learn, for example, in detail how to do such business very well'.[23] This unmediated, uncensored contact with the eroticised body strikes the keynote of the sonnets, whose lurid blazons take on

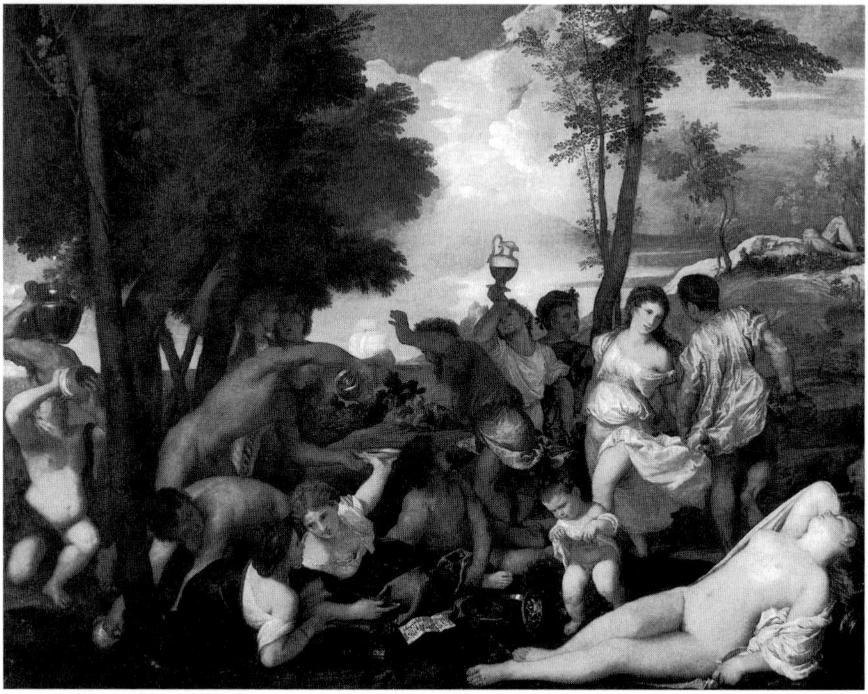

Figure 1.4: Titian, *The Andrians*, c. 1523–4. Museo Nacional del Prado, Madrid.

a distinctly anatomical flavour. Sexual wisdom becomes something best attained, in necrophilic fashion, 'postmortem',[24] and even the empowered female speaker of the third sonnet becomes a willing anatomical specimen, enticing her lover to 'probe well my innermost reaches' (*E trova ben la foia in la matrice*).[25] Aretino's attack on mediatory systems of thought finds embodiment in his satirical swipes at the corruptions of the Catholic Church. Sodomy, the most condemned of all sexual infractions, is 'the food of prelates, who always have had the damnedest taste', a blasphemous inversion of the rite of transubstantiation which must have shocked the audacious sonneteer's contemporaries.[26]

Unlikely as it may at first seem, such reforming sentiments resound with Aretino's *La Humanità di Christo*, produced in the late 1530s, a text in which Pontius Pilate is presented in a sympathetic light and in which the minutiae of theological debate are eclipsed by the example of the afflicted Christ who, in all his suffering humanity, 'resembled a stag about to be dragged down by hounds' at the hands of his worldly persecutors.[27] This idea finds its visual counterpart in Titian's *Ecce Homo* in which Aretino/Pilate stands between Christ and the menacing mob while pointing decisively towards the wounded body of the thorn-crowned man. What historians of anatomy have to date overlooked is the fact that this very gesture is eerily recapitulated in Vesalius' title-page in the figure who has attracted the greatest attention among critics, after the dissected woman herself: the bearded man in classical garb who stands prominently to the right of the cadaver.[28] The same figure appears in slightly altered form in the 1555 rendering of the title-page (Fig. 1.5), along with further enigmatic changes which have continued to baffle generations of commentators, including the addition of the skeleton's scythe or pruning-blade and the introduction of a goat among the menagerie of animals.

The venerable man in antique dress certainly shares many of the same characteristics as Titian's Aretino/Pilate. The pointing gesture, the sweep of the beard beneath the turned-back head, the distinctive stance and the placement of the figure at the corner of the stage-like platform, are remarkably similar (compare Figs 1.6a, 1.6b and 1.6c). The classical clothing of this figure also resonates closely with Aretino's preferred method of self-presentation in the propagandist iconography which circulated his image in the title-pages of his own works, including the 1538 Venetian edition of his letters. This motif became popular with other satirists of the time, turning them into descendants of their classical forebears, Juvenal among them, while simultaneously alluding to the imperial glory of the Caesars. It is perhaps significant that in Vesalius' title-page a Latin tag bearing the words '*Cum Caesareo*' ('With Caesar') appears close to the robed man we are considering. While this indicates the publisher's licence to print 'with' the permission of 'the King', it may also function in the same way as the medals which, in imitation of those bearing Caesar's face, circulated with the *all'antica* portraits of both Aretino and Titian, one bronze image of the latter having been inscribed with the honourable title '*Eques Caesaris*'.[29]

If the 1543 title-page of the *Fabrica* included tentative visual references to the figurehead of the intellectual community which had attracted Charles V's favour during this time, it is possible that Vesalius went back and, with more confidence, strengthened these associations having achieved his goal of becoming the king's imperial physician by the time the 1555 edition had hit the presses. Could the sudden addition of the goat which actually touches the mysterious bearded man in the later version of the title-page – the attribute of the Satyr with which Aretino was so closely identified – be an insider's joke intended to raise a chuckle among the courtly initiates who recognised the reference to the notorious satirist? Could the antique figure, given such prominence in the foreground as he gestures towards the open female body before him, really be a deliberate allusion to Aretino?[30] Is he a speaking picture

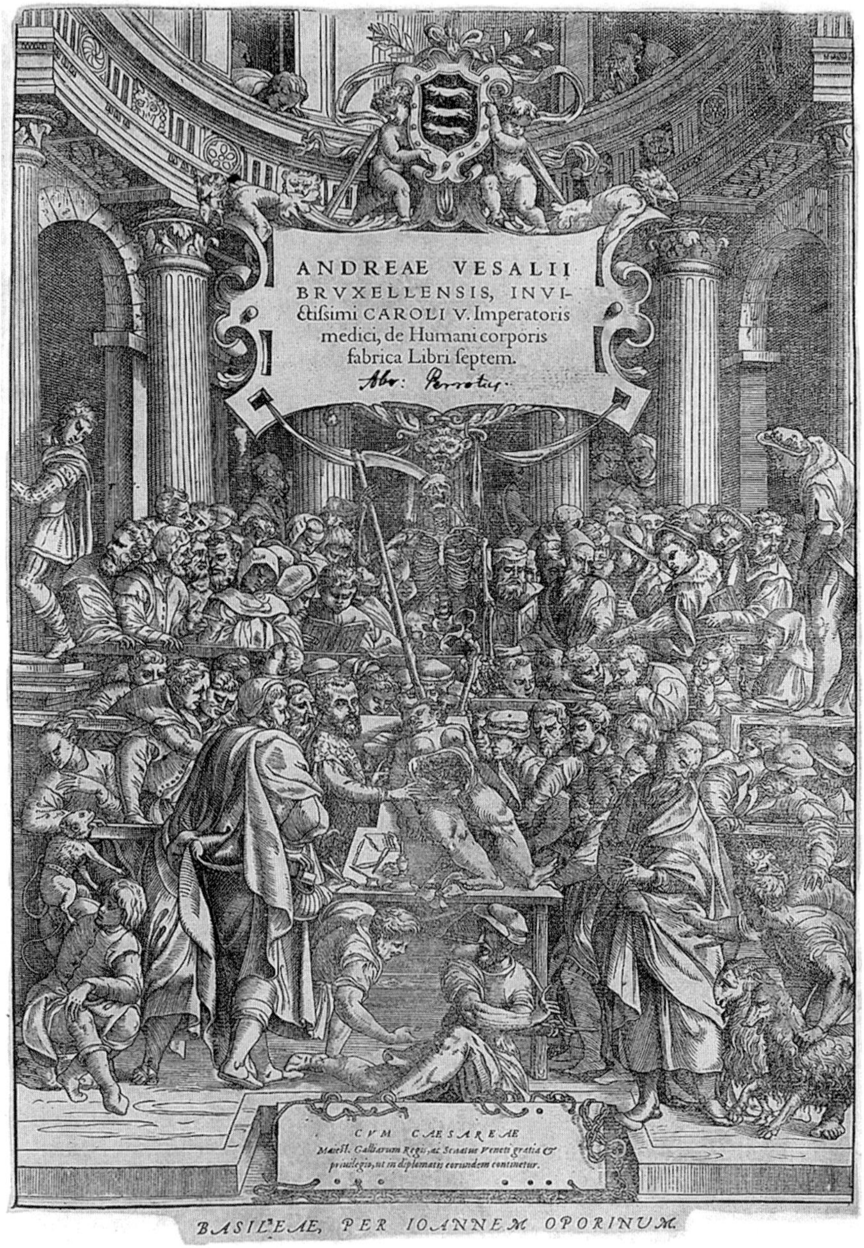

Figure 1.5: The title page of Vesalius' *De Humani Corporis Fabrica*, 1555. Wellcome Library, London.

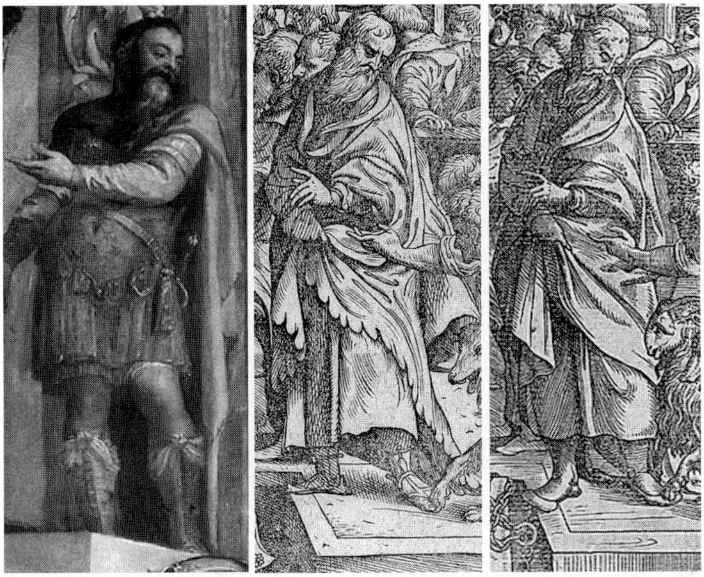

Figures 1.6a–1.6c: Details from Titian's *Ecce Homo* of 1543 and the 1543 and 1555 editions of Vesalius' *Fabrica*.

telling the viewer, like his counterpart in the *Ecce Homo* painting, to 'Behold the Woman'? If a few elite viewers of the image were expected to make this connection, then perhaps Vesalius was adding his voice to that of Aretino through a recognised satiric topos, a pictorial encomium on the womb, which stressed the anatomical regime's willingness to transgress any limits of propriety in the pursuit, and uncensored dissemination of, anatomical and sexual knowledge.

Whether or not the title-page of the *Fabrica* alludes specifically to Aretino, I suggest that Vesalius' strategies for establishing the professionalised status of the new anatomical regime borrow from the emblematic devices – Satyrical, sacrificial and pornographic – which formed the satiric repertoire of the cutting-edge humanist circle that gathered around Charles V. In particular the sexualised idiom of the pagan sacrifice may have informed Vesalius' self-presentation as much as it did Aretino's.[31] The most influential of such pictorial references appeared in Aldus Manutius' Venetian edition of the best-selling romance, the *Hypnerotomachia Poliphili* (1499) by Francesco Colonna. The woodcut of the Worship of Priapus (Fig. 1.7) shows a sacrificial scene presided over by the phallic god in his guise as priapic satyr, carrying the emblem with which he is often associated, the pruning-scythe.[32] This scene forms a striking visual analogue to the 1555 title-page of the *Fabrica* in which the skeleton seems almost to

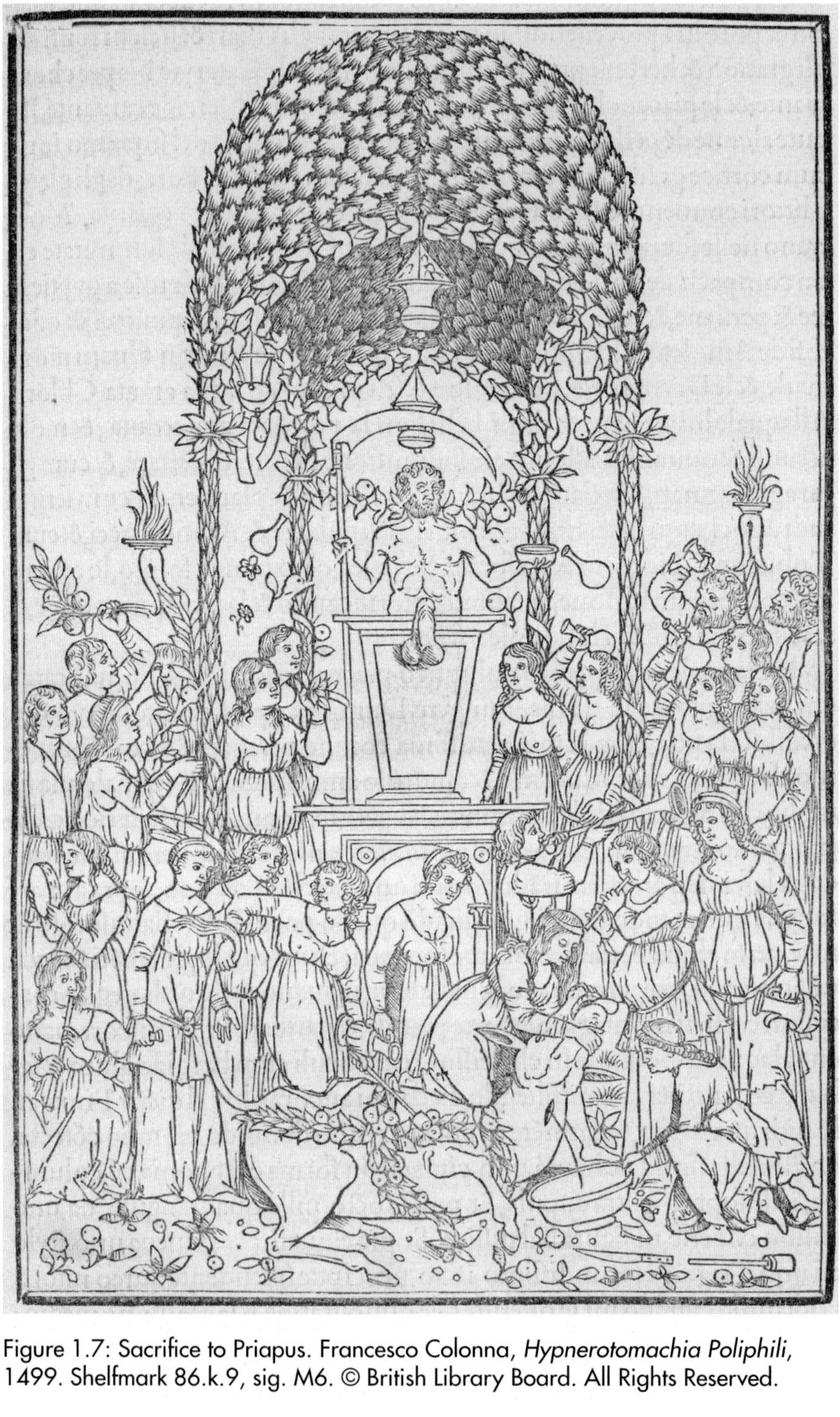

Figure 1.7: Sacrifice to Priapus. Francesco Colonna, *Hypnerotomachia Poliphili*, 1499. Shelfmark 86.k.9, sig. M6.

take the place of Priapus. The image's compositional features – the classical dress of the worshippers, the animals being readied for sacrifice before an altar upon which the presiding deity is placed in elevated position, and the Bacchic or Satyric elements – are staple features of the sacrificial scene which are strongly alluded to in the *Fabrica*'s title-page. More significantly still, accorded a central place beneath the cartouche which bears Vesalius' name is the governing symbol of Aretinian satire: the Satyr's mask.

That Vesalius' title-page alludes to this tradition is suggested by the inclusion of a decorated architectural frieze which could easily have been lifted from Book IV of Sebastio Serlio's *Architettura*, first published in Venice just five years before the *Fabrica*. This describes the interior of classical pagan temples 'set, cut, or grave[d], [with] Oxe heads, [and] with Dishes', motifs which, Serlio explains, were 'not without secret signification. For in ancient time, when the unbeleeving folke sacrificed Oxen, they also used Dishes, & Platters thereunto, placing such things round about their Temples for ornaments'.[33] By staging his dissection in a temple-like structure, replete with reminders of pagan sacrifice, Vesalius forges a new anatomical theology in which the womb becomes the locus of a salvific narrative. The elevated pagan god to whom a sacrifice would traditionally have been offered is replaced by an altogether more disturbing titular deity: the figure of Death, eerily placed in physical and semantic proximity to the Satyr's mask. With its reminders of the fall which rendered humanity mortal, the Christian *memento-mori* undertone of the image both alludes to and challenges the prohibited nature of the knowledge promised by the opening of the maternal anatomy.

The commensurability of these Christian, pagan and anatomical elements is a common feature of contemporary works of art in which the paraphernalia of pagan sacrifice appear as adjuncts to the display of Christ's wounded body.[34] An image which Vesalius may well have seen in his adopted city of Padua is that included on the Paschal candlestick, created by Andrea Briosco in 1515 for St Anthony's Basilica (Fig. 1.8). Figures in classical attire perform an animal sacrifice before an altar upon which stands the bleeding Christ whose open body comes to occupy the same semantic space as the slaughtered Paschal lamb. By presenting us with a sacrificial scene in which the dissected woman takes the place of the suffering Christ, Vesalius forces us to re-orient our understanding of the anatomical ritual. The maternal body, sacrificed on the altar of learning, becomes the locus of an authentic and redemptive truth. Vesalius is at once both priest-like confessor, drawing out the fallen body's darkest secrets, and daring sexual connoisseur, whose

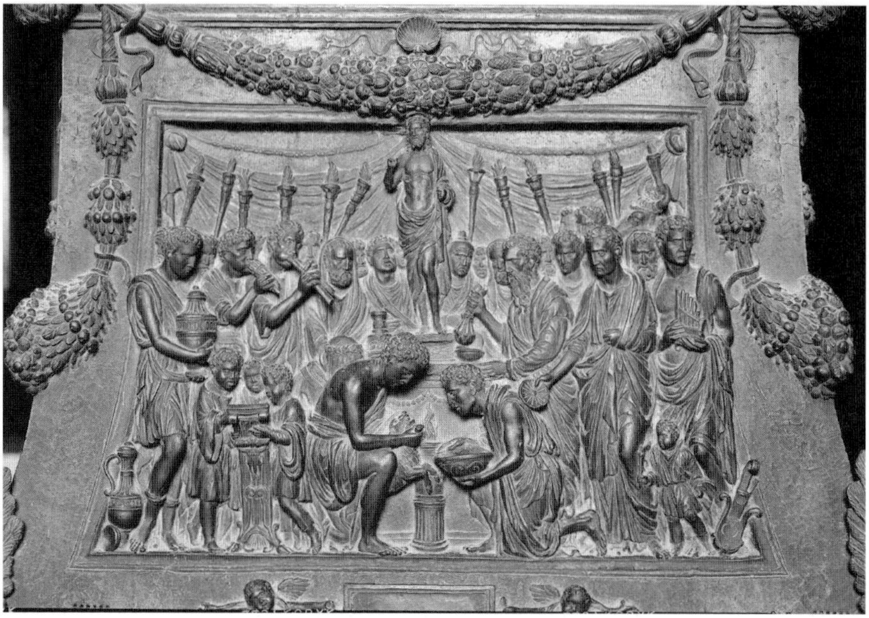

Figure 1.8: Andrea Briosco, *The Paschal Candlestick*, 1515, Basilica of St Anthony, Padua. Fototeca del Centro Studi Antoniani.

charismatic personality animates a masculine camaraderie cemented through an appreciation of the sexualised reproductive anatomy.[35]

The concern with recovering a direct, unmediated anatomical knowledge is precisely what governs Vesalius' employment of the *Fabrica*'s satiric machinery as a whole. And once again it is to the satirical idiom made so popular by Aretino that we should look in order to understand better how Vesalius and his contemporaries were engaging with, and overcoming the limits of, their own pedagogical culture. In a particularly famous letter, penned in 1537, Aretino recounts a dream which satirically targets those who mindlessly reproduce the hackneyed phraseology of their Petrarchan forebears:

> I also saw several fellows who, having given back what belonged to others, were left with blank sheets of paper . . . The conclusion of the dream was that I found myself in a market, as I thought, where the starlings, the magpies, crows and parrots were imitating geese on Hallowe'en. And along with these birds were several pedagogues, bombastic, bearded and bothered because they had to teach the birds to babble by the phases of the moon.[36]

Aretino locks horns with a humanist community dangerously prone to the uncritical recapitulation of inherited forms of expression. It is with this satirical lexicon that Vesalius and his contemporaries revised the ideological scaffolding which had underpinned the study of anatomy in medieval Europe. The earliest surviving records of anatomical demonstrations suggest that up until the fourteenth century dissections for pedagogical purposes were largely conducted on animals. Characteristic of the twelfth-century texts compiled at the medical school of Salerno, for example, is the *Anatomia Magistri Nicolai Physici*, which explains that 'in particular the female pig . . . shows the greatest likeness to the human structure in all internal organs, including the uterus'.[37] Such manuals were succeeded by those which took the human body as their object of enquiry, the first of which was the *Anatomia* of Mondino dei Liuzzi (d. 1326), published in 1316.[38] The purpose of these early procedures was not to make new anatomical discoveries but merely to confirm the writings of Galen and his Arabic commentator, Avicenna.[39] As such the ritual of anatomy was a highly stratified affair in which the actual practice of incision was undertaken by a barber-surgeon lower down the medical hierarchy while the lecturer, refusing to sully his hands with the surgeon's ignoble craft, would merely read out the lesson from a prescribed Galenic text.[40] This method was critiqued by one of Vesalius' contemporaries, the anatomist Niccolo Massa (1499–1569), who practised medicine and dissection in Venice and had regular access to bodies from the hospital of Saints Peter and Paul. In his *Liber Introductorius*, published in Venice in 1536, he censured those anatomists who did not 'care about making actual incision itself', but who 'clouded the brightest light of the sun with manuscripts accepted from others, [and] corrupted by age'. These *medici*, Massa went on to say, 'are like little birds who utter in song the things they hear and by their chirping delight the ears of certain people'.[41] While Massa's concern was the resurrection of a more authentic Galenic text, one less 'corrupted' by the inaccuracies of contemporary interpreters, Vesalius went further in his condemnation of those who exhibited a slavish adherence to past authorities and, in a manner reminiscent to that of Aretino, decried:

> that detestable procedure by which usually some conduct the dissection of the human body and others present the account of its parts, the latter like jackdaws aloft in their high chair, with egregious arrogance croaking things they have never investigated but merely committed to memory from the books of others.[42]

The *Fabrica*'s title-page becomes a visual manifesto intended to flesh out these very ideas. Presented in the act of touching the body, a scalpel poised like a pen in his hand, Vesalius turns the womb into the very wellspring of textual production, the direct experience of which is an indispensable catalyst for the new body of anatomical knowledge he is engaged in assembling. This project did not, however, constitute a violent break with tradition so much as an augmentation of emerging trends in medical practice which mobilised the maternal body as an ideologically freighted medium for the professionalising of the discipline. The origins of this enterprise inhere in the *Fasciculus Medicinae*, doubtfully attributed to Joanne de Ketham, a medical compendium which included Mondino's text, and which was first published in 1491 in Venice with a striking gravida figure (Fig. 1.9). Poised in the Mariological attitude of benediction, this figure reproduces those of medical compendia which focused on healing the diseases of women, like that delineated in a manuscript produced around 1420 in which the womb, marked 'embrio', is depicted in an impossibly elevated position (Fig. 1.10).[43] The most sacred part of the Mariological body, the womb, distanced from the cervix, is resistant to sexual opening. Preserving the indissoluble mystery of the incarnation, the image is designed to deflect a precise apprehension of the process of impregnation.

That this kind of anatomical iconography could have served a dual purpose, functioning also as a meditative aid to prayer, can be seen in its proximity to a feature of monastic writing which sought confirmation of the divine presence in the feminised open body. The Cistercian, Bernard of Clairvaux, in his series of sermons *On the Song of Songs*, described the process of Incarnation as a form of sacred injury, for

> the living and active Word of God that cuts more keenly than any two-edged sword . . . not only pierced Mary's soul but penetrated through and through, so that even the tiniest space in her virginal breast was permeated . . . [and she] who brought forth in visible flesh him whom she conceived visibly . . . experienced through her whole being a wound of love.[44]

Bernard's disciple, Guerric of Igny, similarly described the workings of the Holy Spirit in terms of visceral dissection in his *Liturgical Sermons*:

> It was not enough for that supreme mercy not to close the bowels of his compassion to the wretched. He draws them into his very bowels and makes them his members . . . Unspeakable are the groans and inexplicable the affections to which the spirit gives birth as if impregnated by the incomprehensible. The human heart is too narrow for them and therefore it is torn and pours itself out. The ardor which it conceives but cannot contain it breathes forth and spreads abroad in what ways it can, by tears, groans, sighs.[45]

The maternalised body of medieval anatomy, commensurate with its divine prototype, serves to demonstrate the limits of human knowledge when confronted with God's supreme creative powers, which are '[u]nspeakable . . . inexplicable . . . incomprehensible'.[46] In images like

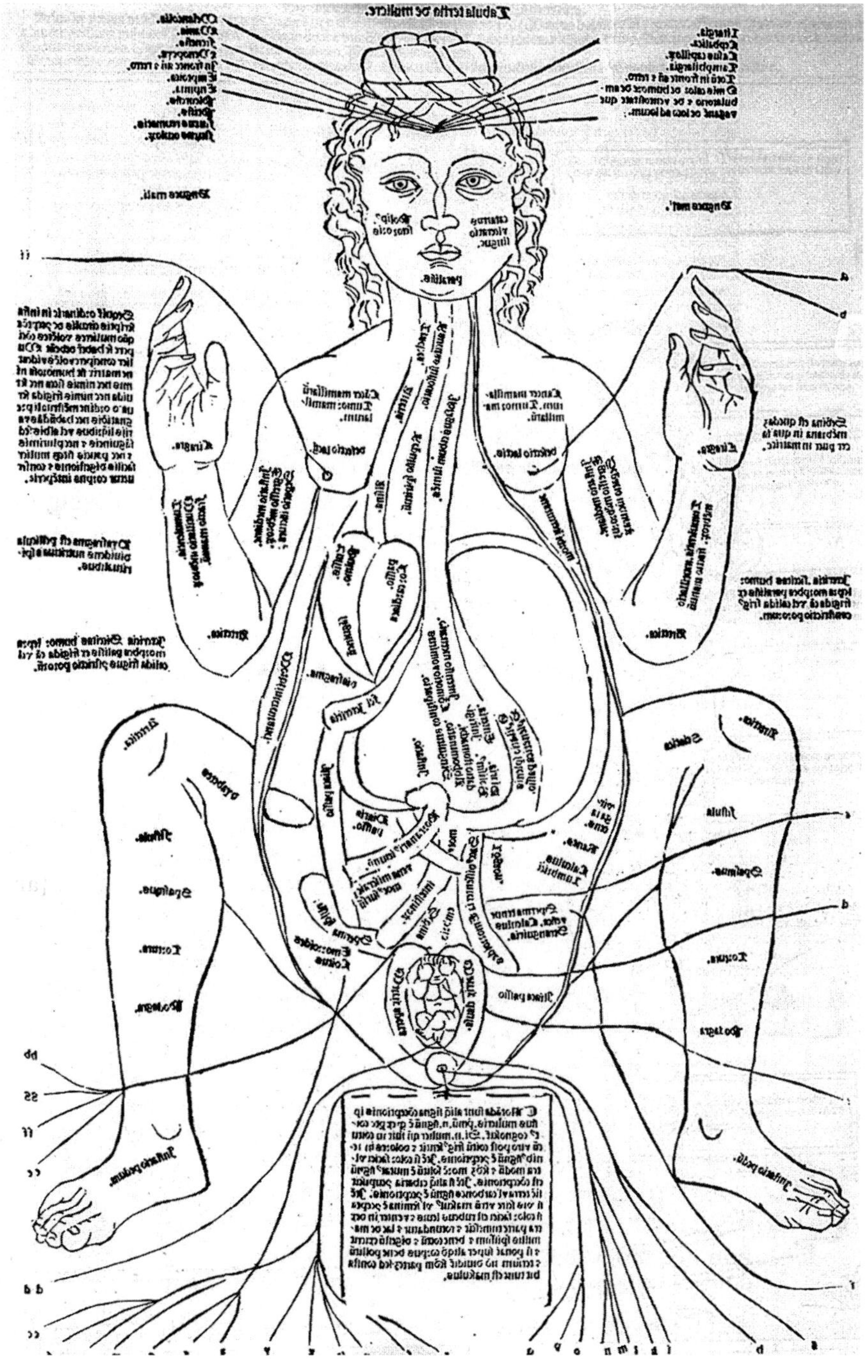

Figure 1.9: Gravida figure. Joanne de Ketham, *Fasciculus Medicinae*, 1491. Wellcome Library, London.

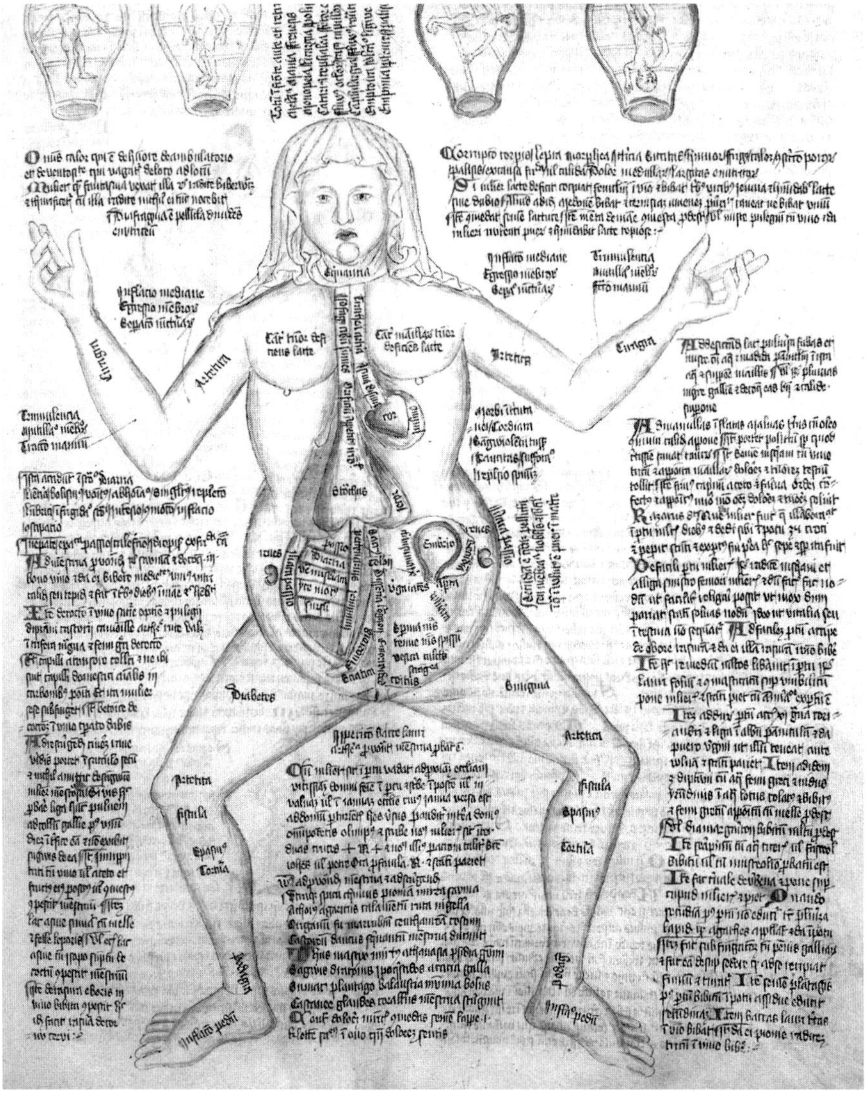

Figure 1.10: Gynaecological receipts; pregnant woman. Western MS 49 *Apocalypse*, c. 1420, f. 38. Wellcome Library, London.

the gravida of the 1491 *Fasciculus* we find a contemplative silence where we would expect to see a wholehearted disclosure of the reproductive anatomy. The *Fasciculus* was, however, reissued in 1493 with an adapted template for the uterine system. In the new edition an illustration by Gentile Bellini (for whom Titian was said to have served as apprentice before entering the workshop of his brother Giovanni), or his brother-in-law Andrea Mantegna,[47] replaces the Mariological pose of the gravida with the rhetorical gesture indicating speech (Fig. 1.11). Embellished with classical touches, the anatomised woman is poised in a manner which correlates her capacity for speech – her *confessional* posture – with her sexual openness.[48]

The iconographic trajectory of de Ketham's manual was also adopted by Berengario da Carpi (1460–1525), lecturer of anatomy at Bologna from 1502 to 1527.[49] Some of the explicitly Christian prototypes which provided the templates for anatomical diagrams in his *Commentaria* (1521), including a flayed man portrayed in the attitude of the crucified Christ,[50] were removed from his later *Isagogae Breves* (1535). This text introduced illustrations of a classicised female anatomy which tapped into the archaeological ethos of contemporary aesthetic theory, the vogue for collecting and displaying antique fragments.[51] One of a series of anatomised women, who appear like miraculously animated statues descending from their plinths, is presented in a demeanour which seems to equate the lifting of her veil with the revelation of hidden truths (Fig. 1.12). But these truths are not to be derived from textual sources. Stepping upon a set of closed books she points to an extracted uterus which has taken the place of the statue as object of scrutiny. The gesture at once dispels the antiquated myth of the seven-celled uterus, illustrating that it in fact 'has a single cavity or cell, which somewhat near its fundus is divided into two parts, as if two uteruses terminated in one neck'.[52] Berengario is mindful to attribute this discovery to personal experience, claiming that he 'saw a diseased uterus extracted completely in the town of Carpi by my father'.[53] While Berengario exhibits a respect for the classical world, fitting for this one-time pupil of Aldus Manutius, his appeal in the *Commentaria* to 'let those who write books on anatomy also not trust in authorities but in their sense perception as I do' makes sense when set against the visual programme he carefully cultivates: the antique fragments of the ancient body give way to the flesh and blood of the empirically-conceived maternal anatomy.[54]

This culture of dissection was reproduced in the cheaper printed broadsides which brought anatomical models to a wider audience from the early sixteenth century. Taking their cue from the iconographical programme instituted by Vesalius and his immediate precursors, these incorporated the reformist thinking which, I suggest, was instrumental in spreading an awareness of the commensurability between satirical and anatomical forms of utterance across Europe and into England.[55] This is clear from the earliest anatomical sheets which were being issued in Strasbourg by the engraver Heinrich Vogtherr the Elder.[56] In 1539 a Latin version was printed by Jean Ruelle in Paris, the *Perutilis*

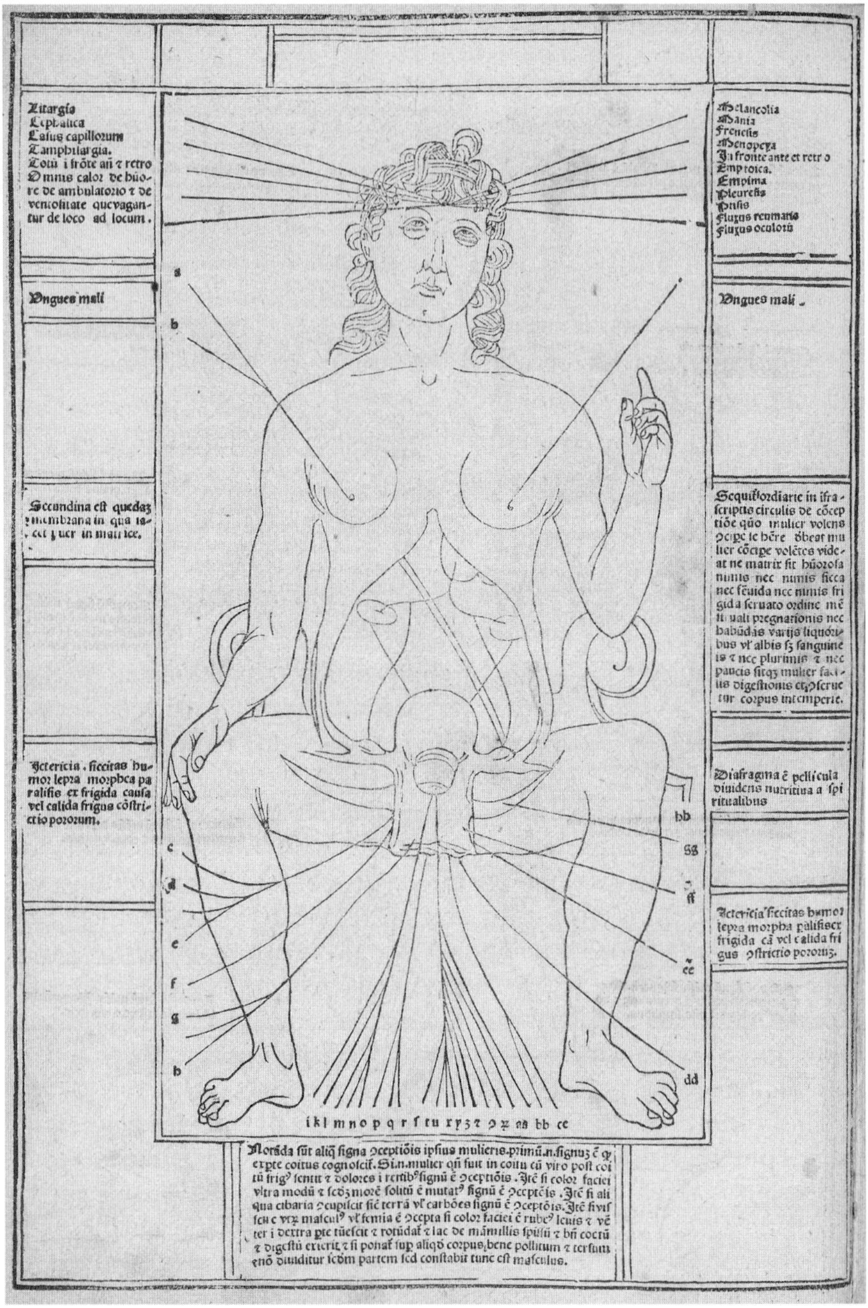

Figure 1.11: Gravida figure. Joanne de Ketham, *Fasciculus Medicinae*, 1493. Wellcome Library, London.

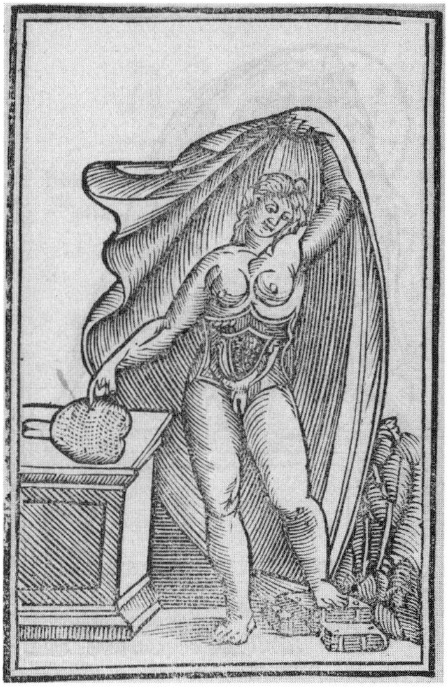

Figure 1.12: Dissected woman pointing to an extracted uterus. Berengario da Carpi, *Isagogae Breves*, 1535. Wellcome Library, London.

Anatomes Interiorum Mulieris. Poised like a statue on the edge of a plinth, the female body can be opened to reveal a tiny foetus (Figs 1.13a and 1.13b).[57] Such anatomical broadsides were often reproduced in centres of Reformation activity, by printers like Johann Schott, who played an important role in advancing the Protestant cause in Strasbourg during the 1520s.[58] The stress they place on verification by personal experience is consonant with the reformist insistence on a faith unmediated by hierarchical authority. Under the aegis of Protestantism, therefore, anatomical knowledge became an important adjunct to spiritual salvation. Those who wished to redeem themselves before God were required to do so in body as well as spirit. A sheet by Giles Godet printed in London around 1559 declares that 'The Anatomie of the inward Partes of wooman, [is] very necessarie to be knowen to Phisitians and Surgians and all other that desyre to knowe them selves.' The seminude female adorning the broadside is complicitous in her own anatomisation, clutching a sign which bears the Delphic dictum '*Nosce teipsum*' (Fig. 1.14).[59]

In 1573 anatomical sheets conveying more detailed embryological information were printed in Wittenberg, one of the intellectual

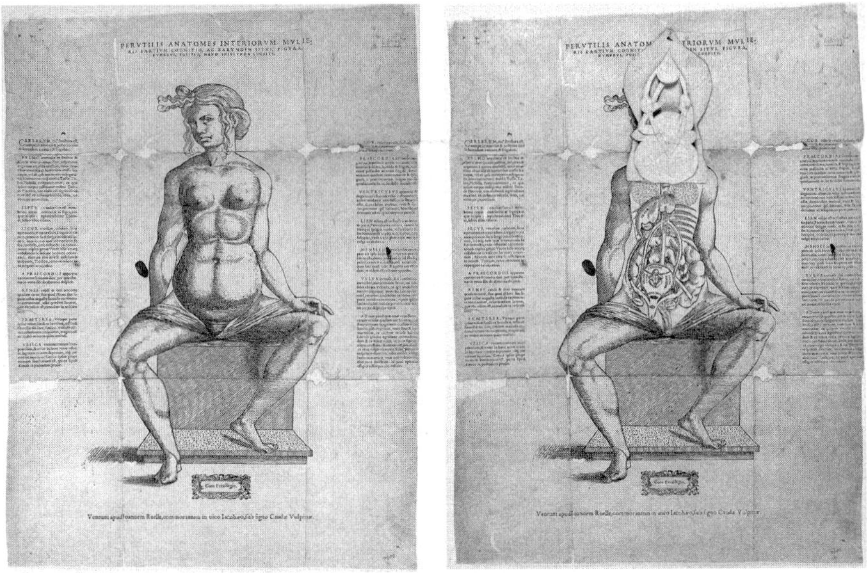

Figures 1.13a and 1.13b: Jean Ruelle, Anatomical Fugitive Sheet (shown right with anatomical flaps raised), *Perutilis Anatomes Interiorum Mulieris Partium*, 1539, EPB 289. Wellcome Library, London.

powerhouses of the Reformation. The series incorporating the *Tabula Foeminae Membra Demonstrans* was intended as a teaching aid to accompany Philip Melanchthon's *De Anima* (1540), a Lutheran reinterpretation of anatomical knowledge, revised in 1552 in response to advances introduced by the *Fabrica* (Figs 1.15a and 1.15b).[60] The fact that the male figure in the series bears an uncanny resemblance to Vesalius (compare his portrait in the *Fabrica*'s title-pages, Figs 1.1 and 1.5), suggests that the methodological principles instituted by his monumental work could be readily adapted to fit reforming sentiment.[61] As Melanchthon insisted in the *De Anima*, a true *agnitio Dei* could be achieved only through a rigorous process of self-examination, through which 'the external limbs are seriously persuaded to restrain themselves and not rush like the furious or beasts impelled by blind instincts'.[62] This echoes a specifically Lutheran idea of the 'spiritual incapacity of man' in the face of Christ's redemptive grace.[63] In his lecture *On Anatomy*, recited by Jakob Milich before the assembled medical faculty at Wittenberg University in 1550, Melanchthon explained that:

> [t]he very sight of the structure of many parts in us is the nurse of many virtues. And since the foremost virtue is the recognition of the Maker God, the assent to providence is much strengthened when we contemplate the wonderful skill in the entire construction of man.[64]

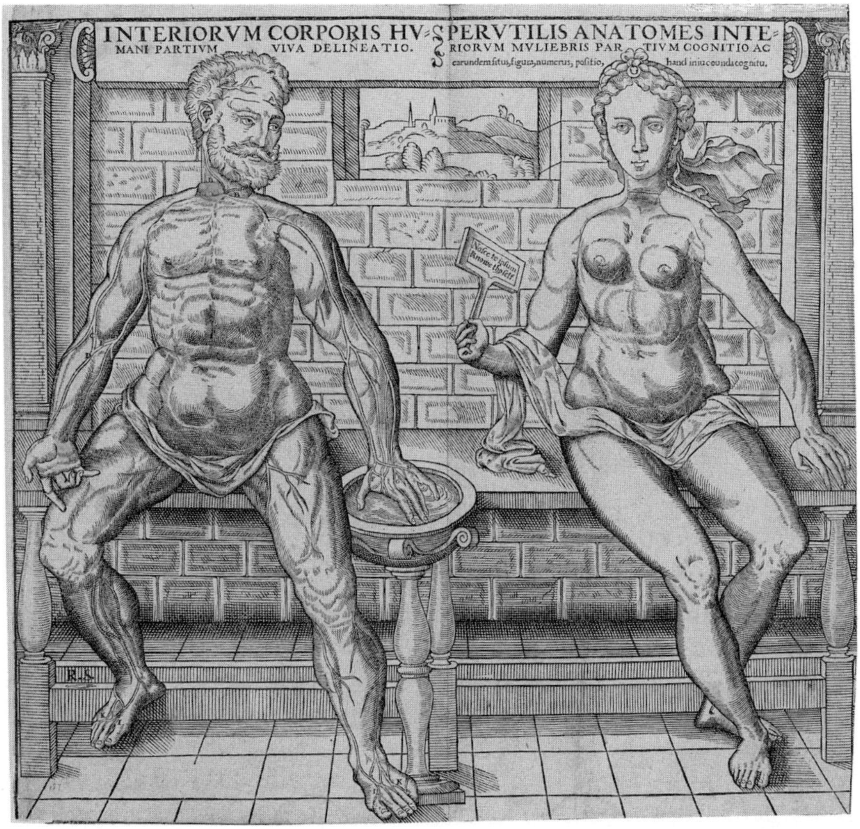

Figure 1.14: Giles Godet and/or Thomas Geminus, Anatomical Fugitive Sheet, *Interiorum Corporis Humani Partium*, c. 1559. Wellcome Library, London.

This 'assent to providence' constitutes a 'recognition of the frailty of this structure of the human body', a realisation which necessarily stimulates a hunger for divine grace. Indeed, Melanchthon's appropriation of Lutheran doctrine provides a means by which sin can literally be read in the body's internal organs, for 'nerves, veins, extremely thin fibres and extremely soft bodies . . . can easily be harmed . . . by intemperance and the inability to restrain . . . desires'. Through this process the very natural faculties with which humanity is inherently endowed turn the body into the 'executor of divine judgement'. Its mediating organ is the heart which, operating in tension with the centre of reason, the 'authoritative part', generates the passions which are an inevitable consequence of the 'depravity of nature'. It is by self-examination which lays bare one's own inward corruption that the 'deadly pain' of guilt arises, the necessary precursor to confession and repentance.[65]

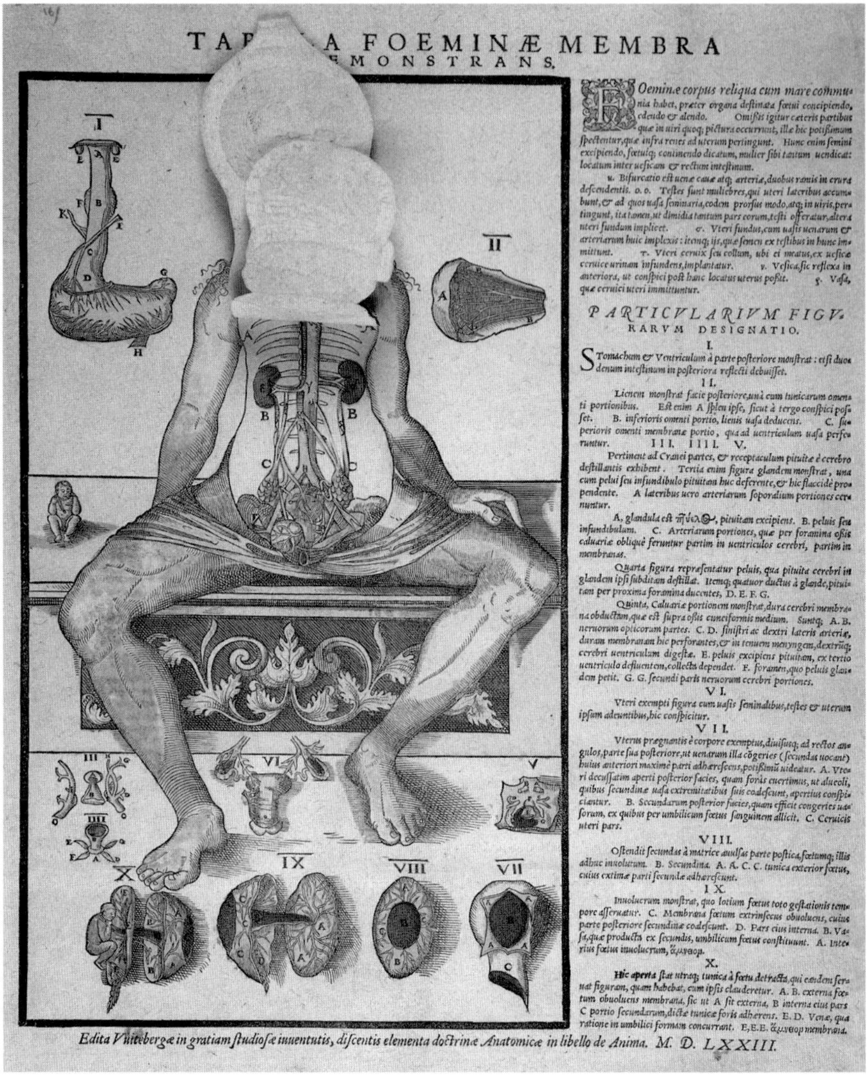

Figures 1.15a and 1.15b: Anatomical Fugitive Sheets, *Tabula Foeminae Membra Demonstrans* (shown above with anatomical flaps raised) and *Tabula Exhibens Insigniora Maris Viscera*, 1573, EPB 298.17. Wellcome Library, London.

Melanchthon's visceral theology maintains that the soul's heart of darkness, the vagaries of the human will itself, can be visibly exposed through the opening of the fallen body. In the same way the sexually declarative, confessional postures introduced by the new Vesalian anatomy function to excite an awareness of the body's frailty, its physical capacity for sin and depravity.[66] That the flap-anatomies which

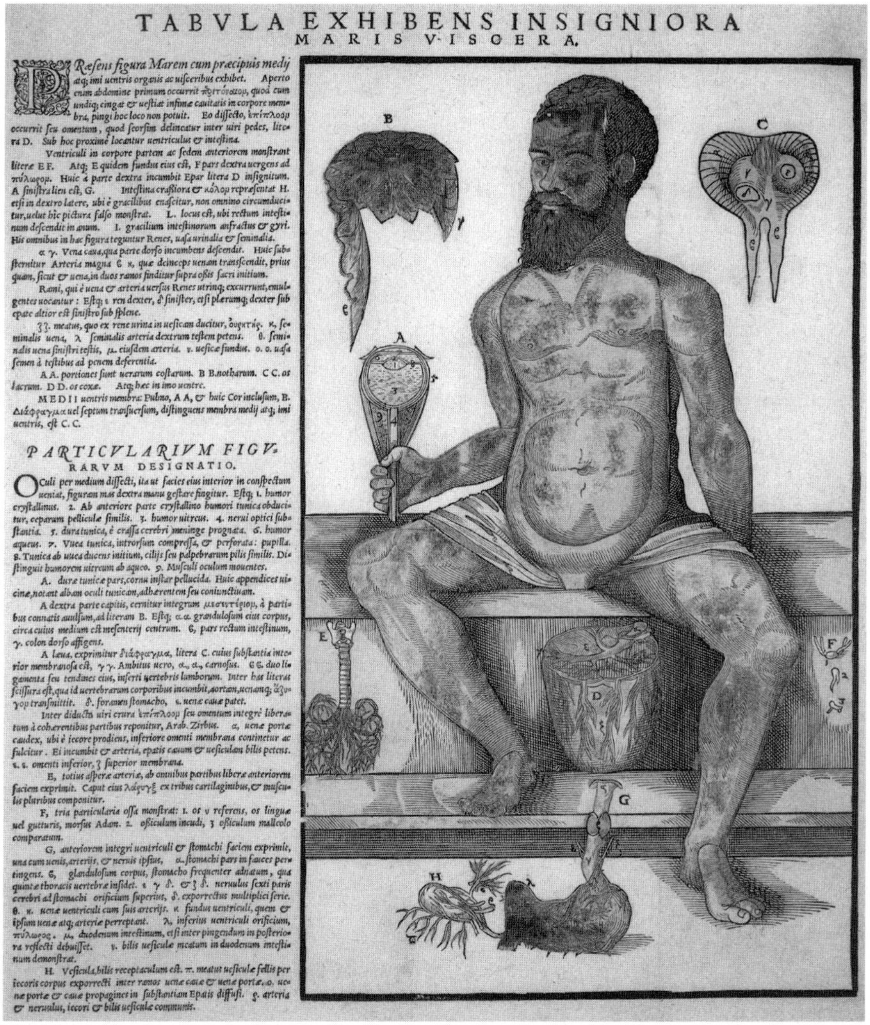

Figure 1.15b

circulated in early modern Europe were popularly known as Adam and Eve figures suggests the peculiarly reforming theology they encapsulated. Anatomy theatres, such as that in Leiden and the Domus Anatomica in Copenhagen,[67] contained three-dimensional reminders of the fallen pair, a biblical topos which accompanied the setting of anatomy in England since it is known that the Barber-Surgeons' theatre also housed a morbid show-piece consisting of '2 Humane Skins on the Wood Frames of a Man and a Woman in imitation of Adam and Eve'.[68] This iconography was reproduced in midwifery manuals like Jacob Rueff's *De Conceptu et Generatione Hominis*, published in Zurich in

1554 and later in Frankfurt in 1580, both centres of Reformation activity.[69] It is no coincidence that Rueff was himself a Lutheran and that his most notable forebear in the field of midwifery was Thomas Raynalde, publisher of Richard Jonas' translated work *The Byrth of Mankynde* (1540), who also issued, among other texts by noted reformers, a book of prayers for women in childbirth which encouraged expectant mothers to identify with Eve in their sufferings rather than the Virgin Mary.[70] It is possible, therefore, to suggest an iconoclastic dimension to the new visual culture of dissection. The solemn countenance of the medieval gravida figure, with its subtle evocation of the Mariological body, gives way to the more erotic pose of the Renaissance anatomy with its classical and statuesque beauty. The corporeal state it represents is not that of the second, redeeming Eve, but of the first fallen woman.

For those who attended anatomy theatres, spaces which could be infiltrated, as we saw in the Introduction to this study, by rituals of carnival and social inversion, the process of dissection – whether physically practised or merely orally reproduced through pedagogical disquisition – could potentially become amenable to the kinds of satirical thinking which engaged with the corpse in moralised terms.[71] Perhaps it would have seemed as if what was being offered was nothing less than a dissection of original sin itself, or rather of the originary mother who gave birth to Death. This is indicated by the anatomies conducted by Alessandro Benedetti (1460–1525). His *Anatomice*, first published in Venice in 1502, and later in Strasbourg in 1528, staged the body's gradual unveiling as a step-by-step revelation of inward depravity, providing a study of the way in which 'intemperance often troubles that portion of us which is divine and unjustly pushes away our spirit'. In particular the 'genital members' of women, through which 'God has placed [in them] the marvellous desire and incredible love of giving birth to their kind', must be explored:

> These members are by no means to be despised although often in women they fatally hinder the conceived creature from being born. When we have examined these parts we shall condemn those who pursue the wantonness of the stomach and the violence of lust since (as Plato tells) we see how they demonstrate that such people not unseasonably degenerate into the forms of various beasts.[72]

Faced with the anxiety stimulated by the potentially erotic connotations of the naked body in such settings, the deployment of a Juvenalian satirical discourse provides the justificatory moral engine for the voyeuristic impulses of the male academic community. It is no coincidence that Aretino himself became lauded, in many of the works which bore his image, with the motto '*Acerrimus Virtutum ac Vitiorum Demonstrator*', the word '*Demonstrator*' or '*Demonstrans*' particularly associated at this time with popular anatomical works, like the *Tabula Foeminae Membra Demonstrans*.[73] More significant still, the *I modi*, with which Aretino would become so closely associated, served as templates for another set of erotic engravings by Jacopo Caraglio, the *Gli Amori Degli Dei* ('Loves of the Gods').[74] Caraglio had struck up a friendship with Aretino in Venice during the 1530s and had produced an *all'antica* portrait of the satirist which was circulated in the latter's printed works. Caraglio's daring plates participated in the same visual culture as the Bacchic and Satyric motifs which proved so popular with Aretino, Titian and their followers, framing the sexual act with mythological scenes such as that showing Jupiter's dalliance with Antiope while disguised as a Satyr (Fig. 1.16) in which Antiope appears as a re-oriented version of the posture recorded in one of the original *I modi* engravings (compare the fragment shown in Fig. 1.3). Charles Estienne (c. 1505–64), who hailed from a family of printers with strong reformist sympathies, adopted these pornographic plates for his anatomical manual, the *De Dissectione Partium Corporis Humani*. This was produced in its early stages with the collaboration of the surgeon Estienne de la Riviere and completed before Vesalius' *Fabrica*, despite its later Parisian publication date of 1545.[75] In the hands of Estienne, Caraglio's sexually provocative courtesan-like women became anatomical models. The form of Antiope, for example, served to divulge the mysteries of the uterine anatomy (Fig. 1.17).[76] The violent fragmentation of these notoriously Aretinian pornographic prototypes, visible in the inset anatomical blocks which reproduce the act of cutting and opening on these paper bodies, constitutes a moralised re-orientation of the erotic gaze. This includes a dissection of the uterus which overlays the erotic postures of the *Loves of the Gods* with the possible biblical allusion to David and Bathsheba (Fig. 1.18).[77] The reformation of the fallen woman's maternalised anatomy, subjected to the disciplines of surgical intervention, turns on the violent incongruity between apparently classical models of sexual knowledge and the new body of anatomical wisdom which is supplanting them.

Vesalius' engagement with the female reproductive system, I suggest, participates in a similar dynamics of fragmentation which emerges from the humanist culture of archaeological recovery.[78] The *Fabrica*'s renderings of the exposed viscera, and particularly the uterine anatomy, are superimposed onto fragments of antique sculpture (Fig. 1.19). These are reminiscent of some of the most significant archaeological discoveries of the Renaissance: the *Belvedere Torso* and the *Laocoön*, sculptures whose highly dramatic torsion proved particularly influential to the

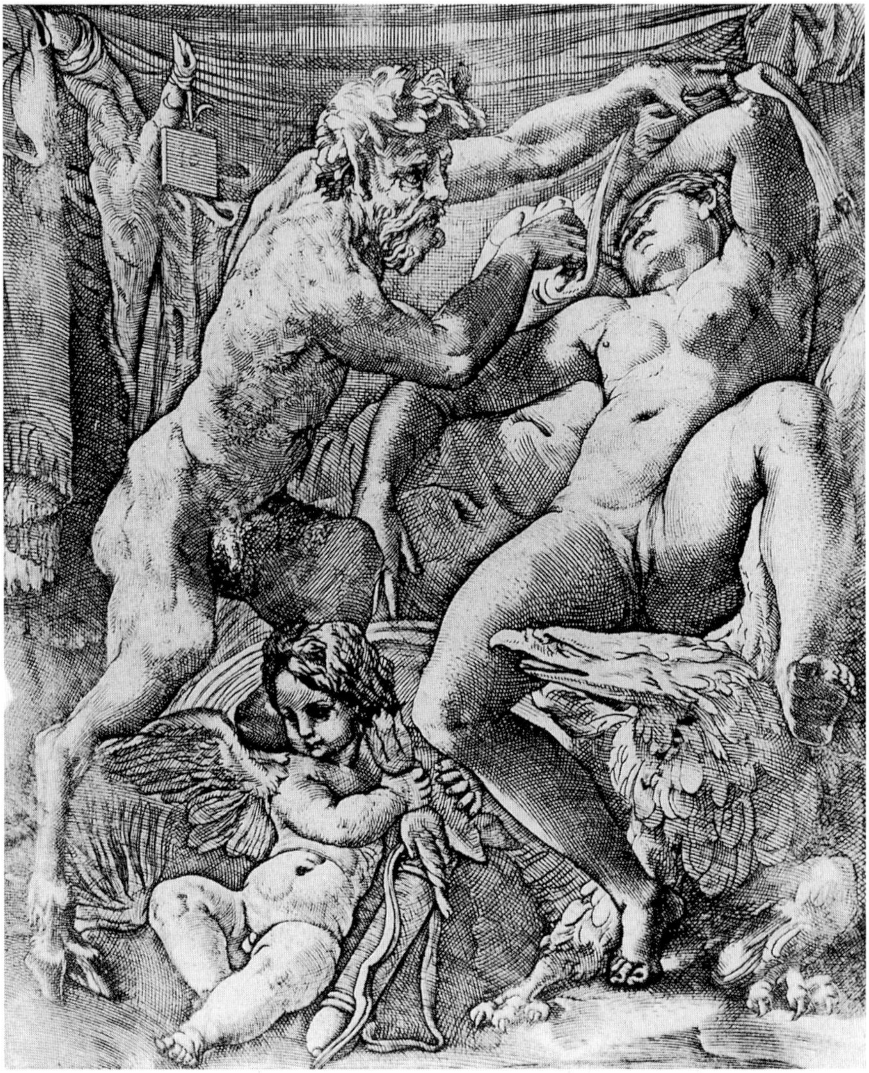

Figure 1.16: Jacopo Caraglio, after Perino del Vaga, *Loves of the Gods*, Jupiter and Antiope. The Albertina Museum, Vienna.

history of anatomical illustration.[79] In his interpretation of the *Fabrica*'s use of classical statuary Glenn Harcourt defines these stone anatomies as expressive of 'a representational strategy that at once belies and elevates the socially problematic practice of physical violation characteristic of the real production of anatomical knowledge'. As such these antique objects constitute a form of 'pictorial evasion' through which 'the locus of anatomical activity is displaced from the hand of the

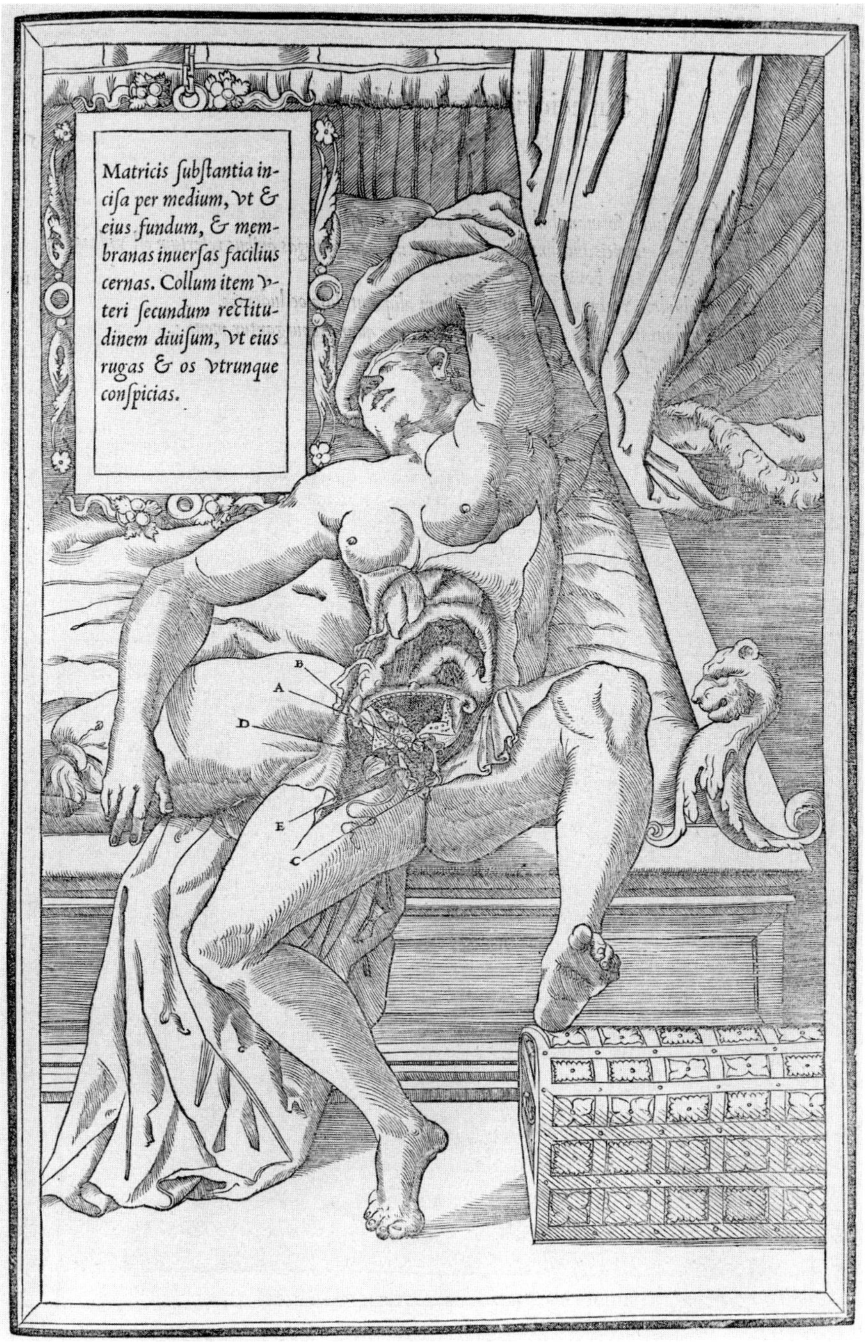
Matricis ſubſtantia in-
ciſa per medium, vt &
eius fundum, & mem-
branas inuerſas facilius
cernas. Collum item v-
teri ſecundum rectitu-
dinem diuiſum, vt eius
rugas & os vtrunque
conſpicias.
B
A
D
E
C

Figure 1.17: Dissected Woman. Charles Estienne, *De Dissectione Partium Corporis Humani*, 1545. Wellcome Library, London.

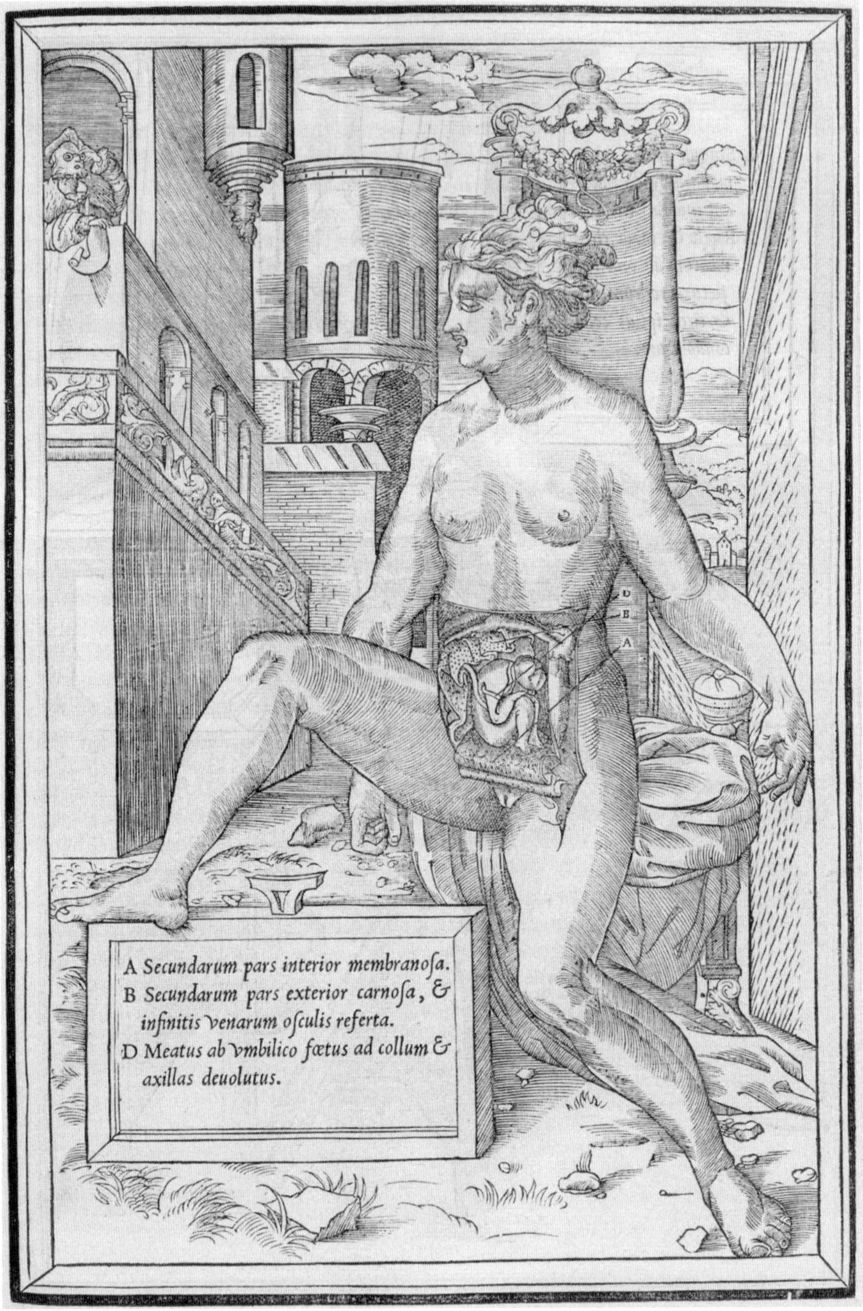
A Secundarum pars interior membranoſa.
B Secundarum pars exterior carnoſa, & infinitis venarum oſculis referta.
D Meatus ab vmbilico fœtus ad collum & axillas deuolutus.

Figure 1.18: Dissected Woman. Charles Estienne, *De Dissectione Partium Corporis Humani*, 1545. Wellcome Library, London.

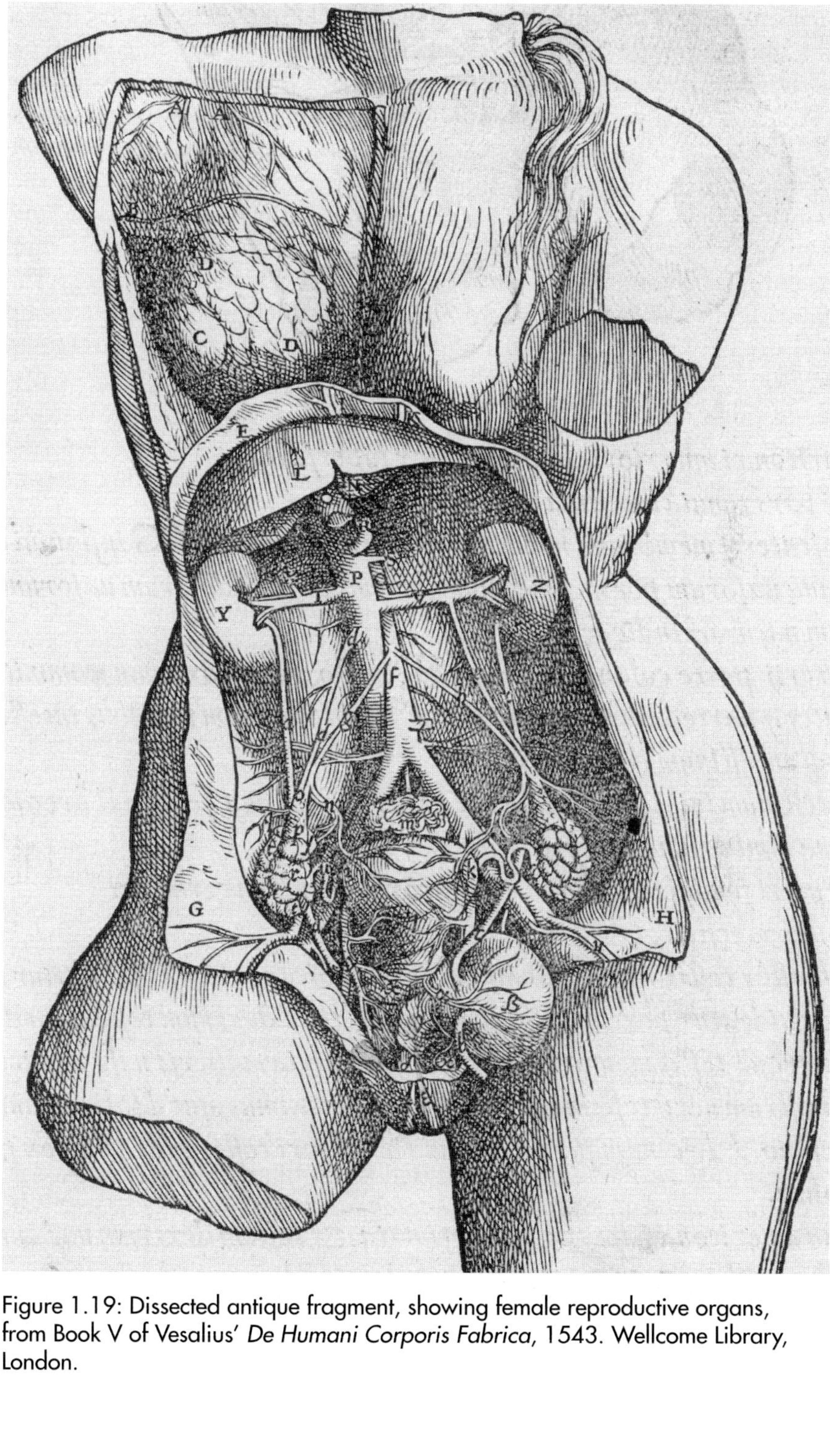

Figure 1.19: Dissected antique fragment, showing female reproductive organs, from Book V of Vesalius' *De Humani Corporis Fabrica*, 1543. Wellcome Library, London.

anatomist to that of the draftsman'.[80] I would like to argue that in fact the opposite is the case. If we read these archaeological remains *satirically*, it becomes clear that far from decentring the work of the hand they form a striking pictorial critique of those physicians who, in Vesalius' words, 'abstain from the use of the hands as from a plague'.[81] That we should understand the archaeological elements of the *Fabrica* in this way is evident from the frequency with which antique fragments became a medium for satiric utterance in the Renaissance, particularly within the immensely influential intellectual circle of Titian and Aretino. The most significant example of this is the broken Hellenistic statue (second century BC) known as the *Pasquino*, which stood in the Palazzo Orsini in Rome. This inaugurated a satirical language of its own, for it was upon this stone fragment that citizens would attach scurrilous satirical verses which came to be known as *pasquinades*, publicly attacking figures of authority in Church and government and claiming to root out the sources of corruption in the state. An engraving from Antoine Lafréry's *Speculum Romanae Magnificentiae* (1598) shows the verses affixed to the statue below which are displayed the symbols of the satirist in his guise as Satyr: a club (symbol of Priapus), a pair of Satyr's horns, faun's or Satyr's ears, and the whip of the satirical scourge of humanity's ills (Fig. 1.20). But it was with Aretino that the statue came to be most associated. Using it as a powerful tool for self-promotion, the satirist was noted for his ruthless *pasquinades* and even signed his works with the nom de plume *Pasquino*.[82]

Aretino was not the only Renaissance celebrity to use antique fragments for the purposes of satirical self-expression. In a striking parody of the *Laocoön*, descended in a woodcut copy of c. 1566 by Niccolo Boldrini, Titian displaces the elegant marble figures with a grisly troop of monkeys (Fig. 1.21). It has been recognised that Titian may have been directly engaging in a debate initiated by Vesalius himself who, in his *Fabrica*, indulges in a satirical swipe at the expense of those anatomists whose 'writings are wholly pieced together from Galen's conclusions' and who mindlessly reproduce the unreliable data of a man who 'never dissected a human body; but [was] deceived by his monkeys'.[83] Titian's caricature demonstrates through a *reductio ad absurdum* the dangers of an uncritical acceptance of antiquated forms of anatomical knowledge. Vesalius' own depiction of antique fragments strikes at the heart of the humanist dilemma: the tension between inherited and newly-acquired wisdom. It is the incongruity between palpable flesh and recovered stone, between the fragmented knowledge derived from authorities of the past and the direct experience of once-living tissue and bone, which becomes the satirical fulcrum of the Vesalian programme of anatomy.

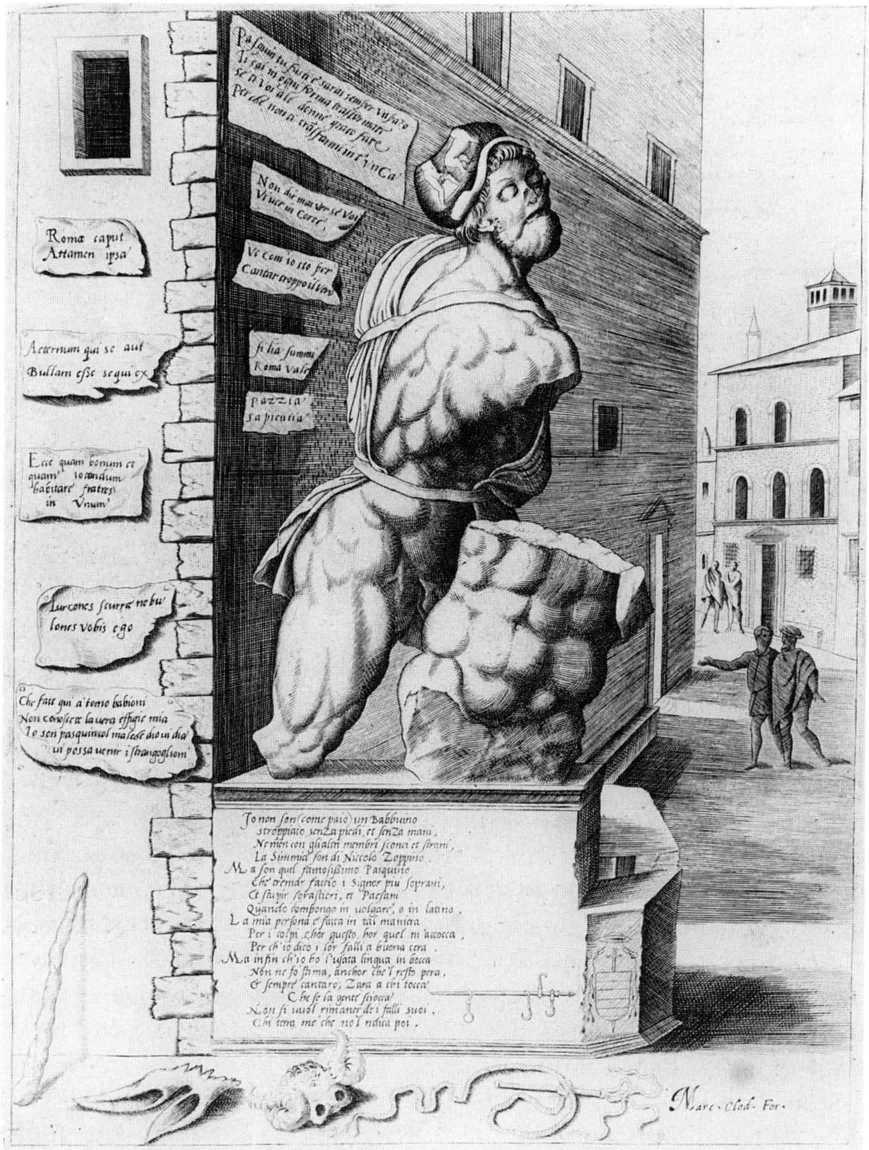

Figure 1.20: Antoine Lafréry, Pasquino, *Speculum Romanae Magnificentiae*, 1598. The Warburg Institute, University of London.

Celebrating the tactile engagement of the hand in the discipline of dissection, Vesalius is condemning those who follow a pedagogical programme divorced from the corporeal matter of the dead body, those who fail to do due service to the anatomist's titular deity of Death.

Vesalius' fragmented female bodies are the visual analogues to the

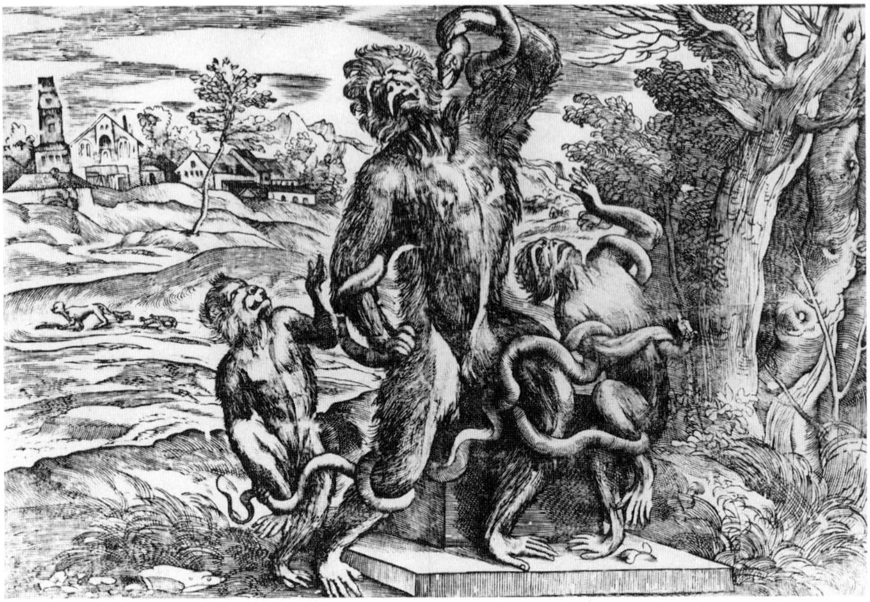

Figure 1.21: Niccolo Boldrini, after Titian, The *Laocoön* group of statues rendered as apes, c. 1566. The Warburg Institute, University of London.

sexually suspicious women – the prostitutes, ambiguous nuns and mistresses of monks – which form part of the *Fabrica*'s satirical narratological apparatus and whose dissections collectively constitute the fleshy anatomical matter which spills out of its reclaimed stone fragments. Vesalius' reformation of the pedagogical culture becomes, therefore, invested with the moral urgency attached to the reformation of manners for which the dissecting act becomes the meaningful corollary. In his antique disposition of satirist, much like his infamous contemporary Aretino, Vesalius is able morally to justify his close attention to the sexualised female body, asserting his value to the king in whose service he is able to expose the hidden corruptions of the state which find their naturalised locus in the fallen maternal anatomy. The popularity of the early modern genre of anatomical satire, I have been suggesting, was not a reaction to the anatomical method but developed as a crucial ideological adjunct to the professionalisation of the anatomical discipline. The reforming impulse with which it infused the unique epistemologies of dissection spread across Europe and into England. It is in Shakespeare's *Hamlet* that this post-Vesalian maternal body receives its most sustained and daring challenge.

Hearts and Hands: The Satirical Disclosures of Maternity in Shakespeare's *Hamlet*

> OTHELLO . . . it is my nature's plague
> To spy into abuses, and oft my jealousy
> Shapes faults that are not . . .
> By heaven, I'll know thy thoughts!
> IAGO You cannot, if my heart were in your hand . . .
>
> William Shakespeare, *Othello*[84]

> [W]ee receive the distinction of Sexe from the Mother . . . besides the nourishment in the Wombe, her paine in Conception and Travell, Milke from her Brests, together with much more Hand and Heart, Labour and Love from the Female Parent.
>
> Samuel Purchas, *Purchas his Pilgrim: Microcosmus or the Historie of Man*[85]

Hamlet marks a point in Shakespeare's dramatic oeuvre in which the formal institutions that govern pedagogical training come under intense scrutiny. Hamlet is a student of Wittenberg University along with his friend and 'fellow-student' Horatio (I, ii, 177).[86] This background renders Horatio the aptest interpreter of the armour-clad apparition who stalks Elsinore, as Marcello suggests when he encourages him to approach the ghost with the words 'Thou art a scholar, speak to it, Horatio' (I, i, 42). Horatio's language during this encounter is characterised by an abiding concern with the amassing of empirical data: 'I might not this believe/ Without the sensible and true avouch/Of mine own eyes' (I, i, 56–8). Carefully weighing his theoretical disquisitions on the spirit's movement 'in sea or fire, in earth or air' against the evidence of his observations he concludes that 'of the truth herein/this present object made probation' (I, i, 135–8). This insistence on verification by direct experience forms an integral component of Hamlet's own scholarly ruminations in a play in which matter is ravelled out, bodily passages responsible for the flow of organic fluids are opened to visual inspection, processes of sexual congress and conception are imaginatively reconstructed, eviscerated corpses and parts of decayed bodies are displayed, and hearts are unpacked, penetrated, wrung and cleaved in two.

Elsewhere in Shakespeare's writing during this period similar concerns find dramatic expression. *As You Like It* is another play in which pedagogical matters take centre-stage. In the very opening scene Orlando mourns that his 'brother Jaques . . . keeps at school [i.e. at university]' while he remains 'home unkept', deprived of 'gentility . . . [and] education' (I, i, 5–19).[87] Jaques finds a ghostly double in his namesake, the self-exiled melancholy courtier Jaques, in whom the occupation of the scholar is satirised in distinctly anatomical terms. An avid dissector of others' failings, Jaques 'most invectively . . . pierceth through/The body of the country, city, court,/Yea, and of this our life' (II, i, 58–60) and claims to provide a restorative panacea for the corruptions he brings to light:

> weed your better judgements
> Of all opinion that grows rank in them . . .
> The wise man's folly is anatomized
> Even by the squandering glances of the fool.
> Invest me in my motley. Give me leave
> To speak my mind, and I will through and through
> Cleanse the foul body of th'infected world,
> If they will patiently receive my medicine. (II, vii, 45–61)

Jaques imitates the kind of promotional machinery which informed popular anatomical manuals like the *Profitable Treatise of the Anatomie of Mans Body* (1548), in which Thomas Vicary maintained that the proper ground of anatomy was to uncover 'greevous wounds, Ulcers, and Fistules, as other hyd and secrete diseases upon the body of man'.[88] Hamlet, seeming to echo his melancholy counterpart in *As You Like It*, defines the world as 'an unweeded garden/That grows to seed; things rank and gross in nature/Possess it merely' (I, ii, 135–7) and in the Second Quarto version of the play ascribes its malignant nature to 'th'imposthume of much wealth and peace,/That inward breaks and shows no cause without/Why the man dies' (IV, iv, 9.17–19).[89] Taking on the role of a surgeon bent on exposing the hidden corruptions of the state, he diagnoses a 'time . . . out of joint' requiring a bone-setter willing to penetrate beneath the surface of the cosmic body in order to 'set it right' (I, v, 196–7). As we will see Hamlet's satirising anatomical postures serve, increasingly as the play progresses, to locate this social and political malaise in the 'matter' of the inwardly diseased and sexually debased maternal body.

An indication of how we should read the crisis that the problematic pedagogies of the reproductive anatomy will prompt in Hamlet can be gleaned from the figure of Jaques who is himself 'full of matter' (II, i, 68), a copious excess of rhetorical sententiae 'crammed/With observation, the which he vents/In mangled forms' (II, vii, 40–2). As well as meaning to expel bodily waste or fluid, 'vent' can also indicate a cut, aperture or gash, thus associating the dissecting process with the fruitless and wasteful production of verbal or textual matter.[90] This is fleshed out in the scatological implications of his name, perhaps a pun on the jakes or privy, a bawdy quibble which Sir John Harington, Queen Elizabeth's godson, exploited in his scurrilous satirical pamphlet *The Metamorphosis of Ajax* (1596). For Harington the jakes becomes an emblem of the foul matter concealed beneath the glittering surface of the eroticised female body, for a 'fine courtesan laden with sinne' is the well-spring of 'a more stinking savour afore God and his holy Angels, then that beastly cart, laden with excrements'.[91] That this text underwent its own dissection in the same year, in C. Traveller's *An Anatomie of the Metamorphosed Ajax*, reveals just how closely the themes of pornography, scatological satire and anatomy were related.[92] In *As You Like It*, Duke Senior's observation that Jaques had 'been a libertine', and is consequently infected with 'all th' embossèd sores and headed evils' he claims to have uncovered in others (II, vii, 65–7), has particular significance when considered in relation to the literary background which invested libertinism with satirical import.

That the source for *As You Like It* is Thomas Lodge's *Rosalynde*, subtitled *Euphues Golden Legacie* (1590), locates the play within a nexus of literary prototypes which draw on the kind of distinctive stylistic features that characterise Lyly's satirical work *Euphues: The Anatomie of Wit* (1578).[93] If indeed the registration or licensing of *As You Like It* was deliberately 'staied', as indicated in a fly-leaf from the Register of the Stationers' company for 4 August 1600, and its publication delayed until the First Folio of 1623, it may have been because its anatomical and satirical elements incurred the attention of the censors.[94] On 1 June 1599 the Archbishop of Canterbury, John Whitgift, and the Bishop of London, Richard Bancroft, sent a decree to the Stationers' Company demanding 'That noe *Satyres or Epigrams* be printed hereafter'. Among the books to 'bee presentlye broughte to the Bishop of LONDON to be burnte' were works by John Davies, who would later author a poem whose title echoed the anatomist's credo *Nosce Teipsum* (1602); John Marston's *Scourge of Villanie* (1598), and *Metamorphosis of Pigmalion's Image* (1598), which was published 'with certaine other Satyres'; and Thomas Nashe's *Anatomie of Absurditie* (1589).[95] What made these texts particularly threatening to the authorities who sought to obliterate them was their participation in a libertinesque discourse which drew from the pornographic and scatological culture inaugurated by none other than Pietro Aretino himself.[96] In his *Scourge of Villanie*, for example, Marston appealed to the '*nursing Mother . . . /Ingenuous Melancholly*' (since both the anatomist and the satirist were popularly thought to be ruled by the melancholy planet Saturn) to endow him with the ability to 'plow/The hidden entrailes of ranke villanie' and expose '*Aretine*'s filth, or of his wandering whore . . . /That stinks like Ajax froth, or muck-pit slime' (XI, ii, 144–7).[97] That Marston became indelibly linked with Aretino is evident in the anonymous play which alludes to this work, the *Returne from Parnassus: Or the Scourge of Simony*:

> Tut, what cares he for modest close coucht termes,
> Cleanly to gird our looser libtertines.
> Give him plaine naked words strippt from their shirts
> That might beseeme plaine dealing *Aretine*:
> I, there is one that backes a paper steed
> And manageth a pen-knife gallantly. (I, ii, 275)[98]

The satirist, in his guise as Aretine, wields a pen as sharp and deadly as a knife. The confluence of images which cast all 'modest[y]' aside, evoking naked bodies and thrusting blades, turns the act of writing into a grisly dissection. This kind of pornographic anatomy formed a general feature of the texts listed in the 1599 censorship which included a ban on any works associated with the so-called Marprelate controversy; a satirical pamphlet war that raged between Gabriel Harvey and Thomas Nashe, which was to earn the latter the infamous title of the 'English Aretine'.[99] Indeed, Nashe courted this reputation, signing his works with the *nom de plume* 'Pasquil' in deliberate allusion to the *pasquinades* with which Aretino had become so closely identified. In his satirical work *The Unfortunate Traveller* (1594) Nashe gleefully recounted Aretino's blood-chilling appellation of '*Il flagello de principi*' ('the scourge of princes'), the motto which made scourging synonymous with the Aretinian style of satire in the European imagination. Nashe's Aretino was a representative of an altogether more subversive educational institution, a 'searcher and chief inquisitor for the college of courtesans' whose 'pen was sharp pointed like a poniard' and whose 'sight pierced like lightning into the entrails of all abuses'. It was in this same text that Nashe offered a satirical vignette of Wittenberg University, that Lutheran bastion which effected a synthesis between the latest anatomical teaching and the emergent reforming theology, as a conglomeration of academics who assembled their scholarship 'by patch and by piecemeal' from the 'entrails' of others' books as if they were 'rags gathered up from the dunghill'.[100]

We should therefore not be surprised to find that Shakespeare, who was writing *Hamlet* at a time of increased sensitivity towards the disruptive potential of the satirical mode, chose to have his scholarly protagonist 'put an antic disposition on' (I, v, 179), as Aretino had done, so that he could more effectively become God's 'scourge and minister' (III, iv, 164) against the wayward King Claudius. This identification places Hamlet within a tradition of satirical anatomists stretching back to the intellectual hotbed that was the Italy inhabited by Aretino, Vesalius and the inaugurators of the new anatomy, as well as to the school of Wittenberg which exploited this satiric potential for its own reforming agenda. As we have seen, the maternal body provided Hamlet's continental precursors with a powerful symbol of self-ratification and a means of engaging satirically with the dichotomies of the humanist endeavour which relied heavily on the accumulated fragments of received wisdom on the body. If Vesalius and his contemporaries therefore emphasised the importance of a direct engagement with the matter of the maternal interior by satirically critiquing the very humanist agenda which supplied so much of the scaffolding for the new anatomy, Shakespeare's *Hamlet* would take this process to its logical conclusion, throwing into crisis the sufficiency of an anatomical discipline whose justification depended on the disclosure of women's reproductive mysteries; mysteries which can never be directly *known*.

Early in the play Hamlet identifies his vengeful agenda with the removal of all 'baser matter' (I, v, 104) from his mind which, once purified, shall henceforth be occupied with the remembrance of his father alone. The Ghost's appeal that he 'Let not the royal bed of Denmark be/A couch for luxury and damnèd incest' establishes a conflicting demand on Hamlet's imagination however, providing a corporeal locus for the pornographic fantasy in his mother's concealed interior which is infested with 'those thorns that in her bosom lodge/To prick and sting her' (I, v, 82–91). This stimulates in Hamlet a fixation with 'matter' which increasingly takes on the moralised burden of the maternal body. In Act III, for example, Shakespeare moves deftly from the 'country matters' of Hamlet's jovial repartee with Ophelia (III, ii, 108) to a more intricate pun on mother/matter, *mater* (Latin for 'mother') still providing the root of the word *mater*nity: 'My wit's diseased . . . as you say, my mother. Therefore no more, but to the matter. My mother, you say . . ./O wonderful son, that can so astonish a mother!' (III, ii, 303–10).[101] Similarly Hamlet associates Claudius' 'wanton' desire to 'tempt . . . [Gertrude] to bed' with his ability to seduce her into confessing her deepest secrets, making her 'ravel all this matter out' (III, iv, 171–5). Weighted with the hierarchical sexual biology of Aristotelian embryological theory, which defined the female contribution to conception and gestation as gross 'matter' acted upon by the masculine motive principle of generation,[102] Hamlet's imaginative penetration into the anatomical reaches of the womb turns it into the origin of the 'corruption' which plagues the state:

> So, oft it chances in particular men
> That, for some vicious mole of nature in them –
> As in their birth, wherein they are not guilty,
> Since nature cannot choose his origin,
> By the o'ergrowth of some complexion . . .
> Carrying, I say, the stamp of one defect . . .

His virtues else, be they as pure as grace . . .
Shall in the general censure take corruption
From that particular fault. The dram of evil
Doth all the noble substance over-daub
To his own scandal. (I, iv, 18.7–22)[103]

The 'fault' responsible for the 'scandal' of human depravity is linked to the material determinants of childbirth through its etymological closeness to the French *foutre*, indicative both of the sexual act and, more specifically, of the female genital organs.[104] Hamlet's peeling back the layers of the fallen body to reveal that 'vicious mole of nature' which is stamped upon it from the time of conception may allude to the congenital defect to which many Renaissance manuals referred as the 'mole', or Mola. Believed in some instances to grow in the 'likenesse and similitude of a piece or lump of mishapen flesh' this was, according to Jacob Rueff in his *Expert Midwife* (1637), most likely to develop in 'those women which are somewhat more lascivious than others are'.[105] In his *Sicke Womans Private Looking-Glasse* (1636), John Sadler, in terms very similar to those used by Hamlet, labels the 'mole' a 'vicious conception' which is commonly thought to be 'ingendred of the menstruous blood'.[106] Hamlet's anatomical critique plays upon the idea that the opening of the body, the exposure of its secret 'fault', provides material evidence of the matrilineal transmission of 'evil'. This is precisely the kind of vocabulary we find in Donne's *Progress of the Soul*:[107]

Man all at once was there by woman slain,
And one by one we're here slain o'er again
By them. The mother poisoned the well-head,
The daughters here corrupt us, rivulets . . .
She sinned, we bear; part of our pain is, thus
To love them, whose *fault* to this painful love yoked us. (91–100, my italics)

Donne chooses to identify his work as a '*poema satyricon*', a satirical unpacking of the postlapsarian world beginning with humanity's fateful dalliance with the Tree of Knowledge, that 'Prince of the orchard' (81). The poem ends with a double anatomisation in which the opening of Eve's womb, with its blazon of embryological detail, becomes a dissection of Themech, 'Sister and wife to Cain', whose 'hardened . . . heart' is discovered when the 'sinewy strings which do our bodies tie,/Are ravelled out'. The anatomising process reveals an incestuous body whose 'every part' carries 'some quality/Of every past shape, [for] she knew treachery,/Rapine, deceit, and lust, and ills enow/To be a woman' (498–510).

It is this very language, which recapitulates the misogynistic dictum 'frailty, thy name is woman' (I, ii, 146), which underpins the Ghost's argument for revenge in *Hamlet*. Beginning with a tale of origins in which there is a 'falling-off', the Ghost purporting to be Old Hamlet casts his 'seeming-virtuous queen' in the role of Eve who was seduced to 'incestuous . . . shameful lust' by a 'serpent that . . ./Now wears his crown' (I, v, 39–47). The account of Old Hamlet's death in the 'orchard' becomes an anatomy in which we venture 'through/The natural gates and alleys of the body' (I, v, 59–67) as we witness the effects of the poison which 'with a sudden vigour . . . doth posset/And curd, like eager droppings into milk,/The thin and wholesome blood' (I, v, 68–70).[108] In another of his satires, which serves as a companion piece to his *Anatomy of the World*, Donne describes the consequences of the Fall upon the body by employing an almost identical image:

> Think but how poor thou wast, how obnoxious;
> Whom a small lump of flesh could poison thus.
> This curded milk, this poor unlittered whelp
> My body, could, beyond escape or help,
> Infect thee with original sin . . . (163–7)[109]

For Donne the human anatomy, from its conception, is an infectious mola, a 'lump of flesh' which carries the taint of the first Mother's 'original sin'. Old Hamlet's rehearsal of the milk-curdling 'leprous distilment' whose 'lazar-like' infection caused an 'instant tetter' of 'vile and loathsome crust' (I, v, 71–2), reveals a body whose core is equally replete with the signs of a diseased femininity, emanating from the instance of the fall.[110] It is infused with milk, that most defining feature of the reproductive body, as well as with newly thickened blood which is evocative of menstrual fluid. Indeed, not only was it believed that menstrual blood had the power to curdle milk directly, but it was also thought to be one of many reasons why, as Rueff suggests, a developing embryo could be 'corrupted' in the womb in the same way 'as creame or the fatnesse of milke, although it be congealed and clotted together, notwithstanding with some motion is troubled and spoiled . . . that some deformed and mishapen birth must follow'.[111] The 'menstruous bloud', as Jacques Guillemeau maintains in his *Childbirth, or the Happy Deliverie of Women* (1612), 'is grosse and thicke, unfit for the framing of a child',[112] and as late as 1671 Jane Sharp circulated the persistent myth that a child conceived during the time of purgation 'will be Leprous, and troubled with an incurable Itch and Scabs as long as they live'.[113] That the 'leprous' poison passes through the 'natural gates and alleys' of Old Hamlet's body may also carry an echo of the kind of anatomical lexicon that was often used to define the womb itself. In his *Birth of Mankynde* (1564), Thomas Raynalde explained that 'the extreme end, or th[e] fyrst entraunce of this privie or wombe passage, ye shall name the passage port: for because that it is the port gate, or entraunce of that passage'.[114]

The description of the changing consistency of Old Hamlet's blood may owe something to contemporary theories of male menstruation. Renaissance anatomists like Vesalius had dissected male bodies said to have been endowed with the propensity to evacuate blood from the 'portal vein'.[115] Male menstruation was often linked to the positive traits of virility and fecundity and since, as Gianna Pomata suggests, there was 'no connection here between male bleeding and effeminacy' early anatomists believed its 'flow should not be inhibited but encouraged'. Any attempts to block the passage of this fertile blood would foster the breeding of internal diseases and, in both men and women, obstructed menstruation could result in bleeding from other orifices, including the nose, the mouth and the anus, organs which take over the biological functions of the womb.[116] The infection which penetrates the body of Old Hamlet through 'the porches of [his] ears' (I, v, 63) hinders the flow of his 'wholesome blood', evoking a menstruum-filled interiority which disrupts the parthenogenic fantasy of the menstruating male. While he is 'Cut off even in the blossoms of [his] sin' (I, v, 76), the moral weight of these crimes is diffused through a wayward biology defined as distinctly feminine, even maternal. The evisceration of Old Hamlet's 'dead corpse', which Hamlet identifies with the Ghost (I, v, 31),[117] centres on the ear, the portal-veins, and the corrupted blood- and milk-producing conduits, body parts whose allusion to the perverted function of the womb connotes the lecherous, mola-producing woman. The medical lesson which the Ghost offers Hamlet becomes, therefore, a form of politicised pornography which conflates a diseased body politic, tainted by the act of usurpation, with the sexually debased anatomy that is the legacy of Eve.

Contemporary texts which purported to be anatomies often recapitulated this process by adopting the moral framework of continental, Melanchthonian anatomy and did so in explicitly Juvenalian terms. John Woolton, one of the first authors to adopt the anatomical method in his *Newe Anatomie of Whole Man* (1576), maintained that 'although it be accompted of some, an yrksome and cruell thing, to cut and mangle mans lymmes and members: yet the ende and use of the same is both necessarie and profitable'. The good anatomist must 'endever to describe mans excellencie before his fall, and his miserable ruine . . . And then descende in order to Regeneration and restitution of gods Image in man'.[118] Since the sin of the first woman has reduced humanity from 'a bright glasse of justice and holines' to a 'dounghill of the filthy dragon of hell' the universal panacea lies in the masculine appropriation of the functions of childbirth in spiritualised terms:

> Regeneratio[n] signifieth not in this place to returne corporally into our mothers wombe, & to be borne again . . . but a spiritual renewing: and the similitude is taken fro[m] the corporall nativitie. For as man is conceived & borne of his natural mother in sinne: even so in this spiritual nativitie, by the efficacie of gods worde and sacramentes, external instruments, he is regenerate and spiritually made cleane from sinne.[119]

For Woolton, who was responsible for interpreting Melanchthon's Vesalian *De Anima* for an English readership,[120] this 'Regeneratio[n]' relies on an implied homology between the anatomist's hand, with its medical 'instruments', and the hand of God offering His 'worde and sacramentes'. The regenerative agenda of the anatomical method, ideologically buoyed by the reformation of the maternal body, not only provides the rationale for the revenge that must answer Old Hamlet's death, but characterises the wider lexical currency of *Hamlet*. The expediency of this posture is exploited by Claudius who appropriates the sexually suspect maternal anatomy in order to incite Laertes to the killing of Hamlet, a deed which he maintains will proclaim his devotion to Polonius: 'Laertes, was your father dear to you?/Or are you like the painting of a sorrow,/A face without a heart?' (IV, vii, 93–5). The challenge placed before Laertes, that he bring the hidden affections of the heart into view, takes on the significance of self-evisceration:

> There lives within the very flame of love
> A kind of wick or snuff that will abate it,
> And nothing is at a like goodness still,
> For goodness, growing to a plurisy,
> Dies in his own too much . . . But to the quick of th'ulcer –
> Hamlet comes back. What would you undertake
> To show yourself your father's son in deed
> More than in words? (IV, vii, 95.1–98)[121]

Claudius is referring to what was still, during Shakespeare's life-time, a highly contested site of pathological enquiry; the cause of the pleurisy.[122] The visceral immediacy of Claudius' utterance exploits the disjunction between a hidden bodily interior understood 'in words' and one experienced through direct physical action – the penetration and cleansing of the diseased 'ulcer'. Claudius' parthenogenic fantasy depends on the suggestion that Laertes' inability to perform his retributive duty would be evidence that he, as the illegitimate product of the sexually suspect maternal body, has 'too much' of his mother in him. That the flame-snuffing 'plurisy' occupies the same conceptual space as this corrupting maternal influence is crystallised just a few lines later when Laertes admonishes himself for crying with the words: 'When these are gone,/The woman will be out . . ./I have a speech of fire that fain would blaze,/But that this folly douts [i.e. extinguishes] it' (IV, vii, 163–6). The dangerous presence which lies inside the body, and which threatens to sever the patrilineal bond upon which the political order depends, is none other than woman herself. The purging of this pernicious influence requires direct and violent infiltration of the feminised body. Claudius repeats the same strategy in his determination to 'hatch and . . . disclose' that 'O'er which [Hamlet's] melancholy sits on brood'; an aborted birth which will reveal to Claudius' inspecting gaze the 'something-settled matter in his heart' (III, i, 165–74). Hamlet fears that his failure to proceed with his vendetta against Claudius would render him equally incapable of embodying the legitimacy so essential to the parthenogenic reproduction of his patriarchal legacy. Being 'unpregnant of my cause' (II, ii, 556), he casts himself in the posture of the loose woman who can only void waste matter: 'like a whore, unpack my heart with words' (II, ii, 574).

The gendered and highly eroticised aetiology of dissection, popularised, as we have seen, by the satirical postures of Aretino and adopted by Vesalius, Estienne and their contemporaries, provided the Renaissance stage with a forum for the controversial debate surrounding the circulation of sexual knowledge. In Ben Jonson's *Volpone*, Corvino's injunction to Celia to 'Show yourself/Obedient, and a wife' (III, vii, 30–1) by submitting to his peculiar 'physic' and agreeing to 'prostitute' (III, vii, 74) herself, makes her the subject of the voyeuristic gaze accorded the *I modi* by those who had 'read Aretine, [and] conned all his prints' (III, vii, 60–5). Her refusal to adopt this erotic posture results in the anatomisation which, turning her into the living counterpart of one of Estienne's anatomical plates, confirms not her virtuous chastity but her innately lascivious nature as Corvino proposes to 'Cry thee a strumpet through the streets; rip up/Thy mouth unto thine ears; and slit thy nose,/Like a raw rochet [fish]', and administer 'burning corsives' to tear into her 'stubborn breast' (III, vii, 97–105). This amplifies his earlier insistence, in allusion to the Satyrs' insatiable lust, that Celia had been 'gazed upon with goatish eyes' (II, v, 34) and is thus deserving of the worst of punishments: 'I will make thee an anatomy,/Dissect thee mine own self, and read a lecture/Upon thee to the city and in public' (II, v, 66–72).[123] For Hamlet the satirical efficacy of the pornographic blazon turns the maternal body into a contested site through which the relative merits of a textually or empirically acquired anatomical wisdom can be assessed:

> HAMLET For if the sun breed maggots in a dead dog, being a good kissing carrion – have you a daughter?
> POLONIUS I have, my lord.
> HAMLET Let her not walk i'th' sun. Conception is a blessing. But not as your daughter may conceive . . .

POLONIUS . . . What do you read, my lord?
HAMLET Words, words, words.
POLONIUS What is the matter, my lord?
HAMLET Between who?
POLONIUS I mean the matter you read, my lord.
HAMLET Slanders, sir; for the satirical slave says here that old men . . . have a plentiful lack of wit . . . (II, ii, 181–99)

Drawing on the myth that the sun could spontaneously generate life in corrupted flesh, Hamlet places before Polonius an imaginary cadaver whose putrid remains recall Ophelia's sexually opened body. Hamlet's wit depends on the semantic slippage from the physical, possibly erotic matter 'Between' two people (a bawdy allusion which makes sense within the context of the 'breed[ing]' body's disclosure) to the 'matter' of the satirical text. However, Hamlet's 'pregnant . . . replies' (II, ii, 207–8) draw on an implicit disjunction between his own satirical bombast, which he takes to refer to the real 'matter' of Ophelia's body now indeed ready for 'Conception', and the derivative 'Words, words, words' of the 'satirical slave'. The justification for Hamlet's supposed privileging of matter over words rests on the moral probity of identifying an anatomical locus for the transmission of Eve's original sin: 'virtue cannot so inoculate our old stock but we shall relish of it . . . Get thee to a nunnery. Why, wouldst thou be a breeder of sinners? . . . it were better my mother had not borne me' (III, i, 118–25).[124]

This dichotomy similarly becomes the focus of Nashe's *Anatomie of Absurditie* (1589) which has the telling subtitle *a breefe confutation of the slender imputed prayses to feminine perfection*.[125] Having adopted a '*satyricall* disguise', Nashe explains that 'beeing an accessarie to Absurditie, [I] have tooke uppon me to draw her Anatomie'. The condemned female body he is dissecting, however, is the monstrously copious textual output of his contemporaries, comprising those 'who make the Presse the dunguill, whether they carry all the muck of their mellancholicke Imaginations, pretending forsooth to anatomize abuses, and stubbe up sin by the rootes'.[126] These are the very 'bable bookemungers' who profess a desire to search 'into the secrets of nature, when as in respect of deeper knowledge, they seeme meere naturals'.[127] Robert Burton reproduces these concerns in his *Anatomy of Melancholy*, which first appeared in 1621. This opens with a satirical thrust at the very humanist ethos which has left its signature on every page of his encyclopaedic work. Targeted are those who 'pilfer out of old writers to stuff up their new comments, scrape Ennius' dung-hills . . . "that not only libraries and shops are full of our putrid papers, but every close-stool and jakes" '.[128] Ventriloquising Democritus, one of history's most famed anatomists, he claims a moral mission to 'anatomize and cut up these poor beasts, to see these distempers, vanities, and follies' and to expose those iniquities which have infected the body politic with 'base flattery . . . parasitical fawning, and colloguing, etc., brawls, conflicts, desires, contentions, [that] it would ask an expert Vesalius to anatomize every member'. Like Hamlet he finds a root cause for this malaise in humanity's first ancestors for 'we are stony-hearted, and savour too much of the stock'. The dangerous overproduction of textual excreta, which obfuscates rather than clarifies understanding of the human body, is associated therefore with the sexual excesses of the debased female anatomy. Claiming to reject 'big words, [and] fustian phrases' he insists that 'I respect matter, not words; remembering that of Cardan, *verba propter res, non res propter verba* [words should minister to matter, not vice versa]'. The irony, of course, is that it is Burton's own book which becomes the anatomised and sexualised object, the 'prostitute . . . muse', whose copious reproduction of fragmented ancient wisdom and pedagogical tracts will 'bring forth this confused lump', giving birth to a monstrous textual mola.[129]

Hamlet attempts to avoid such crises of conception – the recognition that his knowledge may not necessarily be any less monstrously obtuse than that of the satirists upon whom he models himself – by making the matter/*mater* with which he satirically engages the site of essential moral truths. This strategy is more clearly delineated in Thomas Rogers' *Anatomie of the Minde* (1576) in which a debased maternity again becomes the controlling metaphor for a spiritual myopia, since whoever cannot 'subdue his coltishe affections, and make them to abyde under the yoake of reason' is likened to 'Laodice, which to live in adulterie murthered her owne sonnes'. An intimate knowledge of the body's 'internal motions' will inevitably impress one truth upon the would-be anatomist: 'Know thy selfe, and thou shalt not offend . . . forget thy selfe, and thou art a Nero for crueltie . . . forget thy selfe, and what art thou but a beast'.[130] While Rogers' Nero represents anatomical ignorance, for other anatomists of the age, the embryologist Hieronymous Fabricius among them, the example of 'the emperor Nero . . . [who] wished to look into the corpse of his dead mother and gaze upon that first domicile of man' is an apt emblem of their ability to discern the 'provident and elegant' design of nature from knowledge of 'a single fetus'.[131] Hamlet's most engrossing dissection of the maternal body is caught in between these two interpretations:

Now could I drink hot blood,
And do such bitter business as the day
Would quake to look on. Soft, now to my mother.

O heart, lose not thy nature. Let not ever
The soul of Nero enter this firm bosom.
Let me be cruel, not unnatural.
I will speak daggers to her, but use none . . .
How in my words somever she be shent,
To give them seals never my soul consent. (III, ii, 373–82)

It was the infamous Emperor Nero who, as Geoffrey Chaucer reminds us in *The Canterbury Tales*, murdered his own mother Agrippina and 'hire wombe slitte to biholde/Where he conceyved was'.[132] The story is graphically brought to life in a miniature from a Flemish manuscript of the *Roman de la Rose*, executed around 1500 (Fig. 1.22).[133] The half-open eyes and mouth suggest a body in pain, a victim to be pitied, and this accords with the medieval renderings of the Nero myth which usually remain silent about Agrippina's moral character, while focusing almost exclusively on the emperor's tyrannical nature.[134] It is not until the Renaissance that a central aspect of the Suetonian classical narrative is restored, bringing to light Agrippina's own turpitude; the crime of incest.[135] Since she was recognised as the subject of Nero's dissecting gaze, this may have been due in fact to the post-Reformation ethos of anatomy which made the opening of the maternal body naturally coterminous with the revelation of original sin. In Edmund Bolton's *Nero Caesar, or Monarchie Depraved* (1624), she is presented as the instigator of the most shameless acts of sexual depravity:

> She was a mother . . . whom it was no shame for a sonne to a kill . . . because her selfe was rather an infernall furie then a matron . . . who meerely for prowd ends did most alluringly offer her body to the lustfull embraces of him who scarcely twenty yeares before was bred therin . . . having formerly traded her self in manifold incests with Caligula Caesar her brother & with her uncle Claudius.[136]

It is possible that Shakespeare found in the Nero story a fitting analogue to Hamlet's overwhelming and almost incestuous fascination with the sexual dalliances of his 'aunt-mother' and 'uncle-father' Claudius (II, ii, 371). Though Hamlet attempts to distinguish himself from the classical emperor, he indulges in a Nero-like anatomical investigation of his mother which brings him close to characters like Giovanni, in John Ford's *'Tis Pity She's a Whore*, who undertakes a dissection of the 'corrupted bastard-bearing womb' (IV, iii, 14) of the incestuous Annabella, becoming a Nero-figure, a 'happy monarch of her heart' (VI, vi, 46) whose 'dagger's point ploughed up/Her fruitful womb and left to me the fame/Of a most glorious executioner' (VI, vi, 32–4).[137] Hamlet similarly seeks evidence of his mother's crime in a vivisection of her body: 'You go not till I set you up a glass/Where you may see the inmost part of you'

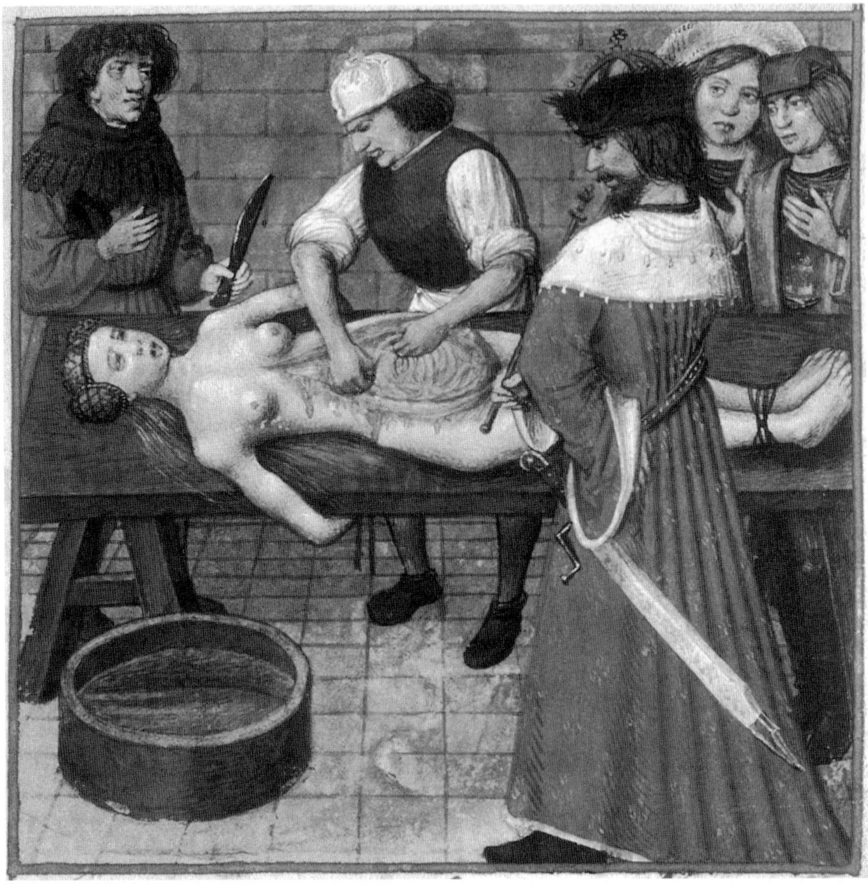

Figure 1.22: Nero dissects his mother's womb. Flemish Manuscript of the *Roman de la Rose*, c. 1500, Harley MS 4425, f. 59. © British Library Board. All Rights Reserved.

(III, iv, 20–1). Those who had seen pictorial renderings of *Anatomia*, the titular deity of the dissecting art, on the title pages of anatomical manuals like Julius Casserius' *Tabulae Anatomicae* (1627), would have been familiar with her defining emblems: the mirror and the skull. Like Hamlet, John More attempts to define his role as dissector by alluding to this dual symbolism in his *Lively Anatomie of Death* (1596):

> [I]t will not be amisse (if according to my skill) I shew you some Anatomie, in which you may see (as in a glass) the originall of Death, and from whence it came, what it is by nature, with the power, strength, and sting thereof: and what through Christ to the faithfull . . . for by Sinne, Death entred, and Death is the wages thereof.[138]

More explains that the cause of Death, proceeding from the 'originall' mother, lay 'hidden' from view until the inception of 'Gods lawe', when 'sinne . . . shewed it selfe: all our spots did then appeare, which before were darkened . . . by our fall'. Through the unravelling of His redemptive scheme God becomes an anatomist who 'opened the inward man with all his concupiscence', revealing 'how all things both within us . . . were corrupted . . . all our members, both head, handes, and heart'.[139] In a similar vein, Hamlet's moralised partitioning of his mother would impel her to cry, 'O Hamlet, speak no more./Thou turn'st mine eyes into my very soul,/And there I see such black and grainèd spots/As will not leave their tinct' (III, iv, 80–3). His penetration to the 'Rebellious hell' which 'actively doth burn' in her 'matron's bones' (III, iv, 74–9), associates her spiritual malaise with the symptoms of syphilis. This is expanded in his pornographic evocations of the bodily fluids involved in sexual congress, the 'rank sweat of an enseamèd bed, stewed in corruption' (III, iv, 84–5), and of inwardly festering disease: 'Lay not a flattering unction to your soul . . . It will but skin and film the ulcerous place/Whilst rank corruption, mining all within,/Infects unseen' (III, iv, 141–5). This comes close to Philip Stubbes' own dissection of 'Whoremongers and Fornicatours' in his *Anatomie of Abuses*, in which he follows Melanchthon's catalogue of the corporeal effects of lust: 'it infirmeth the sinewes, it weakeneth the joyntes, it exhausteth the marowe . . . it bryngeth consumption, it causeth ulceration, scabbe, scurffe, blaine, botch, pockes and byles'.[140] Similarly Burton's disclosure of the lustful woman who is beneath 'her skin . . . all loathsomeness . . . bones, nerves, sinews . . . full of filthy phlegm, stinking, putrid, excremental stuff', is intended to stimulate the viewer's need for divine grace for 'a desire of grace in the want of grace, is grace itself; a constant and earnest desire to believe, repent, and be reconciled to God, if it be in a touched heart'.[141]

Throughout his encounter with his mother Hamlet asserts the immediacy and directness of his engagement with his mother's body, promising to 'wring her heart . . ./If it be made of penetrable stuff' (III, iv, 36–7), a process to which Gertrude succumbs with the admission 'thou hast cleft my heart in twain' (III, iv, 152). If Hamlet asks his 'Mother, for love of grace, [to]/. . . Confess yourself to heaven;/Repent what's past' (III, iv, 140–6), emphasising the role of 'reason' (III, iv, 80) and 'judgement' (III, iv, 71) in this endeavour, this is because, as Roland Mushat Frye maintains, 'the Prince "smites" his mother in the ways that might be expected of one who was educated at Wittenberg'.[142] While Frye is referring specifically to Luther's teachings, I would go one stage further by suggesting that Hamlet is accessing the Melanchthonian appeal to the reasoning faculty, the 'authoritative part' which, as the 'executor of divine judgement', was thought to instil a love of grace in the sinful 'heart'.[143] The dual appeal to the body and soul which characterised the Wittenberg curriculum and its Melanchthonian school of self-knowing finds, as we have seen, its English counterpart in Woolton, but is also echoed by John Davies, whose poem *Nosce Teipsum* (1602) defines the task of understanding the 'inward self', the operations of 'the clocke within our breasts', in maternalised terms, as synonymous with the operations of the rational soul whose '*quickening* power in every living part,/Doth as a Nurse, or as a Mother serve'.[144] If the anatomist justifies his craft by claiming to expose the incorrigibility which naturally inheres in the human fabric as a consequence of its maternal origin, then the dissecting process itself gives the anatomist – or the self-knowing penitent who agrees to take on the dissecting role for themselves – powers akin to those of the ideal, conceiving mother.

Hamlet's own attempts to expose and stem his mother's 'compulsive ardour' (III, iv, 78) reproduce the salvific trajectory of the Wittenberg anatomical lecture. By inculcating in her the need to eviscerate her own corrupted heart and 'throw away the worser part of it' (III, iv, 153) she will come to incorporate the traits of proper maternal conduct which are the certain signs of divine grace. This finds dramatic articulation in his stage-managing of the *mother's blessing*;[145] a ritual which affirms the divinely sanctioned nature of the maternal role: 'when you are desirous to be blest,/I'll blessing beg of you' (III, iv, 160–1). However, this blessed state is always to be deferred, and the apparently reconciliatory tone of Hamlet's parting words to his mother is rudely shattered by his drawing attention to the eviscerated body of Polonious which has been on display throughout the entire mock-dissection scene: 'I'll lug the guts into the neighbour room./Mother, good night indeed. This counsellor/Is now most still, most secret, and most grave' (III, iv, 192–4). It is the spectacle of the open bleeding body which throws into ironic relief Hamlet's imagined anatomical penetration of his mother. In the early modern anatomy theatre the corpse on display served as a repository of physical evidence intended to *flesh out* the medical lecture. The new body of knowledge generated by the Vesalian process of anatomy was therefore *comparatively* conceived, privileging the dissected cadaver over the theoretical component of the lesson. The stubbornly 'secret' and 'grave' body of Polonious, however, refuses to lend credence to Hamlet's aping of the Vesalian and Melanchthonian dissector which the play's full rhetorical and satiric machinery has, up until this point, worked to solidify.

It is this disjunctive and unsettling process of comparative anatomisation which, in the play's climactic graveyard scene, foregrounds the limits of the satirical mode of dissection. This makes sense when considered against Hamlet's fraught engagement with the classicising ethos which traditionally informed the humanist scholar's pedagogical training.[146] Hamlet's persistent resurrection of classical maternal figures, including Niobe (I, ii, 149), Hecuba (II, ii, 546–7) and Nero's mother, serves as a counterpoint to his visceral engagement with the 'matter' of the reproductive anatomy which he believes his 'antic disposition', his *satiric* postures, will afford him. In this stance, which formed, as we saw in the first part of this chapter, the adopted mode of the Vesalian and post-Vesalian anatomists, Hamlet seems to embody the Menippean satirist, a figure who displays a distrust of generic intellectual, aesthetic and pedagogical formulae indicative of the Greek Cynic Menippus and who therefore maintains, in the words of W. Scott Blanchard, a 'resolutely anticlassical posture'. The Menippean satirist indulges in a 'mock-lecture' or aping of 'the learned treatise' in order to target the 'premise . . . that one unifying concept (melancholy, vanity, envy) can explain, through a reductio ad absurdum, all human behaviours', a task particularly suited to the anatomical method of satire:

> Menippean satire . . . exposes its readers to the common ground of a body, which, in its very anonymity, may be the only thing of which humans, in a pre-Cartesian universe, may be epistemologically certain. The false etymological connection of 'satyr' with 'satire' . . . persuaded the humanists of the Renaissance that satire . . . was a form of anatomization.[147]

Hamlet's attempt to secure authoritative knowledge through a mastery of the maternal body results in a transference of the lascivious traits of the 'satyr' to Claudius (I, ii, 140). This process operates in accordance with his scourging role, and is indicative of the English satirical tradition which placed its reforming project in antagonistic relation to the Aretinian Satyr-figure while, paradoxically, exploiting the transgressive potential of the sexual connoisseur so indicative of Aretino himself.[148] This evasive tactic was intended to deflect the probing eye of the censors while offering potential readers the promise of a window to a pornographic fantasy. While Hamlet's anatomising role is coloured by this satirical history the archaeological relics of classical maternity he unearths are not permitted to act as foils against which to promote, in the manner in which they had for Vesalius, Da Carpi and Estienne, the new anatomy's close reforming engagement with the confessional postures of the reproductive body. The inherited forms of maternal knowledge, exemplified by the classical mothers who embody generic extremes of motherhood (Niobe and Hecuba's ideal maternal grief or Agrippina's irremediable evil) fail to give way to the seen and fully-understood 'matter' of the maternal interior. For all Hamlet's probings, neither Gertrude nor Ophelia is made to confess her inner mysteries. Stubbornly resistant to the salvific trajectory of sin and repentance, the mainstay of the Wittenberg anatomy, both die unreformed. This idea is given dramatic force during Hamlet's encounter with the gravediggers. In his hands the bodily relics upon which he meditates increasingly become associated with the fragments of antiquated wisdom which stem back to the classical world of 'Alexander' (V, i, 194) and 'Imperial Caesar' (V, i, 203). His desire to use these once-'breeding' (V, i, 87) bones as material adjuncts to his moralised *sententiae* comes up against the superior forensic knowledge of the gravediggers:

> HAMLET How long will a man lie i'th'earth ere he rot?
> FIRST CLOWN I'faith, if he be not rotten before he die – as we have many pocky corpses nowadays that will scarce hold the laying in – he will last you some eight year or nine year. A tanner will last you nine year.
> HAMLET Why he more than another?
> FIRST CLOWN Why, sir, his hide is so tanned with his trade that he will keep out water a great while; and your water is a sore decayer of your whoreson dead body. Here's a skull now. This skull has lain in the earth three and twenty years. (V, i, 155–65)

The irony of the scene inheres in the fact that the audience knows what Hamlet does not. The 'whoreson dead body', which represents the gravediggers' practical knowledge of the human anatomy, is an analogue to Ophelia's corpse which has succumbed to the putrefying effects of water. This takes on added significance as Ophelia's body is manoeuvred onto the stage, acting as the fleshy accessory to the gravedigger's anatomical lesson.[149] The clownish upholders of 'Adam's profession' (V, i, 30), who seem to become the mocking silhouettes of Hamlet's satirical postures, do not define the body's disintegration as the pretext for a spiritual apotheosis. Rather the 'pocky' status of the corpse, suggestive of syphilitic or sexual diseases, makes the gradual dismantling of the body evocative of a perpetual state of sexual incorrigibility. The skull, the harbinger of a personified Death, presides over the gradual peeling back of the layers of Ophelia's eroticised body, as it does in the *Fabrica*'s title-page (see Figs 1.1 and 1.5). However the scene resists the reforming function of such skeletal specimens – perpetual *memento mori* – as they appeared in the dissecting theatres and anatomical and midwifery tracts of early modern Europe.

What Shakespeare's maternal disclosures are reacting against can be more clearly delineated in Nicholas Hilliard's painting which commemorates the visceral lecture of John Banister (1533–1610) conducted at the Barber-Surgeons' Hall in 1581 (Fig. 1.23).[150] Touching the open corpse while pointing, in a comparative gesture, to the corresponding region on the skeletal double, Banister confirms the new anatomical wisdom enshrined in the book from which he reads: the 1559 *De Re Anatomica* of Realdus Colombus, whose emphasis on the role of the anatomist's hand in dissection reflected the concerns of his one-time teacher Vesalius.[151] The cadaver's reproductive organs, the locus of human passions, are modestly concealed beneath a white sheet, while one of the masters of anatomy draws attention to the dead man's head, the centre of the higher reasoning faculty. With their pristine white sleeves and shining instruments the anatomists demonstrate a privileged access to the secrets of generation which is coterminous with a subtly reforming, even spiritually ennobling agenda.[152] The idea that the discipline of anatomy could be thus legally and politically serviceable to the state would find its way into the barber-surgeons' revised charter, presented by James I on 20 October 1604. This granted to the surgeons exclusive rights in the 'openinge searinge and imbalmeinge of the dead corpes', and condemned:

> . . . the same intruded into by Butchers Taylors Smythes Chaundlors and others of mecanicall trades unskillfull in Barbery or Surgery, And unseemely and unchristian lyke defaceinge disfiguringe and dismembringe the dead Corpes, And so that by theire unskillfull searinge and imbalmeinge, the corpes corrupteth and groweth . . . contagious and ofensive to the place and p[er]sons approachinge.[153]

The catalogue of artisans who exercise an illegitimate and 'unchristian' contact with the 'Corpes' highlights the cadaver's status as a source of contamination within a cultural moment charged with Melanchthon's interpretation of the Vesalian methodology.[154] At the close of the play the gruesome spectacle of 'bodies', as in a theatre of anatomy, 'High on a stage . . . placèd to the view' (V, ii, 330–1) is emptied of such moral connotations, becoming a 'sight . . ./. . . much amiss' (V, ii, 354–5) which underscores Hamlet's dying revelation that 'the rest is silence' (V, ii, 311). As we have seen, under the regimen of dissection the gradual confession and eventual reformation of the incorrigible maternal body provided the justificatory machinery for a satirical assault on those who refused to respect matter over words, a direct engagement with the reproductive biology over the mere repetition of the classical models which made up inherited bodies of knowledge. In *Hamlet* Shakespeare dramatises the failure of this satirical posture. Hamlet may indeed echo the roguish, pornographic, scatological, melancholic and necrophilic associations of his Aretinian and Vesalian predecessors but he is unable

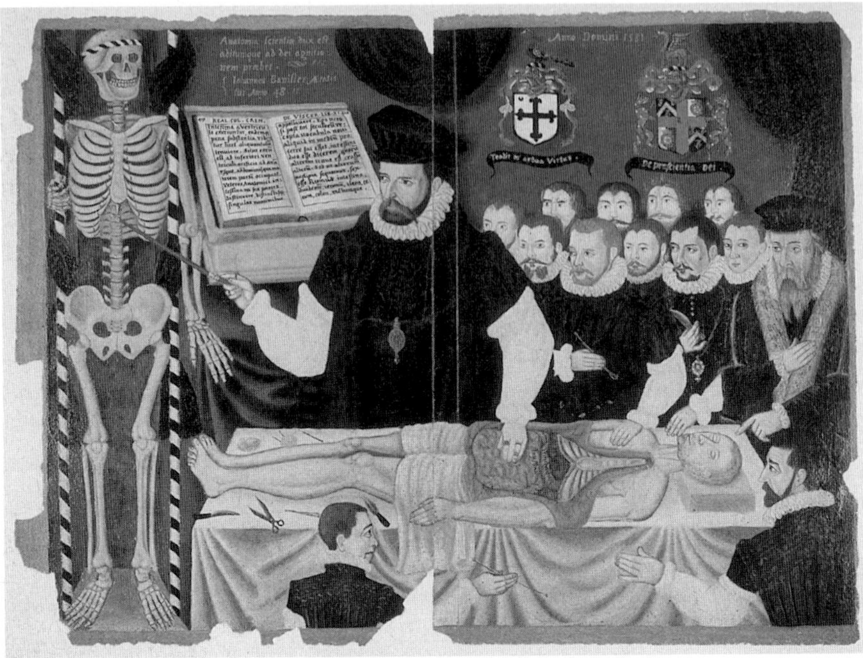

Figure 1.23: Nicholas Hilliard, *Master John Banister's Anatomical Tables with Figures*, double page showing Banister presiding over a dissection, Hunter MS 364 (V1.1), f. 1. By kind permission of Glasgow University Library, Special Collections.

to find in the maternal body the authoritative knowledge which, he believes, would allow him to get to the heart of the 'matter' if only he could hold it with his hand.[155]

Notes

1. *John Donne: A Critical Edition of the Major Works*, ed. John Carey (Oxford: Oxford University Press, 1990), p. 404.
2. All quotations from Vesalius' works are taken from C. D. O'Malley's *Andreas Vesalius of Brussels 1514–1564* (Berkeley: University of California Press, 1964), which includes useful appendices containing translations of his medical treatises and letters.
3. O'Malley, *Andreas Vesalius*, p. 64; pp. 161–2 of the *Fabrica* (1543).
4. O'Malley, *Andreas Vesalius*, pp. 222 and 201.
5. Ibid., p. 222.
6. Ibid., pp. 113–14; p. 538 of the *Fabrica*.
7. Ibid., p. 60; p. 538 of the *Fabrica*. For a list of Vesalius' female cadavers see p. 436, n. 7 of O'Malley's text.
8. Ibid., p. 201.

9. The literature on the *Fabrica*'s title-page is vast. Particularly useful accounts include: Andrea Carlino, *Books of the Body: Anatomical Ritual and Renaissance Learning*, trans. John Tedeschi and Anne C. Tedeschi (Chicago and London: University of Chicago Press, 1994), pp. 39–53; Hillary M. Nunn, *Staging Anatomies: Dissection and Spectacle in Early Stuart Tragedy* (Aldershot: Ashgate, 2005), pp. 9–19; and Jonathan Sawday, *The Body Emblazoned: Dissection and the Human Body in Renaissance Culture* (New York and London: Routledge, 1995).
10. O'Malley, *Andreas Vesalius*, p. 143; p. 221 of the *Fabrica*.
11. On anatomists' difficulty in obtaining female bodies for dissection see Katherine Park, *Secrets of Women: Gender, Generation, and the Origins of Human Dissection* (New York: Zone Books, 2006), pp. 214–15.
12. On the relation of the *Fabrica*'s title-page to forms of prefatorial utterance see Wendy Wall's 'Prefatorial Disclosures: '"Violent Enlargement" and the Voyeruistic Text', in her *The Imprint of Gender: Authorship and Publication in the English Renaissance* (Ithaca and London: Cornell University Press, 1993), pp. 169–226.
13. Titian's involvement in the production of the *Fabrica*'s illustrations is hotly debated. The woodblocks were produced in Venice and could be the work of Titian himself and/or of others in his employ. Jan Stefan van Kalkar, a pupil of Titian's, has also been identified as a possible contributor. For more on this controversy see J. B. deC. M. Saunders and Charles D. O'Malley, *The Illustrations from the Works of Andreas Vesalius of Brussels* (New York: Dover Publications, 1950), pp. 25–9.
14. Giorgio Vasari, *Lives of the Artists*, trans. George Bull, vol. 1 (Harmondsworth: Penguin, 1965), p. 450.
15. It was also in 1543 that Aretino had, famously, acquired the status of one of Charles V's circle of intimates when he was accorded the honour of riding at the right-hand side of the Holy Roman Emperor, in the words of Raymond B. Waddington, 'as if [they had been] equals': *Aretino's Satyr: Sexuality, Satire and Self-Projection in Sixteenth-Century Literature and Art* (Toronto: University of Toronto Press, 2004), p. 105.
16. The best account of Aretino's self-projection as a phallic-Satyr remains Waddington's *Aretino's Satyr*.
17. Pietro Aretino, *Aretino: Selected Letters*, trans. George Bull (Harmondsworth: Penguin, 1976), pp. 156–7.
18. Titian's use of such fragments of antique sculpture within the context of pagan sacrifice and the Satyrical scene can be seen in *The Worship of Venus* (1518–20) and *Bacchus and Ariadne* (1522–3), the latter of which includes a vignette based on the much-lauded *Laocoön* group of statues. See *Art Classics: Titian* (New York: Rizzoli, 2006), pp. 94–7; Ian G. Kennedy, *Titian* (Köln and London: Taschen, 2006), pp. 32–7; and Julius S. Held, 'Rubens and Titian', in *Titian: His World and His Legacy*, ed. David Rosand (New York: Columbia University Press, 1982), pp. 312–20.
19. Bull, *Aretino: Selected Letters*, p. 84.
20. This etymological association was debunked by Isaac Casaubon in his *Prolegomena* to the *Satires* of Persius in 1605. See Peter E. Medine, 'Isaac Casaubon's *Prolegomena* to the *Satires* of Persius: An Introduction, Text and Translation', *English Literary Renaissance* 6 (3) (Autumn 1976), pp. 271–98.

21. The connection between satire and pagan sacrifice may also have emerged from the possible etymological roots of the word *satura* (denoting a 'mixture' of different things). Sacrificial offerings of first-fruits made to the gods were known as *lanx satura*. Satire had in fact little to do with Satyrs or Satyr-plays in its original etymology. See Gilbert Highet, *The Anatomy of Satire* (Princeton: Princeton University Press, 1962), pp. 231–2. See also pp. 24–41 of the same work for the differences between Horatian and Juvenalian satire.
22. Quotations from Aretino's *Sonetti* are taken from Bette Talvacchia, *Taking Positions: On the Erotic in Renaissance Culture* (Princeton: Princeton University Press, 1999) which contains full translations of the sixteen sonnets.
23. Sonnet 15 (Talvacchia, *Taking Positions*, p. 223).
24. Sonnet 1 (ibid., p. 199).
25. Sonnet 3 (ibid., p. 203).
26. Sonnet 10 (ibid., p. 213).
27. Quoted in James Cleugh, *The Divine Aretino: Pietro of Arezzo, 1492–1556: A Biography* (London: Anthony Blond, 1965), p. 203. For more on the *Humanità di Christo* see Waddington, *Aretino's Satyr*, pp. 8–10 and 46.
28. Explanations range from an allegory of 'classical authority', therefore a representation of Galen or the Galenic school of anatomy (Sawday, *The Body Emblazoned*, p. 72 and Carlino, *Books of the Body*, p. 48) to a portrait of Vesalius' student Realdus Colombus (Saunders and O'Malley, *The Illustrations from the Works of Andreas Vesalius*, p. 42).
29. For the popularity of the *all'antica* motif with the Renaissance satirists see Waddington, *Aretino's Satyr*, esp. pp. 76, 81 and 100–2. In a letter dated 1545, Aretino expressed his own desire to circulate his image in a way which would render it 'on a par with . . . Caesar', quoted in Talvacchia, *Taking Positions*, p. 100. Katherine Park associates the Latin reference to Caesar on the *Fabrica*'s title-page with national myths of childbirth stemming from Roman and Caesarian traditions: *Secrets of Women*, pp. 240–9.
30. If this is the case, it is not the only instance in which Vesalius based one of his anatomical plates on a well-known painting which includes a portrait of Aretino. The representation of the superficial musculature in Book II of the *Fabrica* (p. 174) appears to be derived from Titian's *Allocution of Alfonso d'Avalos, Marchese del Vasto* (1541) in which Aretino makes another of his cameo appearances.
31. The connection between sacrificial/Satyrical iconography and the satirical treatment of human sexuality may owe something to a text which cemented in the early European imagination the association between satire and the bawdy tales that characterised the classical Satyr plays. Dating back to the first century, Petronius' *Satyricon* includes a description of a sacrifice to Priapus: 'to your altar, holy one, shall come/ . . . a hornèd goat./With it the offspring of a plaintive sow,/A sacrificial suckling will be yours', Petronius, *The Satyricon*, trans. P. G. Walsh (Oxford: Oxford University Press, 1997), p. 135.
32. For the wide influence of the *Hypnerotomachia Poliphili*'s sacrifice to Priapus see F. Saxl, 'Pagan Sacrifice in the Italian Renaissance', *Journal of the Warburg and Courtauld Institutes* 2 (1939), pp. 346–67.

33. Sebastio Serlio, *The Five Books of Architecture: An Unabridged Reprint of the English Edition of 1611* (New York: Dover Publications, 1982), Book IV, f. 16v.
34. Giovanni Bellini, with whom Titian is said to have trained, included a vignette of a Satyric pagan sacrifice in his painting of the bleeding Christ, *The Blood of the Redeemer* (1460–5): National Gallery (NG 1233).
35. For a detailed account of the humanist production of charisma see Lisa Jardine, *Erasmus, Man of Letters: The Construction of Charisma in Print* (Princeton: Princeton University Press, 1993).
36. Bull, *Aretino: Selected Letters*, letter to Signor Gian Iacopo Lionardi, 6 December 1537, pp. 143–4.
37. *Anatomia Magistri Nicolai Physici*, included among the few surviving *Salernitan Demonstrations*, in *Anatomical Texts of the Earlier Middle Ages: A Study in the Transmission of Culture*, trans. George W. Corner (Washington: Carnegie Institution of Washington, 1927), p. 67.
38. Liuzzi conducted the first recorded public anatomy in Bologna: Levi Robert Lind, *Studies in Pre-Vesalian Anatomy: Biography, Translations, Documents* (Philadelphia: The American Philosophical Society, 1975), p. 6. Based largely on the Galenic texts *De Juvamentis Membrorum* and *De Usu Partium* (both of which descended from the same Greek original), the *Anatomia* dominated anatomical teaching for over two centuries: Carlino, *Books of the* Body, p. 10. For an account of the rise of forensic anatomy see Katherine Park, 'The Criminal and the Saintly Body: Autopsy and Dissection in Renaissance Italy', *Renaissance Quarterly* 47 (1994), pp. 1–33, esp. pp. 4–7.
39. Avicenna's *Canon*, translated into Latin between 1170 and 1187, attempted a synthesis of Galenic and Aristotelian theories. This was refined in the fourteenth-century *Conciliator* of Pietro d'Abano of Padua (1250–1316) and, more influentially, in the work of Thomas Aquinas, particularly his *De Anima* (1268). See Roger French, *Dissection and Vivisection in the European Renaissance* (Aldershot: Ashgate, 1999), pp. 8–13 (Aquinas), pp. 50 and 193–4 (Pietro d'Abano).
40. For more on the hierarchical arrangement of the medieval anatomy see Carlino, *Books of the Body*, pp. 9–20; and Jonathan Sawday, 'The Fate of Marsyas: Dissecting the Renaissance Body', in *Renaissance Bodies: The Human Figure in English Culture c. 1540–1660*, eds Lucy Gent and Nigel Llewellyn (London: Reaktion Books, 1990), pp. 111–35.
41. Massa, *Introductory Book on Anatomy*, from the full translation of the text given in Lind, *Studies in Pre-Vesalian Anatomy*, pp. 175–6.
42. From the Preface to the *Fabrica*, trans. O'Malley, *Andreas Vesalius*, pp. 319–20.
43. Wellcome MS 49 [Apocalypse], c. 1420, f. 38. For another anatomical image which derives from this pictorial tradition see the mid-fifteenth-century Pseudo-Galenic *Anathomia* whose English text reproduces the classical homology of the male and female generative organs: 'In the woman for sothe in the stede of the yarde ys the neke of the moder' which is 'yn man[e]r of a yerd or a pyntyl yturned inwarde', Wellcome MS 290, mid-fifteenth century, ff. 31–31v. The image is on f. 52v.

44. Bernard of Clairvaux, *On the Song of Songs II*, trans. Kilian Walsh (Michigan: Cistercian Fathers Series, no. 7, 1976), Sermon 28: 8, pp. 109–10.
45. Guerric of Igny, *Liturgical Sermons*, vol. 1, trans. the Monks of Mount Saint Bernard Abbey (Ireland: Cistercian Fathers Series, no. 8, 1971), Sermon 21: 2–3, pp. 141–2.
46. For more on such birth and maternal imagery in monastic writing see Caroline Walker Bynum, *Jesus as Mother: Studies in the Spirituality of the High Middle Ages* (Berkeley: University of California Press, 1982).
47. K. B. Roberts and J. D. W. Tomlinson, *The Fabric of the Body: European Traditions of Anatomical Illustration* (Oxford: Oxford University Press, 1992), p. 37.
48. My reading of the two *Fasciculae* gravida figures differs from the conclusions reached by Jonathan Sawday who sees the 1491 image as 'not ideal, but fallen', representing 'the curse of Eve', while the 1493 rendering 'echoes, more directly, images of the Virgin', *The Body Emblazoned*, p. 105. My interpretation depends on the opposite assumption; that the sexually provocative pose of the latter figure brings her closer to the more overtly classical representations of fallen woman, particularly of Eve, while the 1491 figure, with *both* hands raised, recapitulates a traditional sign for benediction in the early iconography of the Church, a posture still used today as a hieroglyph for the Virgin Mary in Eastern Orthodox sacred imagery.
49. For more on Berengario da Carpi, including his family's medical connections (his father was himself a surgeon), see Roberts and Tomlinson, *The Fabric of the Body*, pp. 70–7.
50. Jacopo Berengario da Carpi, *Carpi Commentaria . . . Anatomia Mu[n]dini* (Bologna: 1521), BL, 548.f.1.
51. I have used the 1552 edition of the *Isagogae Breves*, Wellcome Library, p. 782.
52. Jacopo Berengario da Carpi, *Jacobo Berengario da Carpi: A Short Introduction to Anatomy*, trans. L. R. Lind (Chicago: University of Chicago Press, 1959), pp. 82 and 78.
53. Ibid., pp. 82–3. In his *Commentaria* Berengario presents an impressive list of personal dissections conducted on pregnant women and also confesses to having bribed midwives in order to obtain aborted foetuses. See also French, *Dissection and Vivisection*, p. 112; and Lind, *Pre-Vesalian Anatomy*, pp. 163–5.
54. Lind, *Pre-Vesalian Anatomy*, p. 10.
55. In contrast Katharine Park, in her *Secrets of Women*, presents the development of the post-Vesalian maternal anatomy without extended reference to the Reformation, as being largely a continuation of the Catholic ethos.
56. Andrea Carlino, *Paper Bodies: A Catalogue of Anatomical Fugitive Sheets 1538–1687*, trans. Noga Arikha, Medical History, Supplement 19 (London: The Wellcome Institute for the History of Medicine, 1999), p. 3.
57. Anatomical fugitive sheet, *Perutilis Anatomes Interiorum Mulieris Partium*, Jean Ruell (Paris: 1539), Wellcome Library, EPB. 289.5.
58. Carlino, *Paper Bodies*, pp. 88–91. As well as Protestant propaganda Vogtherr himself printed illustrations for the vernacular edition of the

Gruninger New Testament and for the Kopfel Bible which was issued in 1530.

59. *Interiorum corporis humani partium* (London: c. 1559). This sheet may also have been produced by, or in collaboration with, Thomas Geminus, the man credited with bringing Vesalius' woodcuts to an English readership through his largely plagiarised *Compendiosa totius anatomie delineatio* (1545), translated into English in 1553 by N. Udall, BL, C.43.h.2. See also Carlino, *Paper Bodies*, pp. 216–17.
60. Anatomical fugitive sheet, *Tabula Foeminae Membra Demonstrans* (Wittenberg: 1573), Wellcome Library, EPB. 298.17.
61. Anatomical fugitive sheet, *Tabula Exhibens Insigniora Maris Viscera* (Wittenberg: 1573), Wellcome Library, EPB. 298.17.
62. Philip Melancthon, *Philip Melanchthon: A Melanchthon Reader*, trans. Ralph Keen, American University Studies, Series 7: Theology and Religion (New York: Peter Lang, 1988), p. 274.
63. Sachiko Kusukawa, *The Transformation of Natural Philosophy: The Case of Philip Melanchthon* (Cambridge: Cambridge University Press, 1995), pp. 103 and 274. Melanchthon was instrumental in establishing the compatibility of Lutheran theology with the new anatomical teaching in the Department of Anatomy at Wittenberg University, a synthesis which he effected through the mediatory influence of Vesalius. See Andrew Cunningham, 'Luther and Vesalius', and Vivian Nutton, 'Wittenberg Anatomy', both in *The Renaissance in Europe: A Reader*, ed. Keith Whitlock (New Haven and London: Yale University Press, 2000), pp. 275–87, and pp. 290–300 respectively.
64. Philip Melancthon, *Philip Melanchthon: Orations on Philosophy and Education*, trans. Christine F. Salazar, ed. Sachiko Kusukawa (Cambridge: Cambridge University Press, 1999), p. 160.
65. Ibid., pp. 161–4.
66. The uniquely private and 'internalised' nature of counter-Reformation confession, exemplified by the development of the confession box in the mid-1500s, may well have been a reaction to Protestant attempts at fashioning a more introspective form of spiritual self-management. See Richard Wilson's *Secret Shakespeare: Studies in Theatre, Religion and Resistance* (Manchester: Manchester University Press, 2004), p. 18. However, confession was, despite its status as a 'collective sacrament' (Wilson, ibid.), just as central to the medieval Church because of its emphasis on priestly mediation (see Eamon Duffy, *The Stripping of the Altars: Traditional Religion in England 1400–1580* (New Haven: Yale University Press, 1992), pp. 54–60), and it is this limitation upon the accessibility of self-knowledge that the new anatomy was able to circumvent by creating a corporealised lexicon which occupied the same semantic locus as confession.
67. The Leiden theatre was constructed inside a church. The religious significance of the anatomy must have been accentuated by its location, particularly since, as William Brockbank maintains, church services were still held in the building up till 1807. See Brockbank's 'Old Anatomical Theatres and What Took Place Therein', *Medical History* 12 (1968), pp. 375–6. For an image of the Domus Anatomica in Copenhagen, see

Guildhall Library ref. 706. This theatre was built around 1640–3 by Simon Pauli, one-time student at Leiden. See Arturo Castiglioni, 'The Origin and Development of the Anatomical Theater to the End of the Renaissance', *Ciba Symposia* 3 (1941), 841–2.

68. Edward Hatton, *A New View of London* (London: 1708), BL, 577.d.1–2.
69. Rueff's text was translated into English and published as *The Expert Midwife, or An Excellent and Most Necessary Treatise of the Generation and Birth of Man* (London: 1637), BL, C.112.c.1.
70. This was *A Newe Boke, Conteyninge an Exhortacio[n] to Prayer. A Prayer with Thankes, at the Purification of Women* (London: 1548). See Mary E. Fissell, *Vernacular Bodies: The Politics of Reproduction in Early Modern England* (Oxford: Oxford University Press, 2004), p. 45 and pp. 29–50 for the Protestant ethos of such early midwifery manuals and the appropriation of Eve as a hieroglyph for reforming ideas about the maternal body. Raynalde's 1545 version of the *Byrth of Mankynde* incorporated plates of the female reproductive function from Vesalius' *Fabrica* of 1543.
71. The *memento mori* references to Death (suggested in the use of skeletal specimens) in anatomy theatres like that of Leiden, Padua and the Barber-Surgeons' Hall may indicate that anatomies could be subtly coloured by the satirical motifs which informed the *Danse Macabre*.
72. Lind, *Studies in Pre-Vesalian Anatomy*, pp. 9 and 89.
73. See also Mizaud Antoine's *Aesculapii et uraniae medicum . . . sive humani corporis cum coelo, paucis figuran et perspicue demonstrans* (Tornaesium: 1550), Wellcome Library, EPB/B and Valverde de Hamusco's *Tabula musculos omnes demonstrans*, early seventeenth century, Wellcome MS 785.
74. The original drawings for this series were executed by Rosso Fiorentino and Perino del Vaga who may have been directly influenced by Giulio Romano's originals for the *I modi*. See Talvacchia, *Taking Positions*, pp. 125–60 and Roberts and Tomlinson, *The Fabric of the Body*, pp. 170–1. Rosso was a pupil of Andrea del Sarto, who was also associated with the notorious Aretino, and had himself planned to compose an anatomy treatise. See Kenneth D. Keele, 'Leonardo da Vinci's Influence on Renaissance Anatomy', *Medical History* 8 (1964), pp. 360–70; and C. E. Kellett, 'Two Anatomies', *Medical History* 8 (1964), pp. 342–53, esp. pp. 344–5.
75. Estienne was lecturer at the Paris medical faculty from 1544 to 1547 and one-time pupil of Jacobus Sylvius (1478–1555) along with his contemporary Vesalius with whom he studied at the University of Paris after moving to the city in 1534: see French, *Dissection and Vivisection*, p. 164. Estienne's *De Dissectione* was the first text to boast an image of the clitoris as a distinct anatomical part in its own right: see Benjamin A. Rifkin, Michael J. Ackerman and Judith Folkenberg, *Human Anatomy: Depicting the Body from the Renaissance to Today* (London: Thames and Hudson, 2006), p. 16–20. For more on Estienne see Gernot Rath, 'Charles Estienne: Contemporary of Vesalius', *Medical History* 8 (1964), pp. 354–9. An overview of Vesalius' theories on the reproductive anatomy appears in Robert Herrlinger and Edith Feiner, 'Why did Vesalius not Discover the Fallopian Tubes?', *Medical History* 8 (1964), pp. 335–41.
76. Charles Estienne, *De Dissectione Partium Corporis Humani* (Paris: 1545), Wellcome Library, 6706.

77. The allusion is suggested in Rifkin et al., *Human Anatomy*, p. 20.
78. For a reading of the pre-Reformation female body and the way in which prevailing concepts of sacred fragmentation enabled women to 'somatize religious experience', see Caroline Walker Bynum, *Fragmentation and Redemption: Essays on Gender and the Human Body in Medieval Religion* (New York: Zone Books, 1992), p. 194.
79. On the wide-ranging impact of these figures on other types of Renaissance art and sculpture see Leonard Barkan, *Unearthing the Past: Archaeology and Aesthetics in the Making of Renaissance Culture* (New Haven and London: Yale University Press, 1999), pp. 1–26 and 190–201.
80. Glenn Harcourt, 'Andreas Vesalius and the Anatomy of Antique Sculpture', *Representations* 17 (1987), pp. 29 and 42.
81. Preface to the *Fabrica*, O'Malley, *Andreas Vesalius*, p. 319.
82. For the significance of the *Pasquino*, and the large body of satirical literature associated with it, see Barkan, *Unearthing the Past*, pp. 210–31. For more on Arenito's association with the statue see Waddington, *Aretino's Satyr*, pp. 19–20.
83. Preface to the *Fabrica*, O'Malley, *Andreas Vesalius*, p. 321. For more on this theory see H. W. Janson, 'Titian's Laocoön Caricature and the Vesalian-Galenist Controversy', *Art Bulletin* 28 (1946), pp. 49–56.
84. III, iii, 149–65. Shakespeare, *Othello*, ed. E. A. J. Honigmann (Surrey: Arden, 1996).
85. Samuel Purchas, *Purchas his Pilgrim: Microcosmus or the Historie of Man* (London: 1619), p. 474, BL, 1113.b.2.
86. Unless otherwise stated, all quotations are taken from *Hamlet*, ed. G. R. Hibbard (Oxford: Oxford University Press, 1987).
87. All quotations are taken from *As You Like It*, ed. Alan Brissenden (Oxford: Oxford University Press, 1993). The hypothesised composition date of the play, entered in the Stationers' Register in 1600, is very close to that of *Hamlet*, around 1599–1600. See *The Oxford Companion to Shakespeare*, eds Michael Dobson and Stanley Wells (Oxford: Oxford University Press, 2001), p. 25.
88. I am using the 1577 edition, Epistle Dedicatory, *A Profitable Treatise of the Anatomie of Mans Body* (London: 1577), BL, C.31.b.20.
89. As this passage is from the Second Quarto of the play, I have chosen to quote from *The Norton Shakespeare*, eds Stephen Greenblatt et al. (New York and London: W.W. Norton and Company, 1997). The scene and line numbers in brackets indicate the Norton edition's interpolations from the Second Quarto. I have choosen not to reproduce the indention and italics as they appear in the Norton text.
90. David Crystal and Ben Crystal, *Shakespeare's Words: A Glossary and Language Companion* (Harmondsworth: Penguin, 2002), p. 480.
91. John Harington, *A New Discourse of a Stale Subject, Called the Metamorphosis of Ajax* (London: 1596), sig. C1, BL, C.21.a.5.
92. C. Traveller, *An Anatomie of the Metamorphosed Ajax* (London: 1596), BL, G.10364.(3). Shakespeare's Jaques has been interpreted by some critics as a parody of Harington. Is there a possibility, however, that Shakespeare identifies the melancholy Jaques with the author of this particular *Anatomie*? The bout of witty repartee with which Rosalind

engages the self-confessed anatomist is highly suggestive, though an explicit connection cannot be proved: 'A traveller! By my faith, you have great reason to be sad . . . Farewell, Monsieur Traveller' (IV, 1, 29–30). There is a possibility that Traveller is in fact a pseudonym for Harington himself (an identification made in the British Library and English Short Title Catalogue records).

93. The Euphuistic style became popular among court wits, and was particularly favoured by Robert Greene, whose dramatisation of Ariosto's *Orlando Furioso* in 1591 supplied Shakespeare with the name which replaced that of Lodge's Rosader. Greene was also the author of two anatomies: *Anatomy of Lovers Flatteries* (1584) and *Arbasto. The Anatomie of Fortune* (1584).
94. On the mysterious history of the play's registration and publication see Brissenden's introduction to his Oxford edition of the play, pp. 1–4, and Katherine Duncan-Jones, *Ungentle Shakespeare: Scenes from his Life* (London: Arden, 2001), p. 125.
95. The bishops' injunction is reproduced in Lynda E. Boose, 'The 1599 Bishops' Ban, Elizabethan Pornography, and the Sexualization of the Jacobean Stage', in *Enclosure Acts: Sexuality, Property, and Culture in Early Modern England*, eds Richard Burt and John Michael Archer (Ithaca and London: Cornell University Press, 1994), pp. 188–9. For more on the ban in relation to Shakespeare's *Troilus and Cressida* and the traditions of satire, see Oscar James Campbell, *Comicall Satyre and Shakespeare's Troilus and Cressida* (San Marino: Huntingdon Library, 1959).
96. On the connection between these satirical works and Aretino see Lynda E. Boose, ' "Let it be Hid": The Pornographic Aesthetic of Shakespeare's *Othello*', in *Othello*, New Casebook Series, ed. Lena Cowen Orlin (London: Palgrave Macmillan, 2003), pp. 22–48.
97. John Marston, *The Scourge of Villainie*, ed. G. B. Harrison (New York: E. P. Dutton and Company, 1925), pp. 11–12 and 113. Harrison has used the 1599 second edition of Marston's text.
98. *Returne from Parnassus: Or the Scourge of Simony*, Part 2, *The Three Parnassus Plays (1598–1601)*, ed. J. B. Leishman (London: Ivor Nicholson and Watson Ltd, 1949). I have omitted Leishman's conjectural character insertions. For more on the connection between Marston and Shakespeare, including the possibility that Shakespeare was satirising 'Jack' Marston through the figure of Jaques in his *As You Like It*, see Felix Pryor, *The Mirror and the Globe: William Shakespeare, John Marston and the Writing of Hamlet* (London: Handsaw, 1992), p. 166.
99. For the anatomical imagery which became a governing topos of the Marprelate controversy, see Devon L. Hodges, *Renaissance Fictions of Anatomy* (Amherst: University of Massachusetts Press, 1985), pp. 43–9. In the pamphlet *Martins Months Minde* (London: 1589) the death of Martin Marprelate is related by 'Pasquin' and is followed by an account of the dissection of his 'wonderfull corrupt carcasse' by 'Phisitians' and his burial on a 'dunghill', sigs. G3v-G4, BL, C.37.d.39.
100. *An Anthology of Elizabethan Prose Fiction*, ed. Paul Salzman (Oxford: Oxford University Press, 1987), pp. 255–7 and 241 respectively.

101. The word 'matter' occurs more frequently in *Hamlet* than in any other work in the Shakespeare canon, and takes on an increasingly corporealised form as the play progresses. For more on matter in relation to the rise of the taxonomic urge in early modern Europe, with reference to *Hamlet*, see Christopher Pye, *The Vanishing: Shakespeare, the Subject, and Early Modern Culture* (Durham and London: Duke University Press, 2000), pp. 130–51. For more on the specific word-play on matter/*mater*/mother, see Patricia Parker, *Shakespeare from the Margins: Language, Culture, Context* (Chicago and London; Chicago University Press, 1996), pp. 254–64.
102. On 'matter' as the 'material cause' of conception in Aristotelian embryology, see Anthony Preus, 'Science and Philosophy in Aristotle's *Generation of Animals*', *Journal of the History of Biology* 3 (1970), pp. 1–52 and, by the same author, 'Galen's Criticism of Aristotle's Conception Theory', *Journal of the History of Biology* 10 (1977), pp. 65–85. Julia Stonehouse offers a succinct introduction to the gendered significance of 'matter' in *Idols to Incubators: Reproduction Theory through the Ages* (London: Scarlet Press, 1994), pp. 13–32.
103. As this passage is from the Second Quarto of the play, I am again quoting from *The Norton Shakespeare*, eds Stephen Greenblatt et al. Francis Bacon justifies the *anatomia comparata* in similar terms:

    > [T]here is no doubt but the facture or framing of the inward parts is as full of difference as the outward, and in that is the cause continent of many diseases; which not being observed, they quarrel many times with the humours, which are not in fault; the fault being in the very frame and mechanic of the part. (*The Advancement of Learning*, Book II, *Francis Bacon: A Critical Edition of the Major Works*, ed. Brian Vickers (Oxford: Oxford University Press, 1996), p. 211.)

    For a contrasting humoral interpretation of anatomy see Robert Fludd, *Utriusque Cosmi* (Francofurti: 1617), BL, 30.g.9.
104. For more on this pun on *foutre* in *Hamlet*, see Janet Adelman, *Suffocating Mothers: Fantasies of Maternal Origin in Shakespeare's Plays, Hamlet to The Tempest* (New York and London: Routledge, 1992), pp. 23–4 in which Adelman exposes the further meaning of 'fall', making the female genital organs the locus of original sin. See also 'fault' (from the Latin past participle *fallere*) and *foutre* in the *OED*.
105. Jacob Rueff, *The Expert Midwife, or An Excellent and Most Necessary Treatise of the Generation and Birth of Man* (London: 1637), p. 139, BL, C.112.c.1. We will go on to explore different types of 'mole' in more detail in the second chapter of this study.
106. John Sadler, *The Sicke Womans Private Looking-Glasse* (London: 1636), pp. 124–5, BL, 1175.a.7.
107. Though the poem was published in 1633 it bears the date 16 August 1601. All quotations from Donne's poems are taken from *John Donne: The Complete English Poems*, ed. A. J. Smith (Harmondsworth: Penguin, 1996). Line numbers are given in brackets.
108. For an account of how this passage engages with contemporary medical and anatomical advances, particularly with reference to the ear, see John Crawford Adams, *Shakespeare's Physic* (London: The Royal Society of Medicine Press, 1989), pp. 33–4.

109. The *Second Anniversary*, first published in 1612. The *First Anniversary* had already been printed a year before to commemorate Elizabeth Drury who died in 1610.
110. In his *Spiritual Phisicke to Cure the Diseases of the Soule* (London: 1600), John Downame described 'the lamentable effects following the sinne of our first parents', as an infection of body and soul caused by 'the fowle spots of original corruption . . . like a contagious leprosie', p. 1, BL, 4406.df.28.
111. Rueff, *The Expert Midwife*, pp. 153–4.
112. Jacques Guillemeau, *Childbirth, or the Happy Deliverie of Women* (London: 1612), p. 14, BL, 1177.d.40.
113. *The Midwives Book: Or the Whole Art of Midwifry Discovered*, quoted in Gail Kern Paster, *The Body Embarrassed: Drama and the Disciplines of Shame in Early Modern England* (Ithaca and London: Cornell University Press, 1993), p. 170. For an earlier account of the consequences for 'a child conceived during the menstrual flow' see Ambroise Paré's *On Monsters and Marvels*, trans. Janis L. Pallister (Chicago and London: University of Chicago Press, 1982), p. 5. Paré's treatise on monsters, the *Des monstres et prodiges* (1573), was translated into English by Thomas Johnson as *The Workes of that Famous Chirurgian Ambrose Parey* in 1634.
114. Thomas Raynalde, *The Birth of Mankynde, otherwyse named the Womans Booke* (London: 1564), f. 7, BL, 1177.h.1.
115. Gianna Pomata, 'Menstruating Men: Similarity and Difference of the Sexes in Early Modern Medicine', in *Generation and Degeneration: Tropes of Reproduction in Literature and History from Antiquity through Early Modern Europe*, eds Valeria Finucci and Kevin Brownlee (Durham and London: Duke University Press, 2001), pp. 109–52. The phenomenon, Finucci maintains, serves as a corrective to the hierarchical structure of the one-sex 'model of sexual difference [which] centered on the male paradigm', revealing that the female reproductive body could also function as the template for constructions of the masculine anatomy: p. 112.
116. Ibid., pp. 119, 130, and pp. 131–41 for an account of the 'unusual pathways' through which 'vicarious menstruation' was believed to occur.
117. For more on the idea of the ghost of Old Hamlet as corpse, as well as on the anatomical, religious and political meanings attached to the corpse in early modern England, see Susan Zimmerman's important study *The Early Modern Corpse and Shakespeare's Theatre* (Edinburgh: Edinburgh University Press, 2005).
118. From the dedicatory epistle to William Moune, *A Newe Anatomie of Whole Man, Aswell of his Body, as of his Soule* (London: 1576), BL, C.130.a.3.
119. Ibid., sigs B7v and D3v-D4.
120. See also Woolton's *The Immortalitie of the Soule* (London: 1576).
121. Second Quarto, quoted from *The Norton Shakespeare*, eds Stephen Greenblatt et al.
122. The hotly-debated nature of the pleurisy constituted a pivotal moment in the conflict between classical or Galenic constructions of the body and those propounded by the new anatomy under the auspices of Vesalius. Even in his first public dissection in Bologna in 1540, Vesalius caused a near scandal by

openly challenging the indomitable Galenist Matthaeus Curtius over the origin of the ailment. Their heated exchange, which took place over the open body itself, was reported by Baldasar Heseler, a Silesian student of medicine who had studied under Martin Luther in Wittenberg. Insisting that 'Galen has erred in this, and this is evident here in these bodies, as also many other mistakes of his', Vesalius explained that 'always here – he knocked with his hands against the middle of the chest – occurs inflammation and pleurisy'. His physical contact with the chest, the very area of the first incision in a visceral lecture, placed the emphasis on a direct contact with the body as the only guarantor of anatomical truth. Baldasar Heseler, *Andreas Vesalius' First Public Anatomy at Bologna 1540: An Eyewitness Report*, trans. Ruben Eriksson (Uppsala and Stockholm: Almquist and Wiksell, 1959), p. 273, and for more on Heseler see pp. 15–19.

123. Ben Jonson, *Five Plays*, ed. G. A. Wilkes (Oxford: Oxford University Press, 1981).
124. On the idea that Hamlet's use of satire against Ophelia acts as a substitute for the 'bitter jibes meant for his mother', see Maurice Charney, *Hamlet's Fictions* (New York and London: Routledge, 1988), p. 137.
125. I am using the 1590 edition, BL, 96.b.15.(10).
126. Nashe, *The Anatomie of Absurditie*, sig. B2. Nashe may be alluding here to Philip Stubbes, who attempted to bring about a 'reformation of manners' with his own *Anatomie of Abuses* (London: 1583), sig. A4v, BL, G.10369.
127. Nashe, *The Anatomie of Absurditie*, sigs A2 and B3v.
128. Robert Burton, *The Anatomy of Melancholy*, ed. Holbrook Jackson (New York: New York Review Books, 2001), p. 23.
129. Ibid., pp. 51, 117, 30–1 respectively. Burton also sites Melanchthon's *De Anima* and 'Vesalius' Controversies' in his discussion of the 'matter of melancholy': p. 173.
130. Preface to the Reader, *A Philosophical Discourse, Entituled, The Anatomie of the Minde* (London: 1576), BL, 1387.a.10.
131. *The Embryological Treatises of Hieronymus Fabricius of Aquapendente: The Formation of the Egg and of the Chick; The Formed Fetus*, trans. Howard B. Adelmann (New York: Cornell University Press, 1942), p. 237.
132. 'The Monk's Tale', l. 2,484, *The Riverside Chaucer*, ed. Anthony Burgess (Oxford: Oxford University Press, 1987).
133. *Roman de la Rose* (c. 1500), BL, Harley MS 4425, f. 59.
134. See Guillaume de Lorris and Jean de Meun, *The Romance of the Rose*, trans. Charles Dahlberg (Princeton: Princeton University Press, 1995), p. 122; Christine de Pizan, *The Book of the City of Ladies*, trans. Rosalind Brown-Grant (Harmondsworth: Penguin, 1999), p. 153; and Boethius, *The Consolation of Philosophy*, trans. V. E. Watts (Harmondsworth: Penguin, 1969), p. 72.
135. Suetonius, *The Twelve Caesars*, trans. Robert Graves (Harmondsworth: Penguin, 1957), p. 228. The *Roman* only briefly suggests the possibility of incest, but the blame for this is placed squarely on Nero, while Agrippina remains a victim of her son's lasciviousness. See p. 122 of Charles Dahlberg's translation.
136. Edmund Bolton, *Nero Caesar, or Monarchie Depraved; an Historical Worke* (London: 1624), p. 23, BL, 196.e.15.

137. John Ford, *'Tis Pity She's a Whore*, ed. Brian Morris (New Mermaids, London: A. and C. Black, 1968).
138. John More, *A Lively Anatomie of Death* (London: 1596), sigs B3v-B4, BL, 1418.c.44.
139. Ibid., sigs C7v-C8v.
140. Stubbes, *Anatomie of Abuses*, pp. 53–4.
141. Burton, *The Anatomy of Melancholy*, pp. 212 and 415.
142. R. M. Frye, *The Renaissance Hamlet: Issues and Responses in 1600* (Princeton: Princeton University Press, 1984), p. 164.
143. See Salazar, *Philip Melanchthon*, pp. 161–4 which was referred to in the first part of this chapter.
144. John Davies, *Nosce Teipsum* (London: 1602), pp. 4, 9 and 40, BL, C.117.b.53.
145. We will go on to look in more detail at the 'mother's blessing' and its use as a marker of divine grace in Chapter 4 of this study.
146. This is reflected in the hackneyed fustian phraseology and worn mythological allusions of *The Murder of Gonzago* (III, ii). For more on the play's association with humanist learning and the interesting idea that the 'To be or not to be' soliloquy was originally an 'intellectual exercise set at Edinburgh University in the early seventeenth century' see Neil Rhodes, 'Hamlet and Humanism', in *Early Modern English Drama: A Critical Companion* (Oxford: Oxford University Press, 2006), pp. 120–9. Rhodes writes, '[W]e can see a conflict acted out in this play, and in Hamlet's mind, between an academic humanism and the version of humanism that emphasizes the authenticity of the inner self': p. 126.
147. W. Scott Blanchard, *Scholar's Bedlam: Menippean Satire in the Renaissance* (London and Toronto: Associated University Presses, 1995), pp. 15, 25, 21 and 30 respectively.
148. See W. J., *The Whipping of the Satyre* (1601), T. M., *Micro-Cynicon, Sixe Snarling Satyres* (1599) and John Davies, *The Scourge of Folly* (1610) which includes a frontispiece showing a personification of Wit scourging Folly while riding Time in the guise of a Satyr whose scythe lies on the ground before him. For an account of this image and of the anatomical aspects of Renaissance satire, see Mary Claire Randolph, 'The Medical Concept in English Renaissance Satiric Theory: Its Possible Relationships and Implications', *Studies in Philology* 38 (2) (April 1941), pp. 125–57.
149. That this contrast may have been deliberately intended at some point in the play's history is indicated in the Second Quarto's instruction that the royal party enter with the 'the cor[p]se' of Ophelia.
150. *Master John Banister's Anatomical Tables*, Glasgow University Library, MS Hunter 364 (V1.1), f. 1. For more information on this painting see D'Arcy K. B. E. Power, *Notes on the Early Portraits of John Banister, of William Harvey, and the Barber-Surgeons' Visceral Lecture in 1581 . . . Reprinted from the Proceedings of the Royal Society of Medicine*, 1912, BL, 10.804.h.19.(2).
151. The book is identified in Carlino, *Books of the Body*, p. 61.
152. For the importance of such accoutrements of sanitation, see prescriptions for the barber-surgeons' conduct at anatomies issued on 5 March 1555, in Sidney Young (ed), *Annals of the Barber-Surgeons of London*, vol. 2

(London: East and Blades, 1890), p. 309 and *Court Minutes 1598–1607*, Barber-Surgeons' Hall MS B/1/3, May 1600, f. 55.

153. Young, *Annals of the Barber Surgeons*, vol. 1, p. 112.
154. Florike Egmond notes that the body used in dissections could potentially 'continue to pollute and endanger the living; it might even provide a means for the dead to return as an evil ghost': 'Execution, Dissection, Pain and Infamy – A Morphological Investigation', in *Bodily Extremities: Preoccupations with the Human Body in Early Modern European Culture*, eds Florike Egmond and Robert Zwijnenberg (Aldershot: Ashgate, 2003), p. 103.
155. Shakespeare would later draw on this bleak vision of the maternalised anatomy in *King Lear*: 'Then let them anatomize Regan; see what breeds about her heart. Is there any cause in nature that make these hard hearts?' (III, vi, 73–5): ed. R. A. Foakes (Surrey: Arden, 1997). It cannot be ascertained how far Shakespeare's understanding of the anatomical process would, at this point, have been influenced by the fact that he had lived just a stone's throw away from the Barber-Surgeons' Hall, on the corner of Silver Street and Muggle Street, from around 1604, possibly as early as 1603. I would like to thank René Weis for pointing this out to me. See also S. Schoenbaum, *William Shakespeare: A Compact Documentary Life* (Oxford: Oxford University Press, 1977), p. 260; and Katherine Duncan-Jones, *Ungentle Shakespeare*, pp. 115 and 207. Michael Wood notes that during his time in Muggle Street Shakespeare lived near to at least two doctors: Dr Gifford, who resided in Silver Street, and Dr Palmer, whose house was situated on the north side of the Barber-Surgeons' Hall, *In Search of Shakespeare* (London: BBC, 2003), p. 247.

Chapter 2

The Cabinet of Wonders: Monstrous Conceptions in the Theatre of Nature

Wonders of Common Things: The Natural History of Maternity and the Renaissance Garden-Grotto

Our eyes are sentinels unto our judgements,
And should give certain judgement what they see;
But they are rash sometimes, and tell us wonders
Of common things . . .
Thomas Middleton and William Rowley, *The Changeling*[1]

When Fynes Moryson (1566–1630), an Elizabethan Englishman abroad, toured Italy in the last decade of the sixteenth century he could not have imagined that the wondrous sights he saw there would soon be reproduced on his own native soil with equal verve. Visiting the lavish gardens of Pratolino just outside Florence he was struck by the many ingenious automata and the breathtaking statuary which adorned an earthly paradise boasting 'a statua of a Giant, with a curled beard, like a Monster, some forty sixe els high, whose great belly will receive many men at once, and by the same are the Images of many Nimphes, all which cast out water abundantly'. These were sentinels to 'a Cave under the earth . . . from whence by many pipes the waters are brought to serve the workes of these Gardens', among which was 'a Fountaine of Jupiter & Iris distilling water'. Reproducing the abundance, fecundity and mystery of the natural world, the Pratolino water-works were 'wrought within little houses, which house is vulgarly called grotta, that is, Cave (or Den), yet they are not built under the earth but above in the manner of a Cave'.[2]

The early modern grotto descended from a classical tradition associated with the Nymphaeum, linking it to the Hellenistic fertility cults surrounding the temples of nymphs.[3] Though an isolated example, England's earliest such construction, the Shell Grotto at Margate, provides some evidence of a possibly medieval English appropriation of this history which draws on some Middle-Eastern influences (Fig. 2.1). This serpentine grotto includes stone- and shell-mosaic depictions of

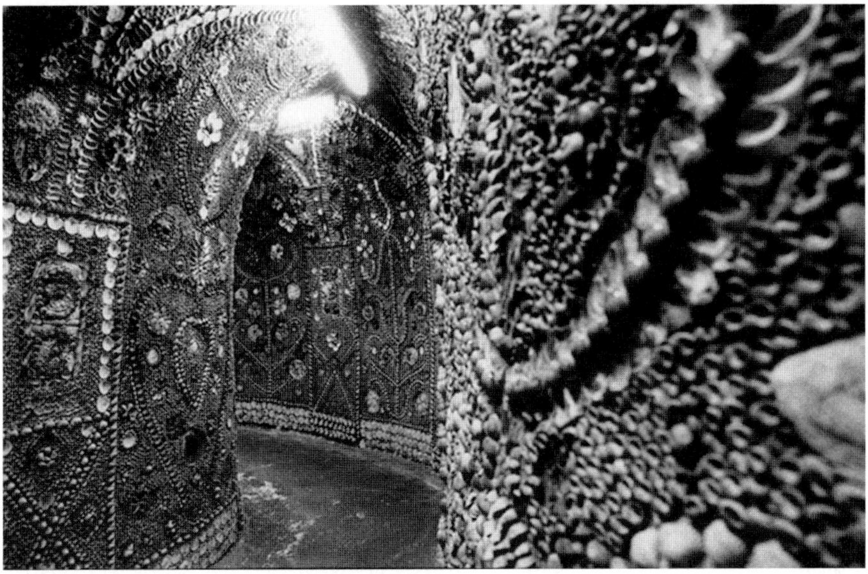

Figure 2.1: The interior of Margate Shell Grotto. By kind permission of the owners of the grotto.

male and female genitalia, insignia connoting the Virgin Birth and even a panel containing a striking anatomical rendering of the womb.[4] The Renaissance grotto was largely, however, a product of the continental influence and reflected an entirely different set of intellectual and social concerns. Such spaces were not merely follies fashioned for recreational purposes.[5] In the hands of Renaissance engineers, architects and gardeners, they would become the fertile testing-ground for emergent geological, hydrological and natural historical theories. They also invited one to ponder on the inventive technologies and natural properties which, channelled through water-pipes, underground conduits, and hydraulic systems, miraculously endowed the mechanised bodies of nymphs, river-gods, monsters, sea creatures and animal and human hybrids with life and movement. This indicates a fundamental anatomical dimension to these rarities.[6] Harnessing the affective properties of *admiratio* through a distinctly theatricalised medium, these grotto-spaces were, as I will show, cabinets of wonders – politicised *Wunderkammer* – on a large scale which distilled ideas about birth, natural reproduction and monstrosity in a specifically colonial context.[7] Recuperating the language of wonder which informed grotto-spaces and cabinets of curiosity will enable us to reconstruct the intellectual and cultural preoccupations of the age that created them, providing rare insights into the treatment of the maternal body in

Shakespeare's *Tempest*. The discipline of natural history consolidated its gradual professionalisation through the disclosure of the inherently monstrous potential of a maternalised nature. While this justified the need for careful, even artful, supervision and management of the natural world under a disciplined regimen of colonial mastery, Shakespeare stages a growing proximity between Prospero, Caliban and Sycorax which unsettles the hierarchical distinction between monster and natural historian upon which this colonial programme depended.

Instrumental in bringing the exotic natural marvels of the world to the domestic culture of the English elite was the Huguenot engineer Salomon de Caus, who entered the service of Anne of Denmark around 1607–8 and was resident in England until 1613.[8] During this period he created elaborate gardens and grottoes for a host of influential patrons, including the grotto for Greenwich Palace which was encrusted with mother-of-pearl, mussels and a shell-decorated rendering of a water-voiding female centaur.[9] The Caus grotto fashioned for Somerset House incorporated an island Mount Parnassus endowed with the flora and fauna of the sea, an artificial cavern and statues of naked gods holding cornucopiae and urns of gushing water in allegorical representation of the rivers of England.[10] What this may have looked like can be seen in Caus' treatise, the *Raisons des forces mouvantes avec . . . grotes et fontaines*, published in 1615 partly to satisfy the 'gentille curiosité' of England's 'Vertuese Princesse' Elizabeth, and which shows the mechanisms which power the grotto's godly *dramatis personae* (Fig. 2.2).[11] This work also includes an illustration of a cave-dwelling monster, a hairy wild man, probably deriving from the Pratolino gardens, which serves as the design for one of the structures Caus produced for Richmond Palace atop a network of grottoes between 1610 and 1612 while under the patronage of Henry, Prince of Wales (Fig. 2.3).[12]

The artificial reproduction of rocks, rivers, islands and inlets in these grottoes, sustained by an elaborate plumbing network of hidden or underground channels, recapitulated a fundamental principle of early modern geology which demonstrated how the earth was nourished and made fertile through the rich properties of subterranean waterways and springs.[13] This knowledge held considerable ideological import as it proved vital to the colonial enterprise. Texts like *A Declaration of the State of the Colony and Affaires in Virginia* (1622) were particularly concerned with the 'rich and exceedingly well watered' spaces which, once rendered 'navigatable', could facilitate the transportation of the many 'Commodities' and 'wonders' found there.[14] In his English translation of Joseph de Acosta's *Naturall and Morall Historie of the*

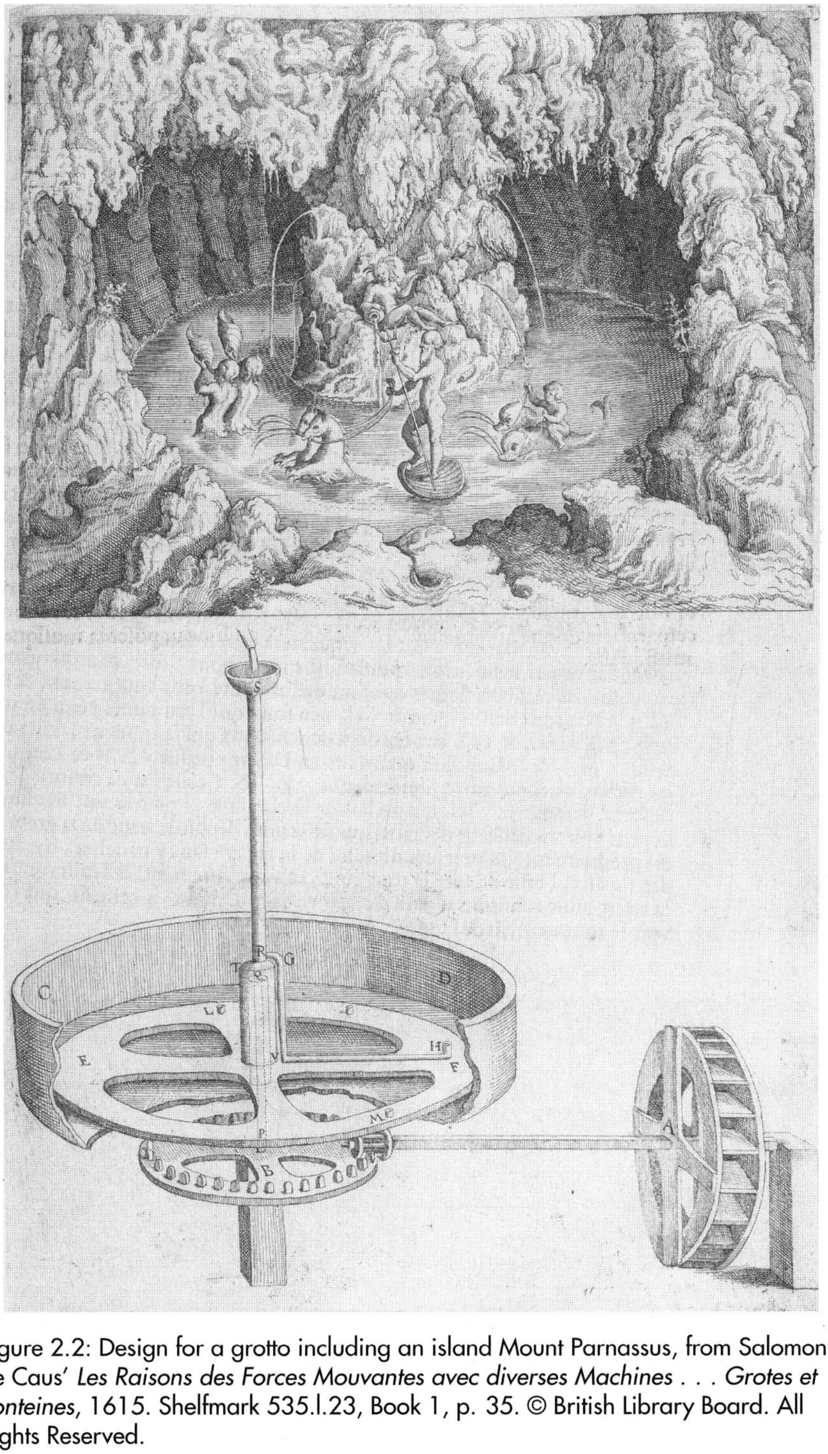

Figure 2.2: Design for a grotto including an island Mount Parnassus, from Salomon de Caus' *Les Raisons des Forces Mouvantes avec diverses Machines . . . Grotes et Fonteines*, 1615. Shelfmark 535.l.23, Book 1, p. 35. © British Library Board. All Rights Reserved.

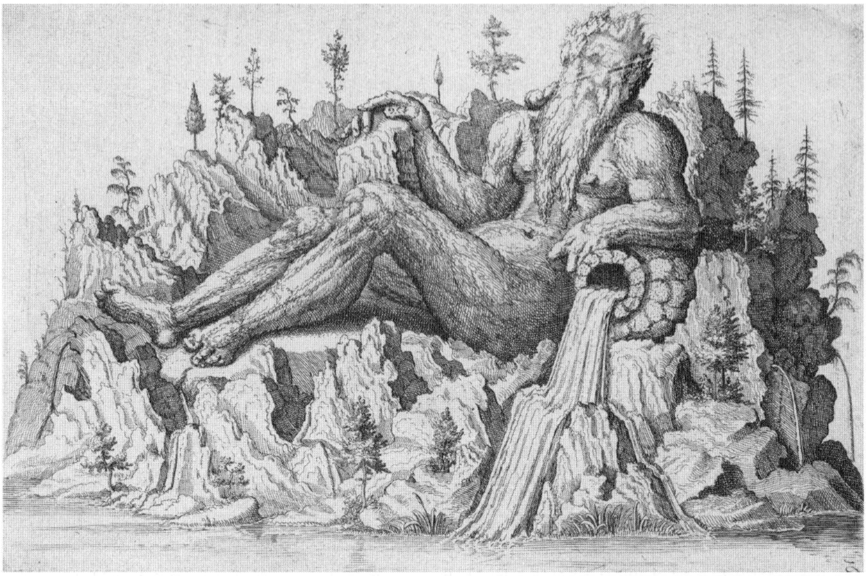

Figure 2.3: Design for a giant/wild man on an artificial island, from Salomon de Caus' *Les Raisons des Forces Mouvantes avec diverses Machines . . . Grotes et Fonteines*, 1615. Shelfmark 535.l.23, Book 2, p. 16.

East and West Indies (1604), Edward Grimeston similarly emphasised the 'great store of springs and fountaines', the 'many lakes, marishes, and such store of rivers' that make the Indies rich and fertile.[15] The discovery of these geological and hydrological features was an important part of what Acosta saw as the ultimate goal of natural history, and one that depended for its unique ideological framework on a re-assessment of older forms of Augustinian wonder which saw marvels and prodigies as a suspension of, rather than an intrinsic motivating force governing, the laws of nature:[16]

> He that takes delight to understand the wondrous works of Nature shall taste the true pleasure and content of Histories . . . He shall comprehend the naturall causes of these workes [of God], then shall he truly occupie himselfe in the studie of Philosophie. But he that shall raise his consideration higher, beholding the gret and first architect of all these marvells . . . shall be divinely imployed. And so the discourse of naturall things may serve for many good considerations, although the feeblenes and weakenes of many appetites are commonly accustomed to stay at things lesse profitable, which is the desire to know new things, called curiositie.[17]

The transitory emotion of wonder, the 'curiositie' which is the catalyst for the discipline of natural history, must be transcended if a true understanding of 'naturall causes' is to be reached. This geologicalising

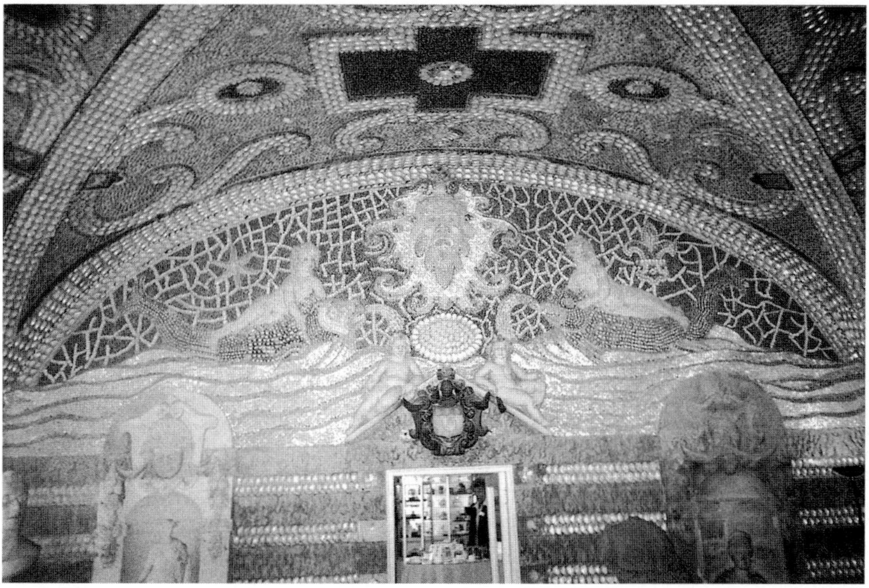

Figure 2.4: Interior of Woburn Abbey Grotto, designed by Isaac de Caus before 1627. Photo: author. By kind permission of His Grace the Duke of Bedford and the Trustees of the Bedford Estates.

impulse, which invests the colonial enterprise with divine authority, would find its material counterpart in the grotto. The strongest evidence for this can be drawn from the rare and precious examples which have survived till today, in whole or in fragments, one of which bears the design fingerprint of Salomon de Caus' brother Issac, who was no less than Inigo Jones' protégé. Thought to have been built some time in the second or third decades of the seventeenth century,[18] the grotto at Woburn Abbey is a piece of fantastical theatre. Against a backdrop of translucent ormer shells and mother-of-pearl, a plethora of exotic creatures and mythological beings indulge in a watery romp; star-fish float above dolphin-riding putti and a stylised human-faced octopus stretches its menacing tentacles towards water-nymphs as they navigate the waves atop giant scallop-shells (Fig. 2.4).[19] Isaac de Caus also designed a celebrated grotto for Wilton House, of which only tantalising fragments survive. Executed under the patronage of Philip Herbert, fourth Earl of Pembroke, one of the two Herbert brothers to whom the First Folio of Shakespeare's works was dedicated, its dazzling vignettes of river-gods and naked nymphs among a fecund sea-world were recorded in Isaac's *Le Jardin de Wilton*, published around 1645 (Fig. 2.5).[20]

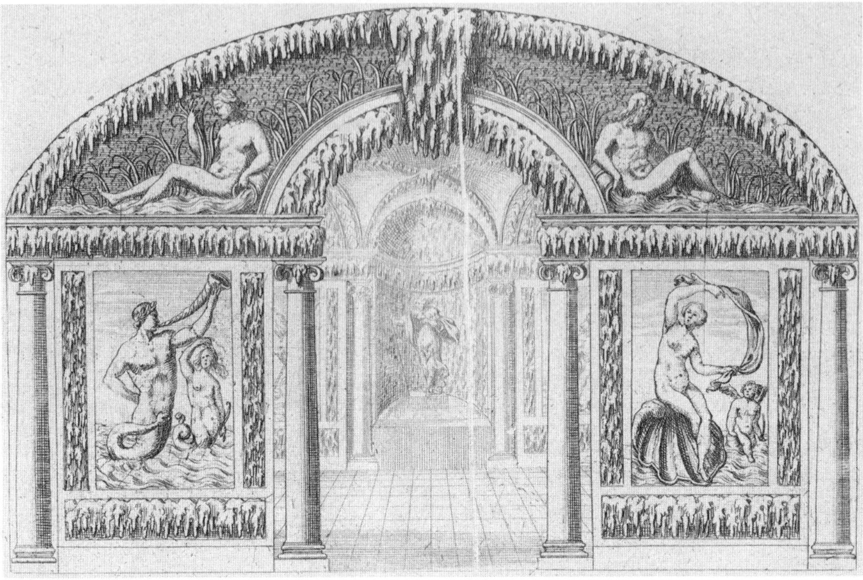

Figure 2.5: Interior of Wilton Grotto, from Isaac de Caus' *Wilton Garden*, c. 1645. Shelfmark 441.g.19, p. 23. © The British Library Board. All Rights Reserved.

These grotto spaces are remarkably similar to some of the theatrical sets designed for masques by Inigo Jones in the early seventeenth century.[21] In Samuel Daniel's *Tethys' Festival*, performed in 1610, very close to the suspected date of *The Tempest*'s composition, the audience was presented with a veritable cornucopia of marine imagery. Queen Anne played the role of Tethys, the 'Queen of the Ocean and wife of Neptune' (59), a casting which was intended to magnify her maternal status on the occasion of her son's investiture as Prince of Wales. Mythological accounts describe Tethys as mother to 3,000 children, the world's rivers, represented in the masque by various ladies in the favour of the royal court. Staging the physical embodiments of the greatest English waterways, the very life-blood of royal hegemony, the histrionic event constituted an anthropomorphised cartography, with the movements of the various actors, marching 'with winding meanders like a river' (304), enshrining current Renaissance hydrological concepts of the natural circulation of water in relation to the great ocean.[22] Indeed, the masque itself was intended to celebrate the royal enterprise of global expansionism through the spectacular setting which accompanied the appearance of Tethys against which the queen and her nymphs appeared in 'niches' amongst 'dolphins of silver', 'sea-horses', 'shells and coral', a 'great murex shell' and 'such artificial stuff as seemed richer by candle than any cloth of gold' (229–42). The royal throne was flanked by 'two cherubins of gold' and topped with 'a great scallop of silver' set among 'a resplendent frieze of jewel glasses or lights, which showed like diamonds, rubies, sapphires, emeralds, and such like'. There was also 'a fountain, with mask-heads of gold, out of which ran an artificial water' and 'a frieze of fishes . . . out of whose mouths sprang water' (244–54). The mask-heads and the water-gushing fish also came to form part of the iconography of the Woburn grotto, as did the emphasis on the manipulation of water:

> [T]here was no place in this great aquatic throne that was not filled with the sprinkling of these two natural-seeming waters. The niches wherein the ladies sat were four, with pilasters of gold mingled with rustic stones showing like a mineral to make it more rock- and cavern-like . . . [B]etween the frontispiece and the arch, was a bowl of fountain made of four great scallops, borne up by a great mask-head which had likewise four aspects, and lying upon this arch, to fill up the concaves, were two figures turned half into fishes . . . Above this were three great cherubins' heads spouting water into the bowl. (257–80)

What the audience would have seen appears to be nothing less than an on-stage grotto, with its presentation of 'cavern-like' structures. The niches described are redolent of that constructed for Woburn Abbey, an in-set space comprising a fountain whose concave wall was carved in imitation of sea-stone, mineral and coral, and placed beneath two large scallop-shells (Fig. 2.6).[23] The emphasis on half-human, half-animal hybrids and metamorphoses is likewise reflected in Isaac de Caus' rendering of a grotto which dramatises the story of Mercury and Europa (Fig. 2.7). It captures a watery domain inhabited by mermaids and river-gods below which appear naked women, allusions to the mythological Daphne, whose fruitful bodies sprout into trees, making them inseparable from the natural landscape. Indeed what Jones' masque-designs share with their grotto counterparts is an Ovidian-inspired visual language. In such spaces a potentially wayward and monstrously copious nature is associated with a feminine fertility subordinated to a colonial project which finds its ratification in the careful manipulation of the emotion of wonder.[24] That *Tethys' Festival* was performed at Whitehall is particularly significant since some time in the early seventeenth century Isaac de Caus designed a grotto for the basement of the Whitehall Banqueting House which no longer survives.[25]

Further evidence for a connection between the grotto and the masque tradition appears in the figure of Lucy Harrington, third Countess of Bedford (1581–1627), who may have commissioned the Woburn Abbey grotto. An enthusiastic patron of the arts, she was known for her

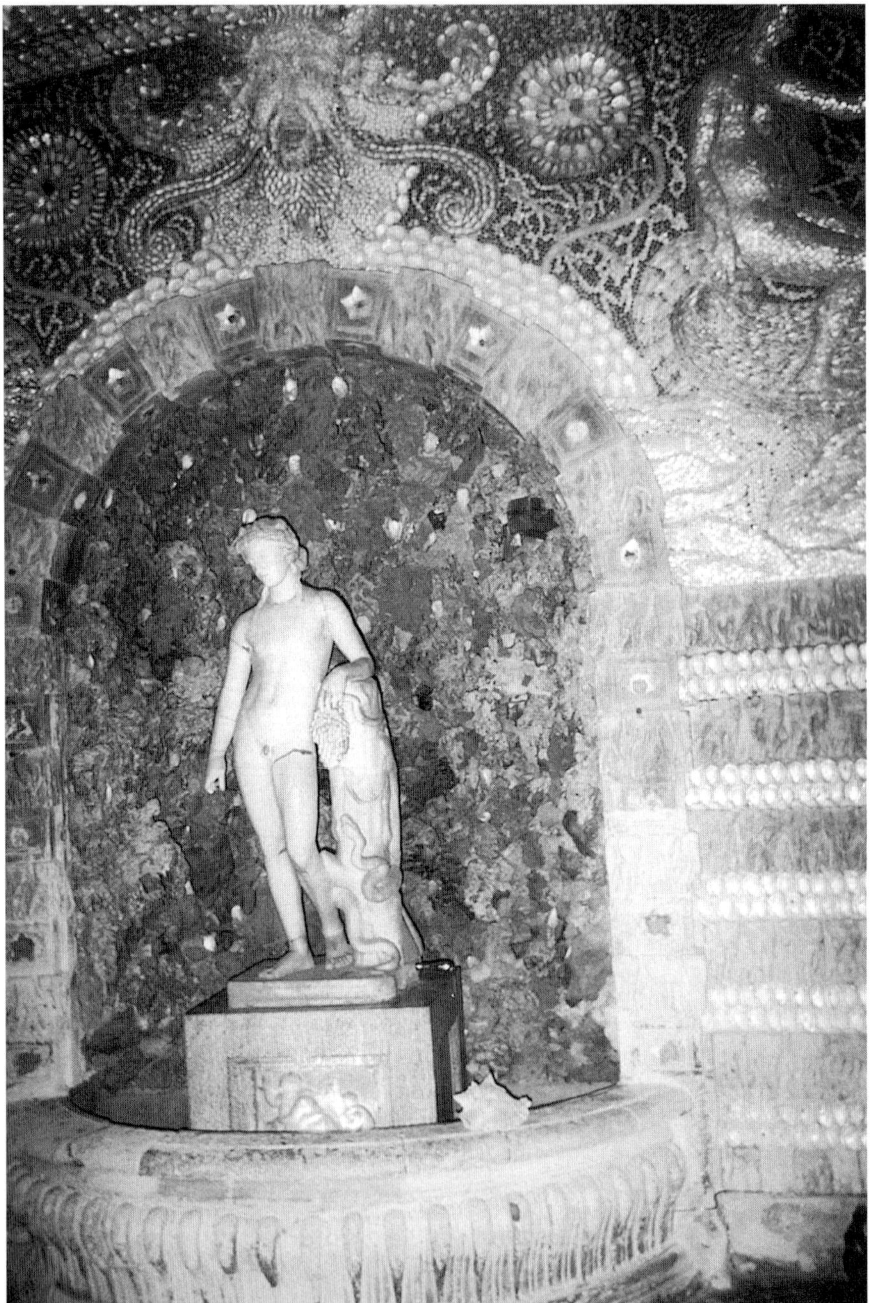

Figure 2.6: Fountain in the Woburn Abbey Grotto, designed by Isaac de Caus before 1627. Photo: author. By kind permission of His Grace the Duke of Bedford and the Trustees of the Bedford Estates.

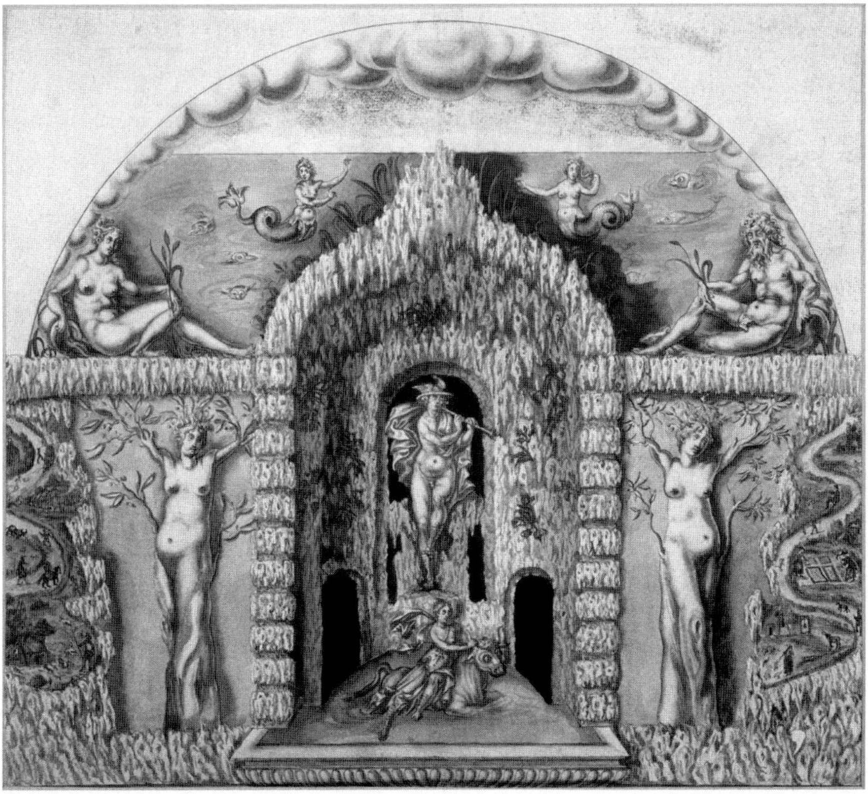

Figure 2.7: Illustration of a grotto by Isaac de Caus dramatising the story of Mercury and Europa. © V&A Images/Victoria and Albert Museum, London.

involvement in court masques and in 1605 she had taken her place among other distinguished ladies at Whitehall in a performance of Ben Jonson's *Masque of Blackness*. In the textual annotations which accompany the masque the aquatic stage-scenery is described as having been constructed for the purpose of 'imitating that orderly disorder, which is common in nature' (24). This suggests something of the way in which the royal gaze was configured in these events. The wonders showcased by the masque embody a concept of creation which posits its incredible variations, even its apparent aberrations and curiosities, as an inherently 'common' part of the fallen world. No longer meaningful anomalies created by God for humanity's moral edification, they are spontaneous generations requiring careful supervision and control. The arts of perspective used in the making of such masques were composed in such a way as to allow the king the best possible view of the unfolding drama, with 'the termination or horizon . . . being the level of the state [i.e. the king's throne]', making 'the whole work, shooting downwards from the eye . . . more conspicuous, and caught . . . [from] afar off with a wandering [possibly also *wondering*] beauty' (67–71). The king, surveying the microcosm of creation into which his court has been transformed before his inquisitive eye, becomes therefore the prototype of the natural philosopher, invested with knowledge of the secrets of nature. However, the masque also presents a warning. The monarch must not be too engrossed, too enraptured, by the spectacles before him, for these are transient, and can lead him not towards but away from his divine calling. The *Masque of Blackness* closes with a dancing measure in which the Oceaniae, the female personifications of the rivers, are joined by the male performers. Their transformation into 'water' and 'earth' reveals that human relations in the physical realm are ephemeral since all the inhabitants of the world's theatre are 'but earth . . . and what [they] vowed was water' (288–93). *Tethys' Festival* closes with a similar note of caution:

> Pleasures only shadows be
> Cast by bodies we conceive,
> And are made the things we deem,
> In those figures which they seem.
> But these pleasures vanish fast,
> Which by shadows are expressed . . .
> Feed apace then, greedy eyes,
> On the *wonder* you behold . . .
> When your eyes have done their part,
> Thought must length it in the heart. (345–60)

The 'pleasures' which the masque stages come to embody a crisis of conception. The apparently material forms which make up its wonders, and by implication the wonders of nature itself, are unstable and cannot provide any epistemological certainties. Seeing should not be consonant with knowing. *Tethys' Festival* dramatises the anxiety which accompanies a recognition of 'the confusion which usually attendeth the dissolve of these shows' (364–5) and attempts to provide a resolution to this sceptical stance by staging a symbolic movement from darkness into light, from the grotto-space into 'a most pleasant and artificial grove' (407). The imaginary journey from grotto to grove which exemplifies this revelatory dialectic actually reproduces the architectural principle which underpinned this room of wonders in the Renaissance house. This spatial symbolism was reproduced in the now lost grotto at Moor Park in Hertfordshire, which has been associated with Lucy Harrington. From the grotto, possibly designed by Isaac de Caus, one could ascend steps leading directly into a tree-lined orchard.[26] The grotto at Skipton Castle,

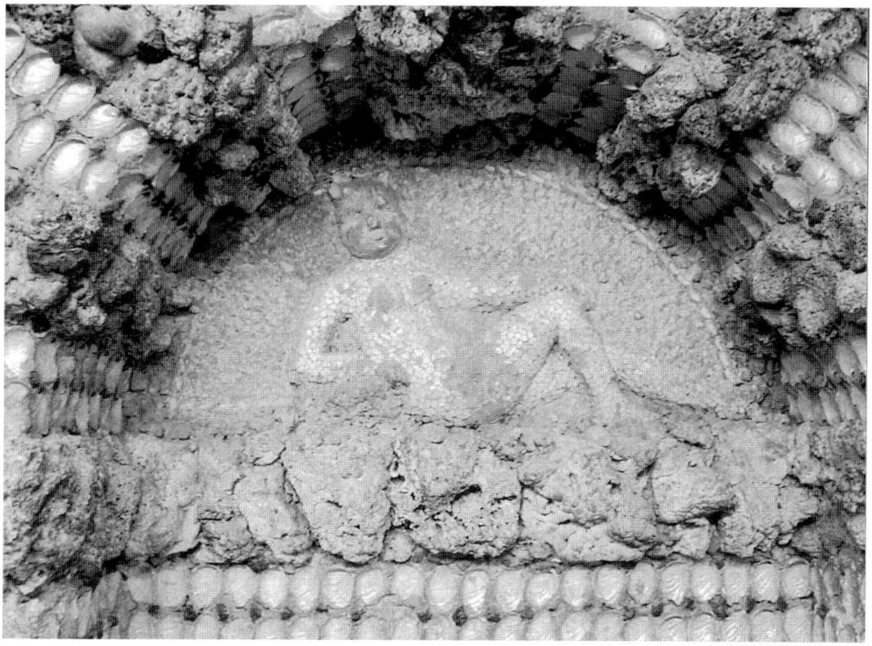

Figure 2.8: Water-Nymph. Skipton Castle Grotto, c. 1626–9. By kind permission of Skipton Castle.

constructed between 1626 and 1629, features Guernsey ormer shells and Jamaican coral possibly collected by George Clifford, the third Earl of Cumberland, an admiral of the English Armada. Also designed by Isaac de Caus, it is attached to an 'artificial' sunken garden and includes mosaics of the elemental deities of earth, air, fire and water (in the form perhaps of a Neptune's mask).[27] The grotto also houses a water-nymph which once presided over a working fountain (Fig. 2.8), recalling those produced for the grottoes of Greenwich and Somerset House. The move from a recognition of the elemental basis of creation, realised in the darkened space of the artificial cave or grotto, to a garden of light provides, I would argue, a peripatetic dramatisation of the kind of neo-Platonic world-view espoused in the romance traditions which stem from Francesco Colonna's immensely influential *Hypnerotomachia Poliphili* (1499).[28] The questing Poliphilo's search for divine knowledge takes him to a 'rare and marvellous fountain' adorned with a niche containing 'an elegant carving' of a water-nymph whose 'breasts . . . spurted streams of water'. He finds himself in a grotto 'beautifully decorated by naked putti . . . [and] aquatic monsters', with walls 'of black stone . . . framed by . . . coral-coloured jasper', inlaid with 'scales of mosaic' depicting 'little fish' and 'Venus-conches', as well as a 'dolphin swimming, with

Poseidon astride it'.[29] The enticing beauties of this grotto-dwelling nymph, which initially evoke a quotidian admiration of earthly forms, must be passed over in favour of the knowledge afforded to those willing to penetrate the surface of the created world, knowledge which, providing 'lofty, sublime and penetrating thoughts', is associated with the 'divine Mother'.[30] This is closely echoed in texts like Robert Basset's *Curiosities: or The Cabinet Of Nature* (1637), which employs its marginal and prefatorial apparatus towards the construction of a specifically feminised, in fact maternalised, image of nature through a similar neo-Platonic medium. An image of the four-breasted goddess 'Natura' on the frontispiece is glossed with a poetical portrait:

> The Goddesse . . . so plac'd on high,
> So open breasted, freely doth descry
> Her love, which heretofore shee long conceal'd
> Wisely, to make thee love what's here reveal'd
> She opens here her closet, richly set
> With high priz'd gemmes, her richest Cabinet.

A rhetorical sleight-of-hand turns the text itself into a cabinet of curiosities, the disclosure of which is compared to the opening of the female body, engaged in the act of nurture-giving. Indeed, the author asserts that anyone wishing to undertake 'the ever-vernant and private walkes of *Naturall Philosophie*' must be 'a Travailer in forraine parts'. These 'forraine parts', it turns out, are directly associated with the enclosed space of the female reproductive system, to which Basset, 'having an eye not incurious', seeks to gain access through the sexualised dissection of 'Natura': 'it being lawfull to enter the very bowels (as I may say) of her secresies, not without infinite pleasure I penetrated her *Arcana*, and opening her *Cabinet* . . . [I found] her full of *Curiosities*'.[31] The sumptuously decked women who appeared as elemental deities in the masques similarly became living curiosities and, in the case of Jonson's *Masque of Blackness*, wore garlands of 'sea-grass . . . stuck with branches of coral' and 'the most choice and orient pearl', performing against a backdrop which included among other 'rare' objects, 'whelks' and 'murex shells', 'huge sea-monsters', and 'a great concave shell, like mother of pearl, curiously made to move on . . . water' (40–65). The use of such words as 'rare' and 'curiously' is not accidental, but points to the conventions of wonder from which Jones and his collaborators were consciously drawing. Indeed, the very objects which made up these masques – the polymorphic coral, glittering jewels, outlandish marine creatures and luminescent shells – were essential elements in the cabinets of any serious collector of curios. And it is to the culture of collecting that we should look for the intellectual framework which made such theatricalised spaces of wonder – with their taxonomies of mineral, vegetable and animal rarities – so amenable to the natural historical project which sought to commandeer the reproductive processes of nature.

When designing the gardens and grotto for Hatfield House, work on which began in 1607, Robert Cecil enlisted the botanist John Tradescant (1577–1638) whose extensive experience as a collector of plant specimens and other rarities enabled him to recreate the wondrous panoply of the natural world in the Hatfield gardens and grotto-spaces. By 1611 Salomon de Caus seems also to have become heavily involved in design-work for part of the gardens. To enrich the fountains and waterworks, statuary of sea-horses and mermaids, Cecil planned to create a spectacular diamond-shaped artificial island. This was to be bisected by a river populated with water-spouting monsters, terminating at one end with a grotto-like Parnassus, work for which was being conducted around 1611–12.[32] The bills for the works, preserved at Hatfield House, are testimony to Cecil's ambitious recreation of the variety of the natural world, and record an order of payment totalling twelve shillings a week for two men, working for four weeks, to complete the 'castinge of leaves, snakes, fishes & c for the rocke and River in the East garden'. Payments were also made for 'moulde[d] pypes to convey the water', for 'openinge the springs', and for 'coulloringe the rocks in the greate sesterne [i.e. cistern] in the East garden and coulloringe the picture [probably a statue or fountain] of Neptune'.[33] Tradescant's work on the gardens, fountains and grotto-spaces took him to Holland, where he purchased 'Strang[e] and Rare' plants, and to France, where he secured 'Rare Shrubs' and 'shells of diverse sorts' to decorate the many waterworks.[34]

Tradescant fashioned his own cabinet of curiosities which he eventually opened to the public.[35] It is likely that he was inspired to do this by perhaps the most renowned collector of curiosities in Renaissance England, Sir Walter Cope. Cope was chamberlain of the exchequer and a member of the Society of Antiquaries as well as master to Cuthbert Burbage, the son of the same James Burbage who became joint partner in the Globe venture in 1597 along with his brother Richard and Shakespeare himself.[36] The Hatfield accounts for the gardens show that Cope had been 'payd . . . in trees' for services to Cecil, perhaps to furnish his own collection of natural specimens.[37] Cope's cabinet was described by Thomas Platter, who visited it in 1599, as 'an apartment, stuffed with queer foreign objects in every corner', 'curios' amassed 'because of the Indian voyage he carried out with such zeal'. Among the plethora of 'strange objects' from domestic and foreign shores were 'An

African charm made of teeth', 'A unicorn's tail', 'An embalmed child (Mumia)' and 'A round horn which had grown on an Englishwoman's forehead'.[38] Similarly decked, Tradescant's cabinet came to be known as the 'Ark' and later formed the basis of Oxford's Ashmolean Museum. In his published catalogue of the museum's holdings, the *Musaeum Tradescantianum: or, a Collection of Rarities* (1656), John Tradescant the younger praised his father's passion for 'The Wonders of the Creatures' of nature and his desire 'to dresse/The worlds great Garden'. The collection was divided into 'Naturall' specimens, which included unknown varieties of 'shell-Creatures, Insects, Mineralls, Outlandish-Fruits', and 'Artificialls', which included what he termed 'utensills' – a word we shall meet again in *The Tempest* – such as 'Householdstuffe, Habits, Instruments of Warre . . . [and] rare curiosities of Art'.[39] Such collections were *de rigueur* well into the late seventeenth and early eighteenth centuries. On 16 April 1691 John Evelyn went to see Dr Sloane's 'curiosities' which he described as a 'universal collection of the natural productions of Jamaica, consisting of plants, fruits, corals . . . animals, insects, & C. collected with greate judgment'. Evelyn saw these fabulous objects as constituting the first steps towards a specifically natural historical process of investigation for, he added, '[t]his collection, with his Journal and other philosophical and natural discourses and observations, is indeede very copious and extraordinary, sufficient to furnish a history of that island, to which I encourag'd him'.[40]

This desire to establish a 'history' of natural productions propelled the empirical endeavours of a small but immensely influential intellectual community working across Europe well before the formation of Dr Sloane's cabinet. In England, the champion of this project was Sir Francis Bacon who, in the July of 1608, had himself sought the advice of his cousin Robert Cecil for the creation of, among other things, a cabinet, a grotto, and a network of artificial islands in his gardens at Gorhambury in Hertfordshire.[41] Bacon realised that in order to make a case for the pedagogical significance of natural history it would be necessary to challenge the syllogistic reasoning which had informed the methodological underpinnings of much medieval philosophy. This included the work of Thomas Aquinas who had insisted in his commentary on Aristotle's *Physics* that 'the order of proceeding in natural science' must be based on 'a consideration of principles', that is 'we must begin with the most universal' before attempting to look at the 'singulars' of nature; a philosophy which subordinated a direct contact with natural objects to the explication of 'moving and agent causes'.[42]

It was in his *Preparative towards a Natural and Experimental History* that Bacon declared the initiatory principle of his inductive method:

'First then, away with antiquities, and citations or testimonies of authors; also with disputes and controversies and differing opinions; everything in short which is philological.'[43] This reorientation of *scientia* required nothing less than the seizing of the determinants of natural reproduction, an endeavour expressed in *The Masculine Birth of Time* in which a feminised nature is violently appropriated for the use of the male intellectual community to which Bacon appeals: 'I am come in very truth leading to you nature with all her children to bind her to your service and make her your slave.' If, as Carolyn Merchant suggests, Bacon effected 'his transformation of the earth as a nurturing mother and womb of life into a source of secrets to be extracted for economic advance',[44] the fulcrum of this new epistemology was the emphasis on the monstrous capabilities of this maternalised nature. In his *Novum Organum* (1620), he insisted that the natural historian must indulge in a close investigation of '*Deviating Instances*; that is, errors, vagaries and prodigies of nature, wherein nature deviates and turns aside from her ordinary course'. Dismantling the Augustinian rhetoric of wonder, Bacon insisted that the early scientist must reject the notion of a direct godly intervention in the natural world, acknowledging instead the inherent tendency of creation to lapse into chaos, for this method of analysis will 'correct the erroneous impressions suggested to the understanding by ordinary phenomena, and reveal Common Forms . . . For he that knows the ways of nature will more easily observe her deviations; and on the other hand he that knows her deviations will more accurately describe her ways.' The study of the potentially monstrous outcome of all reproductive processes, and in particular its place in the oeuvre of the collector, is thus an essential tool in the understanding of all 'Common' natural laws:

> For we have to make a collection or particular natural history of all prodigies and monstrous births of nature; of everything in short that is in nature new, rare, and unusual. This must be done however with the strictest scrutiny, that fidelity may be ensured. Now those things are to be chiefly suspected, which depend in any way on religion . . . and those not less which are found in writers on natural magic or alchemy, and men of that sort; who are a kind of suitors and lovers of fables. But whatever is admitted must be drawn from grave and credible history and trustworthy reports.[45]

Bacon's schema for a 'Natural History' divides the study of nature into 'three kinds of regimen': the examination of 'the *species* of things', which includes the development of nature in its 'ordinary course'; the analysis of '*Pretergenerations*' which refers to 'the perverseness and insubordination of matter', exemplified by the monstrous birth; and the reconstruction of a '*Mechanical* or *Experimental* history' which connotes all '*things artificial*'. These should be interrelated disciplines which have as their pivotal axis the understanding of the aberrant for, he declares, 'I do not make it a rule that these three should be kept apart and separately treated. For why should not the history of the monsters in the several species be joined with the history of the species themselves?'[46] What this tripartite method suggests is an emphasis on the creation of taxonomies, an impulse towards classification which should be distinguished from the 'fabulous experiments, idle secrets, and frivolous impostures' of the alchemist or magus who is too engrossed in the transient effects of wonder to serve the interests of the state.[47] Desiree Hellegers puts the case succinctly: 'Nature, for Bacon, is a recusant subject who must be subjected to a regimen of technological rehabilitation by the natural philosopher acting at the king's behest.'[48] This regimen, however, relies on precisely the kind of panoptic, even histrionic, vision afforded by the grotto-space or cabinet whose taxonomical laying out of nature's copious rarities ratifies the cultivation of a discipline dedicated to the greater understanding and control of a potentially unstable creation, for it is 'by the help and ministry of man [that] a new face or bodies, another universe or theatre of things, comes into view'.[49]

In the first quarter of the seventeenth century Bacon's work came to the attention of a revolutionary society of scholars. This was the Lincean Academy, founded in 1603 by Federico Cesi of Acquasparta, later honoured with the title Prince of Sant Angelo and San Polo. The society's name alluded both to Lyncaeus, an Argonaut famed for the keenness of his vision, and to the lynx, a creature proverbially associated with a highly developed ocular faculty. At the heart of this brotherhood of learning was the figure who was to shake the foundations of early modern cosmology: Galileo, whose ground-breaking *Il Saggiatore* (1623) was edited by members of the academy, including among their number Johannes Faber, Professor of Medicine at the University of Rome, and Cassiano dal Pozzo, who was to acquire Cesi's museum and library after his death in 1630.[50] This was added to his already bulging cabinet of wonders which John Evelyn saw on a visit to his home on 21 November 1644, an event he recorded in his diary in which he described his host as a 'curious man', that is, a gatherer of all kinds of 'fine . . . curiosities', who had amassed a 'rare collection'.[51] While Cesi was still alive Cassiano had expressed to him his desire to have Bacon, whose ideals so closely matched theirs, enrolled in the venerable ranks of the Linceans, praising in particular the contribution his *De Dignitate et Augmentis Scientiarum* (which in a fitting twist of fate was published in the same year as Galileo's *Saggiatore*) had made to the development of the natural sciences.[52]

Acting upon the kind of vision which had fuelled Bacon's own reconceptualising of natural history, the Linceans embarked on an extraordinary and ambitious project to catalogue the vast panorama of nature's varying species. The fruits of these labours can be seen in the thousands of vibrant sketches and colour illustrations they produced, still preserved today in the Royal Library at Windsor Castle.[53] Leafing through page after page of exquisitely executed images of plants, birds, insects and minerals, the eye cannot but linger over certain specimens which, though in some way familiar, seem also to display something of the uncanny, of the strange. Upon closer inspection one realises that these are in fact common varieties of fruit and vegetables which have grown with deformities or abnormalities. Various examples of eccentrically shaped citruses abound, including an orange or tangerine with a tumescent outgrowth (Fig. 2.9) and a 'Siamese' melon (Fig. 2.10).[54] The compilers of this pictorial catalogue seem to have had a particular fascination with a certain type of malfomation; the 'pregnant' fruit. This occurs when one fruit grows inside the other, almost in imitation of a monstrous birth, as demonstrated in a depiction of a citron-lemon (Fig. 2.11).[55] When another citrus-fruit in the collection later appeared in print in Giovanni Ferrari's *Hesperides* (1646) it was labelled 'Pomum Adami Foetum', an explicit reference to this birthing analogy which was repeated in a number of its detailed plates.[56] But the preoccupation with monstrous specimens does not end there. There are representations of deformed animal foetuses, including a chick with four legs (Fig. 2.12)

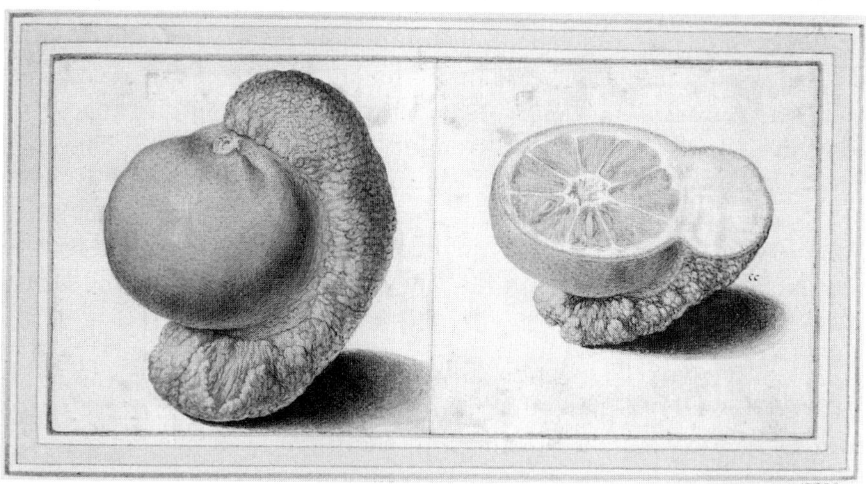

Figure 2.9: Orange or tangerine with a tumescent outgrowth, from the natural historical collection of Cassiano dal Pozzo, Windsor Castle Royal Library, RL19329/RL19330. The Royal Collection © 2007, Her Majesty Queen Elizabeth II.

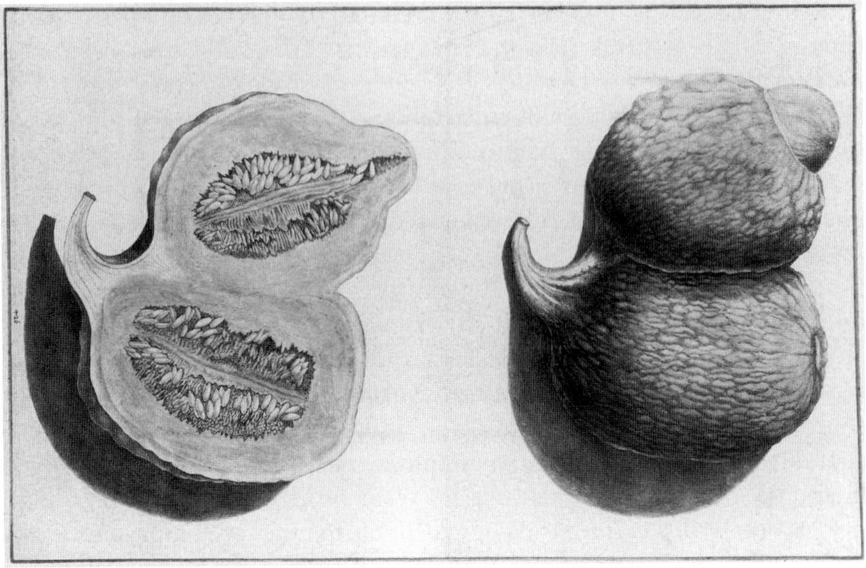

Figure 2.10: 'Siamese' melon, from the natural historical collection of Cassiano dal Pozzo, Windsor Castle Royal Library, RL19365. The Royal Collection © 2007, Her Majesty Queen Elizabeth II.

and, in those papers owned by Cassiano which survive in the Institut de France, we can see a dissected hermaphroditic rat and striking views of a hydrocephalic child (Fig. 2.13).[57] The French manuscripts in particular present one very significant feature: a visually inscribed homology between human and vegetal reproduction, rendered through countless drawings of plants and fungi which resemble male and female reproductive organs and in one case little homunculi with clearly delineated phalluses (Fig. 2.14).[58] That such anthropomorphic motifs appear so often in a natural historical programme characterised by its attention to detail, suggests that this puzzling pictorial vocabulary can only have made sense within an intellectual context which ratified a specifically homological dialectic between microcosm and macrocosm; between the reproductive body and the world. The thrust of this project, therefore, was very closely allied to Bacon's own rewriting of wonder:

> [W]onder is the child of rarity; and if a thing be rare, though in kind it be no way extraordinary, yet it is wondered at. While on the other hand things which really call for wonder on account of the difference in species which they exhibit as compared with other species, yet if we have them by us in common use, are but slightly noticed.[59]

The taxonomical researches of the natural historian reveal wonders of 'common' things, reversing the traditional paradigm which sees

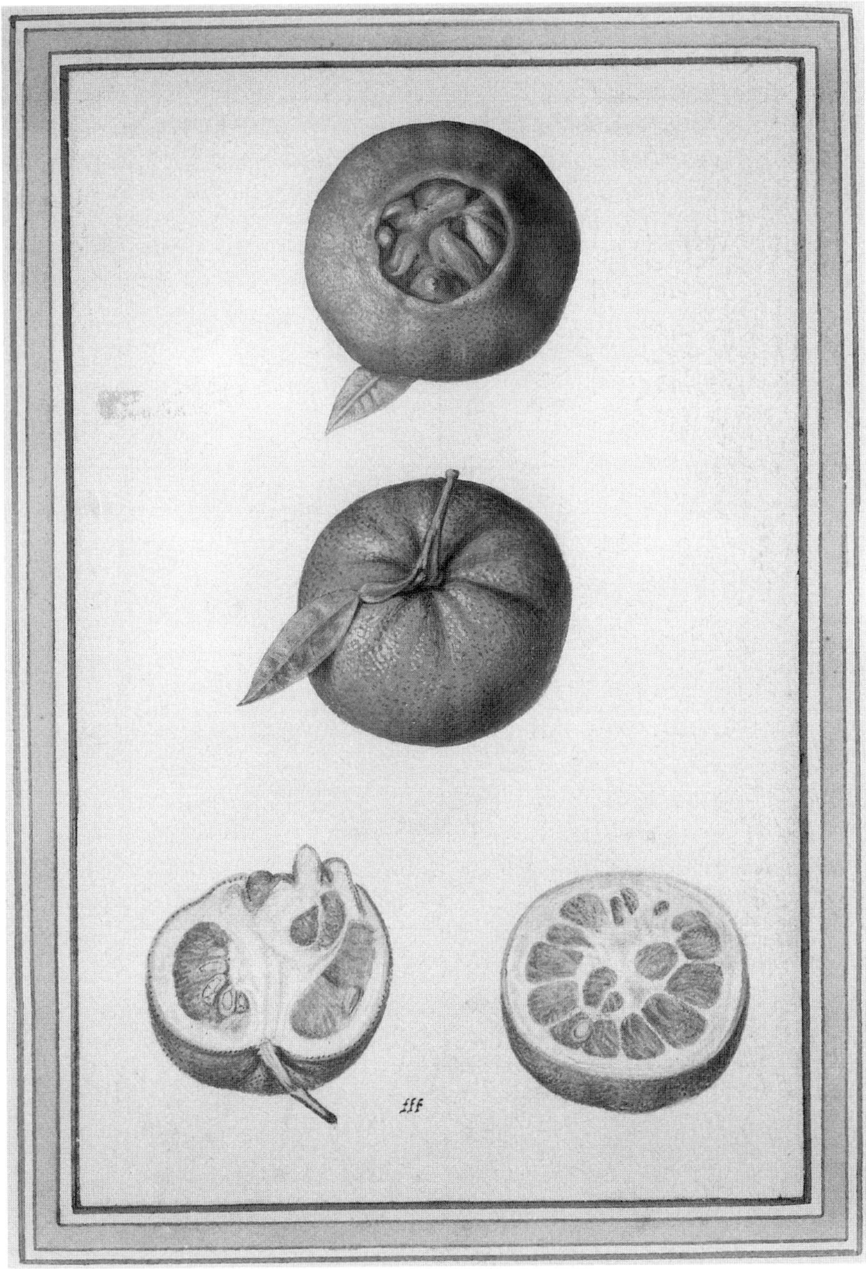

Figure 2.11: 'Pregnant' citrus fruit, from the natural historical collection of Cassiano dal Pozzo. Windsor Castle Royal Library, RL21146. The Royal Collection © 2007, Her Majesty Queen Elizabeth II.

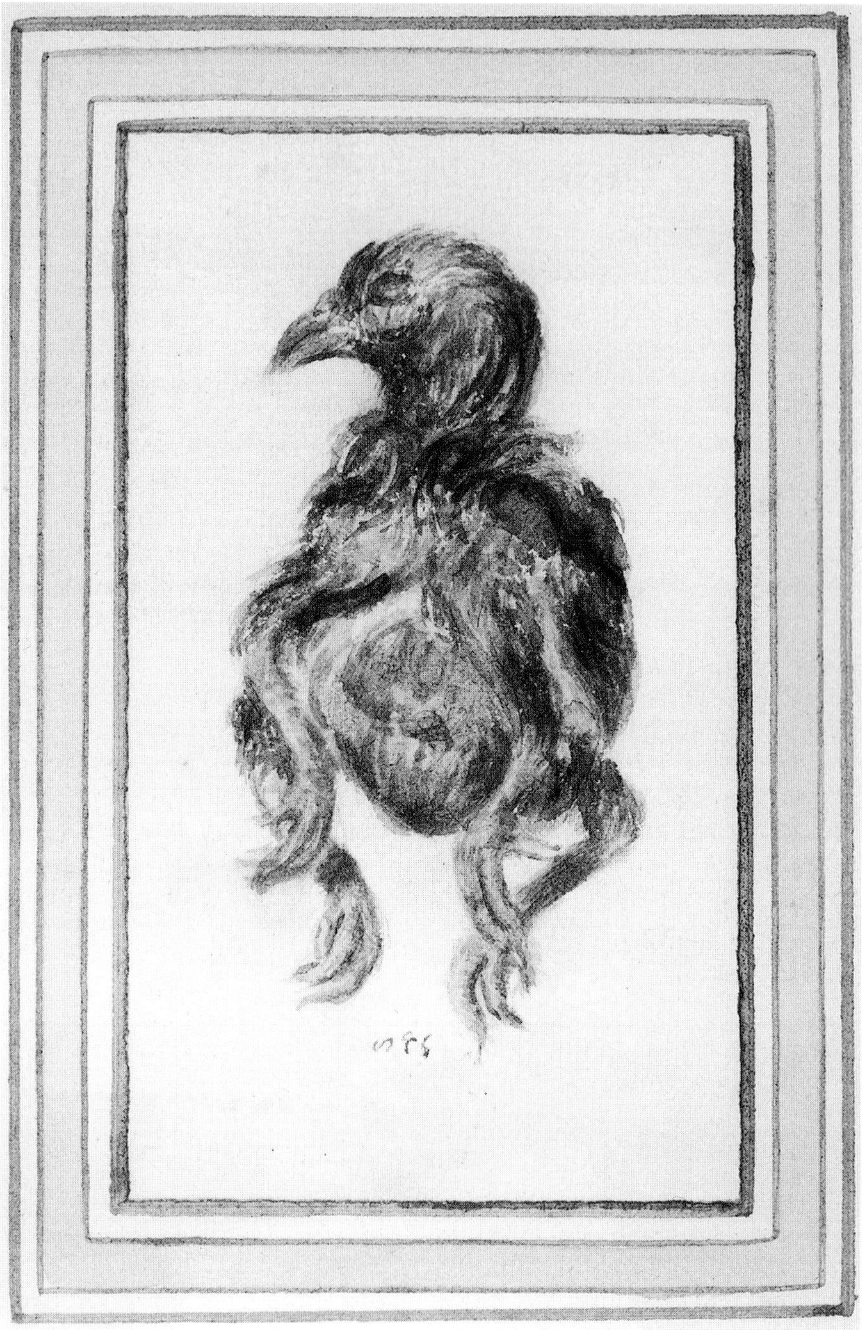

Figure 2.12: Deformed chick foetus, from the natural historical collection of Cassiano dal Pozzo, Windsor Castle Royal Library, RL19431. The Royal Collection © 2007, Her Majesty Queen Elizabeth II.

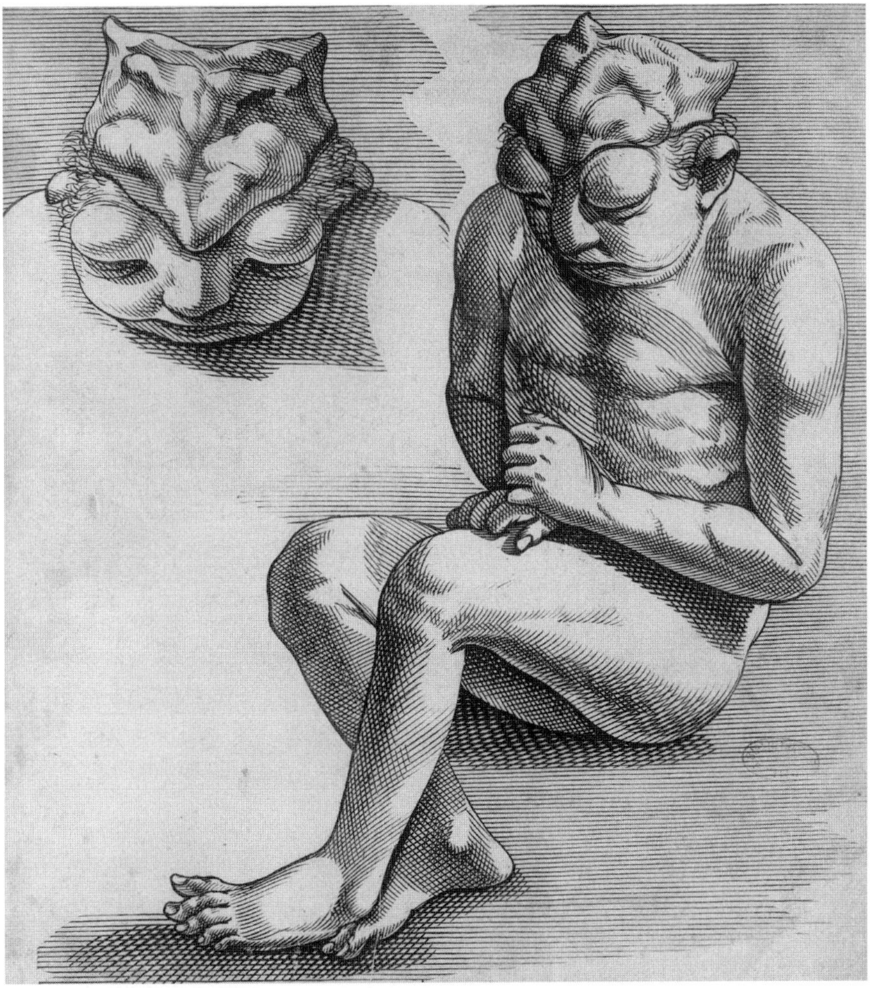

Figure 2.13: Hydrocephalic child, from the natural historical collection of Cassiano dal Pozzo/Federico Cesi, MS 978, f. 361, Paris, Bibliothèque de L'Institut. © Photo RMN/© René-Gabriel Ojéda.

'rarity' as the only identifying mark of wonder. What is truly to be marvelled at is the immense diversity of nature, and it is in this vein that we are to understand the monstrous, not as representing the temporary cessation of the natural order, but as forming an inherent part of a creation whose ordinary workings need not be distinguished from the endless production of autonomous mutations. As early as 1594, in his *Gesta Grayorum*, Bacon had asserted the importance of imposing order on nature's heady bounty through the institution of

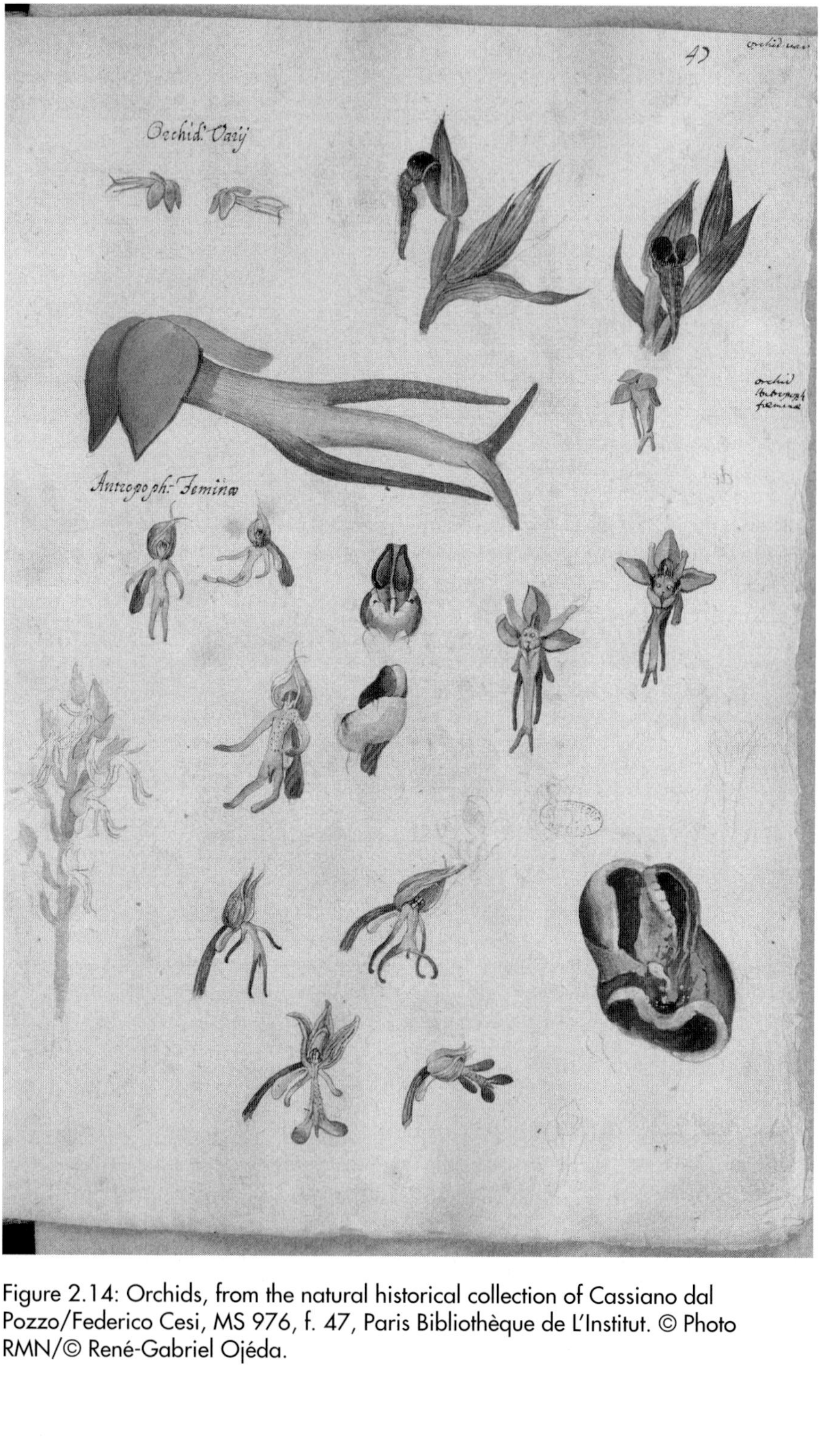

Figure 2.14: Orchids, from the natural historical collection of Cassiano dal Pozzo/Federico Cesi, MS 976, f. 47, Paris Bibliothèque de L'Institut. © Photo RMN/© René-Gabriel Ojéda.

> a goodly huge cabinet, wherein whatsoever the hand of man by exquisite art or engine hath made rare in stuff, form, or motion; whatsoever singularity *chance and the shuffle of things* hath produced; whatsoever Nature hath wrought in things that want life and may be kept; shall be sorted and included. (my italics)[60]

In saying this Bacon was partly returning to an older idea, deriving from Pliny's monumental *Natural History*, which defined 'marvels [*miraculis*]' as products of 'the ingenuity of Nature [made] as toys for herself and marvels for us' [*Haec atque talia ex hominum genere ludibria sibi, nobis miracula, ingeniosa fecit natura*].[61] No other figure before Bacon had so effectively understood the implications of this notion of Mother Nature at play than Bernard Palissy (1510–90). The prototypical natural historian Palissy, more celebrated now as an innovative potter and designer of Renaissance earthenware, presented his *Discours admirables de la nature des eaux et fonteines* in Paris in 1580, writing that:

> to cut the thread of calumny and delusion I have arranged a Cabinet, in which I have put many things note-worthy and monstrous, that I have taken from the womb of the earth, which bear certain witness to my teachings, and no man will be found who will not be constrained to own that they are trustworthy, after he shall have seen things that I have prepared in my cabinet, to give assurance to all those who would not otherwise put faith in my writings.[62]

The cabinet, which Palissy had indeed acquired by 1575, was arranged in such a way as to reinforce visually his theories through the histrionic identification of specimens from the collection during the lectures which took place there. What such a room of wonders may have looked like can be seen in Ferrante Imperato's *Historia Naturale* (1599) which shows a group of men engaged in deep discussion in a room full of natural curiosities including, on the top left hand corner of the curved ceiling, a Siamese lizard with two bodies (Fig. 2.15).[63] Imperato described this cabinet as a 'Theatre of Nature', an appellation which was more than merely metaphorical.[64] The Belgian physician and scholar Samuel Quiccheberg (1529–67) had also produced a treatise on collecting, the *Inscriptiones vel Tituli Theatri Amplissimi* (1565), in which he explicitly referred to the importance of amassing a 'Rich theatre of objects of the whole universe'.[65] Likewise, in his *L'orto dei Semplici di Padova* (1584), Giovanni Porro painted a vivid picture of the botanical garden in Padua as 'this little Theatre, almost a little world, [where] one will orchestrate the spectacle of all of nature's wonders'.[66] As a theatre of the world, a *theatrum mundi*, the early museum was seen as evoking an emotional response every bit as intense and engaging as that which would have possessed the viewer of a stage play. The dynamic

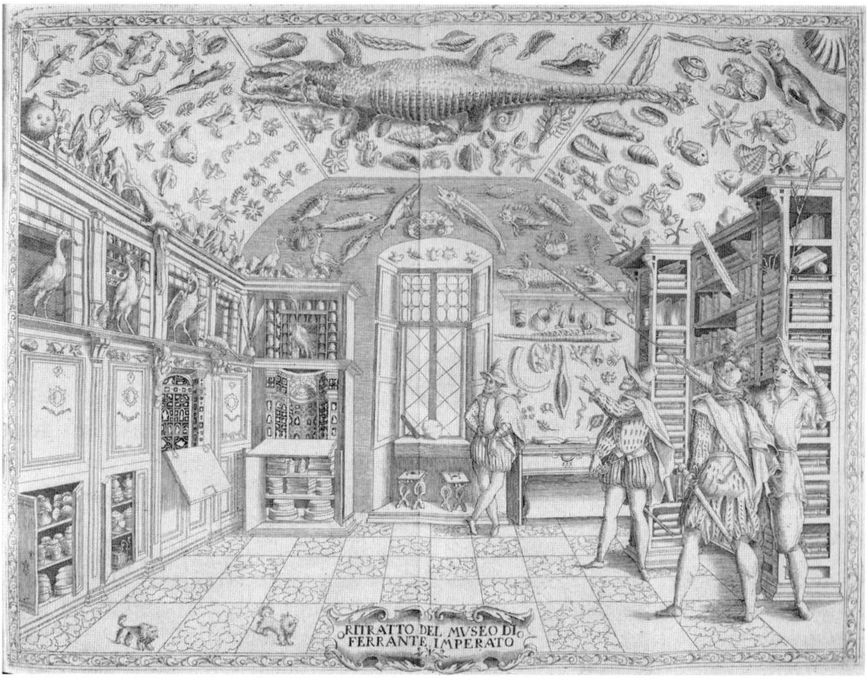

Figure 2.15: The Cabinet of Curiosities. Ferrante Imperato, *Historia Naturale*, 1672. Shelfmark 456.d.16. © British Library Board: All Rights Reserved.

interactions of nature it presented in crystallised form held their own special drama. In Imperato's *Historia Naturale* the force which propels the grand narrative of the *Wunderkammern* is clearly that of water. The emphasis on marine life is noteworthy, with crustaceans, coral and all manner of shells jostling for space.

It was in the production of grottoes and artificial springs that Palissy channelled his natural historical knowledge drawn from the 'womb of the earth'.[67] In particular this homology between the workings of the maternal anatomy and the natural world underpinned his theories on the watery breeding-grounds for life. His treatise on *Waters and Springs* is, he tells his readers, a practical manual on 'the superiority of water derived from springs, which I wish to teach you how to make in the most sterile places', an endeavour which requires 'imitating nature as closely as possible, and following the laws of the great Creator of Springs'. What seems a bizarre insistence on the importance of being able to 'construct fountains' and grottoes is in fact part of a fully-worked philosophy of natural reproduction, which relies on the distinction between the kind of life produced by flowing and 'stagnant water'.[68] The latter he maintains:

> cannot be fit for either man or beast, for it becomes heated by the air and the sun, and engenders and produces, by these means, various sorts of animal life. Frogs, snakes, newts, and vipers are to be found near these ponds . . . I have several times seen snakes and newts lying and wriggling at the bottom of the water . . . therefore, I say, that water so exposed to the air and heated cannot be wholesome, and very often bullocks, cows, and other beasts die, having taken their disease at such infected watering places.

Beneath this seemingly whimsical personal recollection lies a concept of spontaneous generation which Palissy attributes to an entirely natural mechanism. The warmth of the sun and the humidity produced as a result of the enclosure of water by algae or 'green slime' is 'a sign of putrefaction, and that something has begun to generate'. What underpins this principle is the same as that which informs Renaissance theories of reproduction: 'all the while it is cold it [water] cannot engender any animal life, because nothing is ever generated, whether animal or vegetable matter, without damp heat'.[69] Palissy borrows from the kind of embryological idiom that characterised the *Secrets of Women*, a tradition descending from the thirteenth-century natural philosopher Albertus Magnus. Persisting into the Renaissance, these theories asserted the influence of the sun in human conception and on the ill effects of 'gross humidity' in the female body – over and above the necessary heat introduced by the male in conception – which can cause the foetus to become monstrous and 'scaly' like the marine reptiles which usually develop in such natural conditions.[70] The dangerous and 'infected' creatures Palissy describes – the newts, turtles, snakes, frogs and other damp-loving animals – are the very forms of life which are forever enshrined in his famed earthenware (Fig. 2.16). These dishes are therefore not merely decorative artefacts but physically recapitulate Palissy's hydrological theories. In the heat of the kiln, therefore, the process of casting specimens for individual pieces of pottery as well as for the life-like adornments of his grottoes operate in the same way as the formative heat of the impregnated womb.[71] In his essay 'Of Gardens' Bacon reproduced these very sentiments, insisting that the ideal garden should contain fountains of water 'in perpetual motion' since still 'pools mar all, and make the garden unwholesome', breeding 'flies and frogs' and 'putrefaction' when water is left to 'stay, either in the bowls or in the cistern'.[72]

The womb-like grotto-space stages a dramatic interplay between the determinants of monstrosity and hybridity and the masculine motive principle which propels the technologies of flowing water, making the potential fertility of natural forces such a valuable commodity in the colonial context. The coloniser's power rested on his ability to make wonders of common things, to channel the productions of nature for the glories of

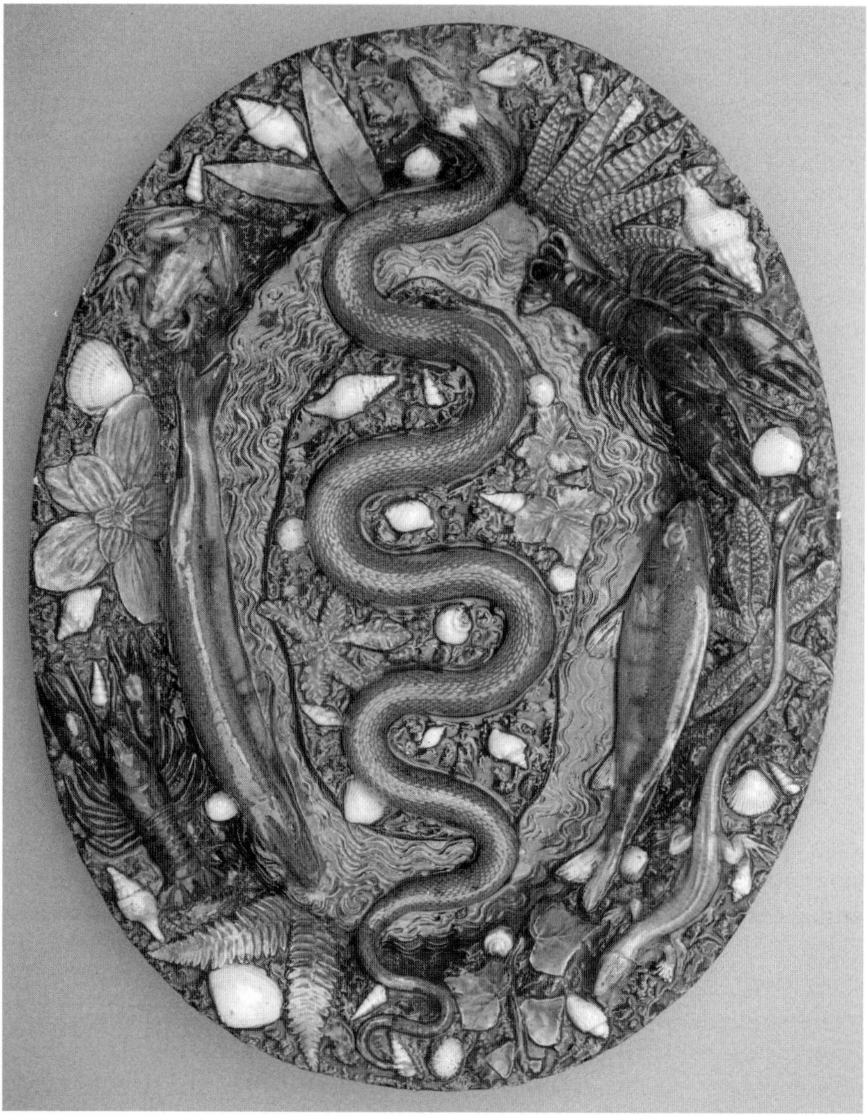

Figure 2.16: Earthenware oval basin, attributed to Bernard Palissy or a close follower, after 1580. Item number C174. By kind permission of the trustees of The Wallace Collection.

imperial dominion. Shakespeare's *Tempest*, which we will shortly turn to, was composed during a period which was slowly giving way to a deeper, more personal, exploration of wonder, of its relation to that which is most 'common' to each of us: ourselves. In his *Religo Medici*, Thomas Browne (1605–82) would lay down the foundations for a natural philosophy which would serve as a mainstay from the crises threatened by the womb, for we are 'subject to the actions of the elements, and the malice of diseases in that other world, the truest Microcosme, the wombe of our mother; for besides that generall and common existence wee are conceived to hold in our Chaos'.[73] For Browne the connection between the natural world and the maternal body means the chaotic anomalies 'common' in nature are also the inescapable legacy of conception:

> I could never content my contemplation with those generall pieces of wonder, the flux and reflux of the sea, the encrease of Nile, the conversion of the Needle to the North; and [therefore] have studied to match and parallel those in the more obvious and neglected pieces of Nature, which without further travell I can doe in the Cosmography of my selfe; we carry with us the wonders, wee seeke without us: There is all *Africa*, and her prodigies in us; we are that bold and adventurous piece of nature, which he that studies wisely learnes in a *compendium*, what others labour at in a divided piece and endlesse volume.[74]

While Browne's interiorisation of the mythical topography of wonder is redolent of the neo-Platonic bias of the grotto-space, it serves to destabilise, rather than shore up the ideological edifice of colonialism. The discourse of monstrosity no longer solely justifies the ownership of the *foreign parts* belonging to a feminised new world, but works as a check against human vanity and the fruitless curiosity which stimulates the search for exotic marvels: '[W]e are what we all abhorre, Antropophagi and Cannibals, devourers not onely of men, but of our selves.'[75] And since 'we are all monsters, that is, a composition of man and beast' those who would pry into nature's secrets 'must endeavour to be as the Poets fancy that wise man Chiron [a Centaure], that is, to have the Region of Man above that of Beast, and sense to sit but at the feete of reason.'[76]

Above the Beast: The Monster and the Natural Historian in Shakespeare's *Tempest*

> We are not ready to believe that wherever such relics of fish or sea animals are found the sea hath had its course. And Goropius Becanus long ago could not digest that conceit when he found great numbers of shells upon the highest Alps.
>
> Thomas Browne, 'On a Bone Dug from a Cliff (to William Dugdale)'[77]

Shakespeare's *Tempest* transports its audience to an artificial island, a world of grotto-like spaces, rocky pools, fertile inlets, streams, underground conduits and groves. At its centre is a cave-dwelling monster – a prodigy of nature – who has made his home in a 'hard rock' (I, ii, 343).[78]

We will never know if the play's staging included the kinds of rarities which made up the cabinets of collectors and the grottoes of the nobility, or the rock- and mineral-encrusted niches, shells, coral, mother-of-pearl, glistening stones, sea-grasses and artificial springs which were incorporated into Inigo Jones' masque-designs for *Tethys' Festival* and *The Masque of Blackness*.[79] The vocabulary of wonder which saturates the play, however, including its ingenious deployment of automata and special effects, is suggestive of the grotto-spaces that provided the theatricalised setting for the hydrological, geological and natural historical theories which, in a specifically colonial context, exploited the ideological potential of a maternalised nature and her rich reproductive capabilities. As the grotto and its allied arts showcased the latest technologies for mastering nature within an aesthetic framework drawn from a classical and Ovidian heritage, the early scientific wisdom it crystallised in its hanging stalactites and subterranean waterways was not incompatible with the cast of wild men, water-nymphs, sea-monsters, chimeras and elemental deities who frolicked mischievously among them. These monstrous productions abound in a play in which the abiding interest in the connection between the wonders of nature and the maternal body find their human counterpart in Miranda, whose very name has its Latin roots in 'admiration' and 'wonder'.

It is Caliban's claim that 'This island's mine by Sycorax my mother' (I, ii, 331) which becomes the fulcrum around which Prospero's own colonial aspirations turn, the fulfilment of which depends on the careful management of his daughter's procreative destiny for the purposes of usurping, and finally expunging the maternal history which haunts the island. That the cave-bound native traces his own familial legacy back to his 'dam's god Setebos' (I, ii, 372), may indicate a lineage descending from the Patagonian giants who were believed to worship this deity.[80] Could this have evoked in audiences' minds the monstrous grotto-dwelling giant or wild man (see Fig. 2.3) which Salomon de Caus designed for Richmond Palace, simply scaled down in size to fit the stage? Caus' monumental creation, an engineering miracle, would have certainly stimulated wide interest since it was said to have been three times larger than its prototype in the famous Pratolino garden-grottoes,[81] and was in all probability erected either in the year of the play's composition or only the year before.[82] Whether or not this was the case, the wild-man as denizen of the cave or grotto was an already widely-circulated motif by this time. In the second half of the sixteenth century King Henri II of France became the recipient of a very unusual gift: a child named Petrus Gonsalvus who was born on Tenerife in 1556 and suffered from a rare disorder which was to earn him and his family the appellation 'cat people'. Receiving the best education, the elegant and engaging Gonsalvus became the darling of the court glitterati, a living emblem of the ruler's ability to tame the wildest of nature's prodigious creations. While residing in the Netherlands, at the court of Margaret of Parma, Gonsalvus married and had children, both of whom inherited his condition, which has since come to be known as hirsutism or hypertrichosis. Portraits of Gonsalvus and his family formed part of Ferdinand II's cabinet of curiosities.[83] Gonsalvus and his son (Figs 2.17a and 2.17b) are both presented before a recessed rocky backdrop suggestive of a cave, the natural environment with which the 'cat-people' were associated, not unlike Caliban who is variously described in the play as 'puppy-headed' (II, ii, 148) and a 'cat' (II, ii, 79), and as a fitting 'present for any emperor that ever trod on neat's-leather' (II, ii, 67–8). Under the aegis of his noble patrons Gonsalvus had, it seems, been permitted to succeed where Caliban was to fail, peopling the court with Gonsalvuses.

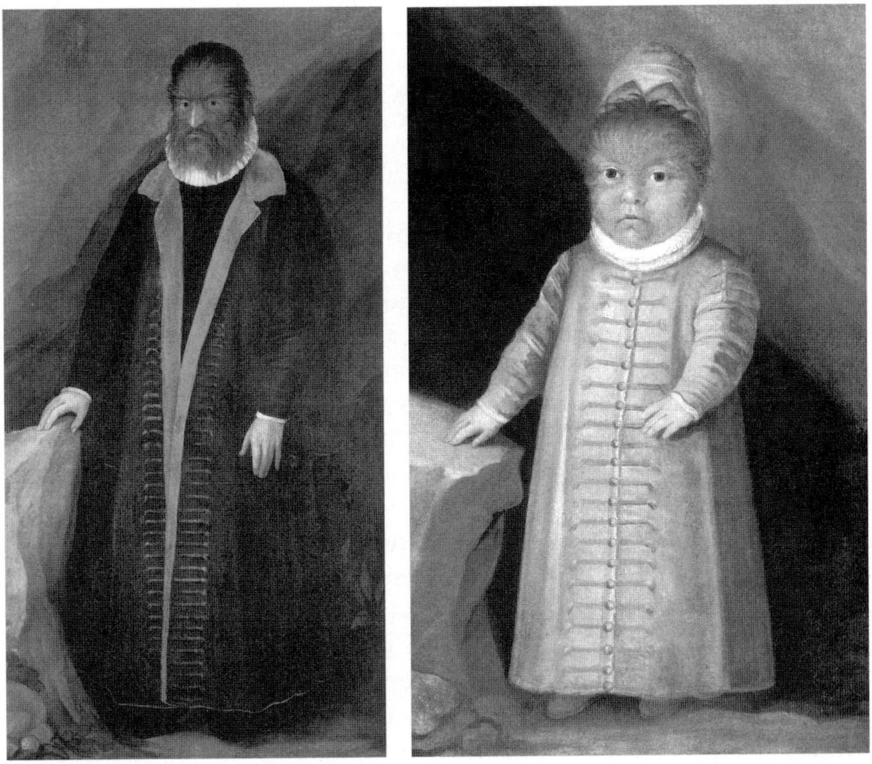

Figures 2.17a and 2.17b: Portraits of Petrus Gonsalvus and his son, Arrigo, Ambras Collection. By kind permission of the Kunsthistorisches Museum, Wien oder KHM, Wien (Vienna).

In referring to his island home as a 'cell' (I, ii, 20 and 39) during his first exchange with Miranda, Prospero turns the stage into a bounded room of wonders in which the 'provision' of his 'art' (I, ii, 28) finds its most miraculous manifestation in the tempest of the play's title. It is the histrionic manipulation of the elements of wind and 'wild waters' which enables him to fashion the 'direful spectacle of the wreck' (I, ii, 26).[84] Prospero's ability to control and contain the potentially chaotic forces of the natural world functions, in the play's symbolic economy, as a precondition for the restoration of the epistemological and political order which he had lost as a result of his absorption in the 'liberal arts' with which he had become perilously 'transported/And rapt in secret studies' (I, ii, 73–7).[85] Prospero's 'priz[ing]' of his studies beyond that which is of more fundamental or 'popular rate', an adequately nurtured political state, is clothed in language evocative of the womb's crises of conception:

> I thus neglecting worldly ends, all dedicated
> To closeness and the bettering of my mind
> With that which, but by being so retired,
> O'er-prized all popular rate, in my false brother
> Awaked an evil nature, and my trust,
> Like a good parent, did beget of him
> A falsehood in its contrary as great
> As my trust was . . . (I, ii, 89–96)

The ruler's misdirected learning is made naturally coterminous with a form of monstrous birth, symbolised by the 'falsehood' Prospero's trust 'beget[s]'. In Renaissance embryological treatises an abnormality in the birthing process was often referred to as a 'false Conception',[86] a term accorded ecological significance by John Donne in his *Anatomy of the World*: 'Th'air doth not motherly sit on the earth,/To hatch her seasons, and give all things birth . . . And false conceptions fill the general wombs.'[87] Prospero's deployment of this vocabulary is part of his preoccupation with the relation between the limits of masculine knowledge and the inscrutability of the maternal body, an anxiety which comes to centre on his own daughter's genetic heritage as he informs her that 'Thy mother was a piece of virtue, and/She said thou wast my daughter' (I, ii, 56–7). Prospero implies that no father can be certain that his wife had not indulged in the kind of carnal excesses which would be a rebuke to both his honour and his lineage, a fact acknowledged obliquely by Miranda as she reflects on Antonio's crime: 'I should sin/To think but nobly of my grand-mother./Good wombs have borne bad sons' (I, ii, 117–19). Regardless of the true extent of a woman's chastity, the womb is always inherently capable of operating outside the bounds of legitimate paternal influence, producing conceptions which stray chaotically from the legitimate form of their progenitor. It is this notion which serves as the justificatory engine for Prospero's control of the island and its inhabitants. Indeed his entrance to this fertile landscape initiates the rewriting of Miranda's origins in parthenogenic terms:

> O, a cherubin
> Thou wast that did preserve me. Thou didst smile,
> Infusèd with a fortitude from heaven,
> When I have decked the sea with drops full salt,
> Under my burden groaned, which raised in me
> An undergoing stomach to bear up
> Against what should ensue. (I, ii, 152–8)

In a tableau of pregnancy, Prospero usurps the role of an expectant mother groaning with the 'burden' of a fruitful womb. His daughter becomes the epitome of the ideal birth, 'a cherubin', similar to the putti who populate countless Renaissance canvases, frescoes and grottoes, and whose exemplification of physical perfection is an apt augury of heaven's 'bountiful' nurture (I, ii, 178). That Prospero's plans to recuperate his former royal power require the strategic orchestration of wonder is revealed in his role in the marriage of Miranda and Ferdinand, the future guarantors of his lineage. Upon their first meeting, the Prince of Naples mistakes Miranda for a 'goddess' and asks 'How I may *bear me* here. My prime request,/Which I do last pronounce, is – O you wonder! –/If you be maid or no?' (I, ii, 422–8, my italics). Ferdinand's ambiguous language suggests his desire to reproduce, to 'bear' himself on the island. That this is Prospero's intention can be seen in his own response to the couple's ritual exchanging of 'hand' and 'heart' (III, i, 89–91), making him witness to a matrimonial pledge: 'Fair encounter/Of two most *rare* affections! Heavens rain grace/On that which *breeds* between 'em!' (III, i, 74–6, my italics). It is the *rarity* of their love which becomes the certain sign and prognostication of the divine 'grace' which will eventually attend their child-bearing, an outcome to which Miranda herself alludes in her partial disclosure of what she 'shall die to want', that which, like a secret pregnancy, 'all the more it seeks to hide itself,/The bigger bulk it shows' (III, i, 79–81).

In his own paean to Miranda, Ferdinand comes alarmingly close to the transporting rapture which Prospero described as 'O'er-priz[ing]' all other considerations: 'Admired Miranda,/Indeed the top of admiration, worth/What's deerest to the world! . . ./So perfect and so peerless . . . created/Of every creature's best' (III, i, 37–48). Miranda appears as a prodigious hybrid of the earth's most marvellous creations. If Prospero 'prompts' (I, ii, 421) the response of wonder in those over whom he holds dominion, it is because he is exploiting an already ingrained cultural leitmotif which provides the justificatory machinery of primogeniture. When Miranda first sees Ferdinand she is moved to question the very foundation of natural law, exclaiming, 'I might call him/A thing divine, for nothing *natural*/I ever saw so *noble*' (I, ii, 418–20, my italics). This finds a suggestive corollary in Henry Peacham's manual, *The Compleat Gentleman* (1622):

> Can we be curious in discerning a counterfat [sic] from the true Pearle . . . and not make difference of lin[e]age, nor be carefull unto what stocke we match our selves . . . Surely, to beleeve that Nature (rather the God of Nature) produceth not the same among our selves, is to question the rarest Work-mistris of Ignorance or Partialitie, and to abase our selves beneath the Beast. *Nobilitie* then (taken in the generall sence) is nothing else then a certaine eminency, or notice taken of some one above the rest.

The equation Peacham makes between the precious and the noble serves as the rhetorical underpinning for the eugenic management of the 'stocke'. To remain above 'the Beast' one must become a connoisseur and learn to distinguish the true rarity from the false, the object genuinely deserving of wonder from that to be discarded. In the wider context for the work Peacham is ratifying, in fact *naturalising*, a set of signs which form the basis for understanding nature as a divinely inspired teleology, making 'blazonrie' an art which, 'sympathizing with every Noble and generous disposition, [is] in substance the most refined part of Naturall Philosophie'.[88] Since nature is a creator of fine artefacts, a 'rarest Work-mistris', the political order can only be safeguarded if its perpetuation is approached in the manner which governs the peculiar ideologies of collecting; with a 'curious' eye.

It is Prospero's interpretation of Miranda as a rarity, demanding the emotion of wonder, that allows him to choreograph her reproductive destiny and regain his imperial power. In contrast Caliban is the foil against which Miranda's brilliance may shine all the more clearly. Merely the progeny of a 'vile race', a 'thing most brutish', (I, ii, 56–7) he is 'not honoured with/A human shape' (I, ii, 283–4). As an 'Abhorrèd slave,/Which any print of goodness wilt not take' (I, ii, 351),[89] Caliban encodes the anxiety surrounding the fragile nature of the printing or copying process which, in embryological discourse, informs the transmission of the paternal principle through the receptive matter of the womb.[90] Had Caliban successfully 'peopled . . ./This isle with Calibans' (I, ii, 349–50), Prospero suggests, the damage caused to the biological and political order, through the contamination of Miranda's ensuing lineage, would have been irrevocable. The play, however, works to dismantle the sufficiency of Prospero's cultivation of curiosity by according dramatic weight to the tension between older conceptions of monstrosity and the emergent natural historical theories which sought to explain nature's prodigious productions. Indeed the ultimately self-serving bias of Prospero's teratological discourse is, I would argue, foregrounded through its parodic treatment in the antics of Stephano and Trinculo, who function as comic mouthpieces for an Augustinian notion of monstrosity as a *meaningful* cessation of natural law, a view which predominated in the popular ballad and pamphlet literature on Renaissance monsters.

When Trinculo first comes across Caliban, who has crept under his 'gaberdine', he mistakes him for a hybrid fish, a 'monster' or 'strange beast' who 'smells like a fish; a very ancient and fish-like smell; a kind of not-of-the-newest poor-john. A strange fish!' (II, ii, 25–30). This reference to 'poor-john', the pungent dried hake,[91] is remarkably reminiscent of Edward Fenton's account of a 'water monster' which he claimed to have seen in Paris along with over 200 witnesses: 'Amongest the things of wo[n]der to be seen in this beaste, it hath chiefly a hydeous heade, resembling rather in figure a horrible Serpent . . . neyther is he so well dried, but he yeldes some savour or smel of fishe.'[92] That Trinculo's discovery of this 'Monsieur Monster' (III, ii, 17) is accompanied by '*A noise of thunder heard*' (stage direction) and a 'storm brewing' (II, ii, 19) would also have conjured in audiences' minds the apocalyptic signs which formed a feature of early modern teratological tracts. On 12 February 1595, for example, a 'monstrous fishe' was washed up on the shores of Outhorn in Holderness, taking its place among other prodigies and 'straunge tokens' of 'sore warning', including 'monsterus birthes, blazing starres . . . and fearefull stormes and tempests', foreboding events created not 'by chance or fortune, but . . . appointed to be the messengers of ensuing plagues which are like to fall upon us, except with repenting harts we turne unto our god and forsake our wicked waies'. The prodigy, whose 'head was in fashion like a great wool-sacke', may remind us of Caliban's head buried under the 'gaberdine', the shape of which may have caused Trinculo to mistake him for a fish.[93] In this vein, Stephano's ensuing description of Caliban as a form of conjoined twin with 'Four legs and two voices', possessing a 'backward voice . . . [in which] to utter foul speeches and to detract' (II, ii, 85–7), mirrors the allegorical repertoire of monster-ballads such as *The forme and shape of a monstrous child borne at Maydstone in Kent* (1568), in which the child's deformities, particularly his 'gaspying mouth' or hairlip, emblematise the 'filthy talke, and poysoned speech' of those who 'Blaspheming God, and Prince reject,/As they were brutish beastes' (Fig. 2.18).[94] Caliban, who had earlier protested to Prospero that 'You taught me language, and my profit on't/Is I know how to curse' (I, ii, 362–3), becomes therefore

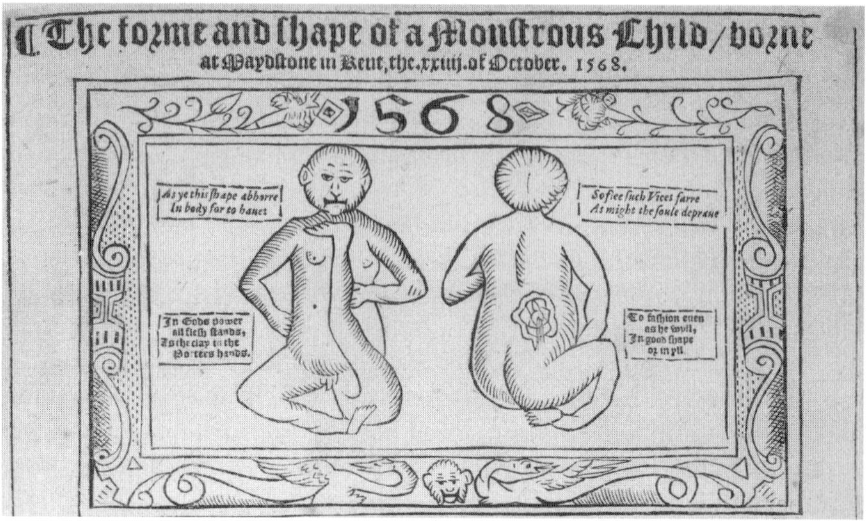

Figure 2.18: *The forme and shape of a Monstrous Child, borne at Maydstone in Kent*. . ., 1568. Shelfmark Huth. 50.38. © The British Library Board. All Rights Reserved.

a descendent of the popular Renaissance allegories of Slander and Detraction, figures representing the monstrous vices which threaten the integrity and stability of the godly political state.[95]

Prospero's morally deterministic use of the kind of wonder literature ventriloquised by Stephano and Trinculo to comic effect, as well as his manipulation of the apocalyptic storm which sets the play's tone, is intended to equate his management of Miranda's maternal capabilities with a providential agenda which finds its most pertinent expression in the threat posed by Caliban's dangerously anomalous nature. The play works, however, to destabilise this process in a manner reminiscent of Thomas Vaughan's own description of Detraction which was published in 1611, the same year as the first recorded performance of *The Tempest*:

> Out of the hearts abundance the tongue speakes. And as abundance of raine causeth rivers to overflow their naturall meeres . . . and breake with a violent deluge over into meadowes and plaine fields: so the heart boyling over with furious motions, will runne quite out of course and temper, except it be suffered to evaporate and vent out by the mouth (which stands like an open sepulchre, or a roaring gulfe) what soever is internally conceived and consopited [sic]. Yea, I have knowne some (like women with childe) sick to the heart, till they were delivered of their suspicious Detractions or monstrous embalons [sic].[96]

While Vaughan's Detraction 'vent[s]' her spleen from the mouth, Caliban is seen by Stephano, in a scatological quip which evokes a parody of a monstrous birth, as having the ability to 'vent Trinculos' (II, ii, 102). Trinculo's explanation that he 'took him [Caliban] to be killed with a thunderstroke' (II, ii, 103) makes an interesting counterpoint to Vaughan's tract, which was composed in response to accusations that his wife had been fatally struck by lightning as a divine punishment for committing adultery. By appealing to embryological theory, however, Vaughan is able to re-assess the processes behind such 'monstrous' effects, thereby laying these 'Detractions' to rest. No longer the work of the divine hand, these wonders are a common part of the inherent operations of the natural world and function in precisely the same way as the maternal body whose own 'closed', or 'internally conceived', environment is responsible for the autonomous production of prodigies and anomalous births. Vaughan echoes the Paracelsan machinery employed by the famous surgeon and dedicated teratologist Ambroise Paré, a member of the Saint-Come Royal College of Surgeons from 1554 and one of the academics who attended Palissy's lectures in his cabinet of curiosities,[97] who explained in his *Des Monstres et Prodiges* (1573) that as the body is a 'microcosm or small portrait of the big world, abridged', it is 'composed of four elements . . . winds, thunder, earthquakes, rain, dew, vapours . . . [and] floods' which can cause monsters in the 'conceiving or pregnant woman'.[98] Vaughan's re-orientation of wonder lies in the connection between the womb and the world within the context of natural historical ideas governing the production of 'rivers' and watery spaces. The same concerns, as we have seen, steered the accumulation, installation and showcasing of wonders in the early modern grotto in a form uniquely suited to a disclosure of the procreative mechanisms of nature. I hope to show that this same value-system is also in operation in *The Tempest* through the manipulation of the very agent that propels the drama of the grotto-space: water or, more specifically, the semantic dynamic existing between the properties of flowing and stagnant water. It is the shared understanding of this natural historical knowledge that increasingly draws the figures of Prospero, Caliban and Sycorax together as the play's action progresses. Shakespeare thus deftly undermines Prospero's procreative regimen which depends for its success on his definition of Caliban as the monstrous object of the curious gaze. As the boundaries between the beast and the natural historian become blurred, the neo-Platonic scaffolding that had shored up the colonial project begins to seem very weak indeed.

In the Ditchley portrait of Elizabeth I, painted by Marcus Gheeraerts the Younger around 1592, the queen stands upon a map of England, the features of which are based upon Saxton's celebrated *Atlas* (Fig. 2.19).[99]

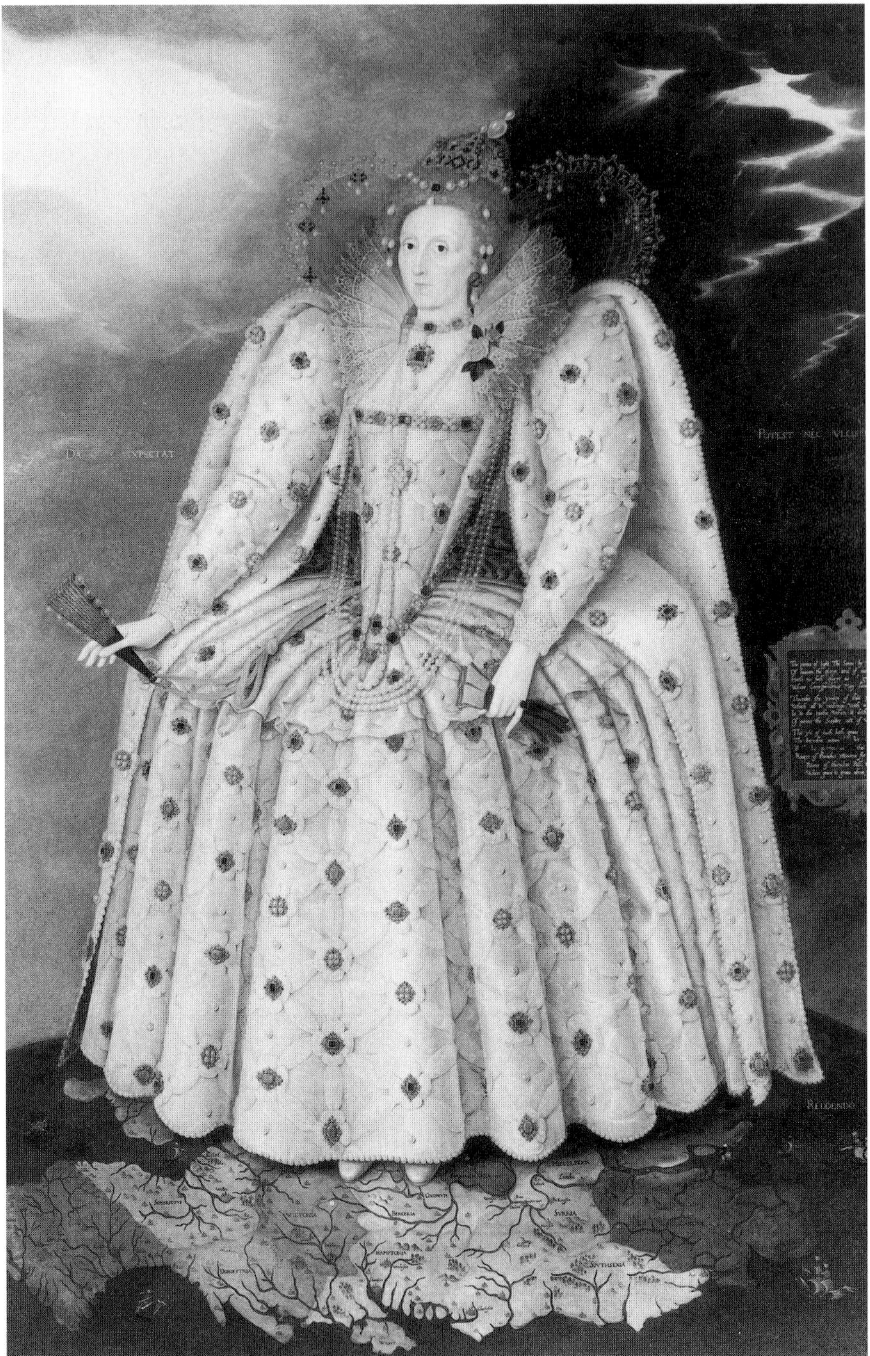

Figure 2.19: Marcus Gheeraerts the Younger, Ditchley Portrait of Elizabeth I, c. 1592. National Portrait Gallery, London.

The hydrographic qualities of the image are emphasised in the clearly-delineated branches of rivers and waterways which meander beneath her feet. Around these, sailing-ships navigate the waters embarking, one imagines, on voyages across the globe. The picture's textual machinery operates in the manner of an emblem:

> This yle of such both grace [and] power [the site]
> The boundles ocean [humb]lye [doth em]brace
> P[eerless] p[rincess vnder] the[arth a]ll [thine]
> Riuers of thankes retourne for Springes [of grace]
>   Riuers of thanckes still to that oc[ean flow]
>   Where grace is grace above, power po[wer below.][100]

This elaborate geological metaphor draws on the belief that the power-house of nature is the network of underground streams which circulate in the womb of the earth. Here these 'Riuers of thankes' animate revivifying 'Springes' while returning to their source of life, who is at once both Oceana/Amphitrite, and Diana/Cynthia/Belphoebe, the driving force behind the flowing waters through which the fruitfulness of nature is made possible. Elizabeth is also 'The prince of light', greater even than 'The sonn[e] by whom thing[s liue]', the corporeal manifestation of the principle of purification which 'doth ayre r[efine]'. These life-giving properties are related to Elizabeth's fantasised role as an empress of the weather and of the seasons, both a mother to her nation and a force of nature: her body is the world itself.

Like Elizabeth I, Prospero seeks to appropriate a geologically-freighted discourse which equates his political dominion with a privileged access to the secrets of nature. It is in particular his desire to master the island's flowing springs and waterways, so vital to its continuing fecundity, which forms the basis for his exploitation of its native inhabitants. Ariel is employed on errands which require a knowledge of the subterranean conduits or mineral deposits which formed an integral component of early modern geological and mining texts.[101] Prospero orders him 'to tread the ooze/Of the salt deep . . . /To do me business in the veins o'th' earth/When it is baked with frost' (I, ii, 253–7). Indeed, his description of Ariel's suffering at the hands of Sycorax, who had caused him to 'vent thy groans/As fast as mill-wheels strike' (I, ii, 280–1), turns the prodigious servant into a water-powered machine. As well as hinting at devices used for the purposes of grinding grain, the image of venting indicates the kind of water- and air-operated pumps which drove the technologies of mining and the fantastical automata which, as we saw in the first part of this chapter, animated grottoes, fountains and artificial islands. The importance of tapping into these 'veins o'th' earth' is suggested by the specifically maternalised ecology which found its way into early embryological tracts such as Thomas Raynalde's *Byrth of Mankynde* (1564), in which the formation of the foetus is equated with the earth's exploitable natural resources:

> [T]horowe the manyfolde and infinite circulatyons of the attracted matter by the conduyctes or vaynes infinetly intricate and wrythed with a thousand revolutions . . . (and all in the litle compasse of the body of the stones) the blood and spirite commixed together, getteth another nature and property . . . [T]hat can she [nature] not do, unlesse she have a mine, shoppe, or workehouse, wherein by continual circulatio[n] of the matter transmutable, she may bryng her purpose to passe . . . even as mettalles and other minerals of the earth, have theyr secrete and invisible vaynes . . .[102]

The 'conduyctes or vaynes' of the maternal body are likened to underground mines which are fed with hidden water-channels and mineral deposits that produce the earth's precious hoard or 'shoppe' of metals. In her moving rendering of Psalm 139 Mary Herbert reflects, in similar terms, on her own gradual formation in the womb 'While yet I in my mother dwelt,/. . . how my back was beam-wise laid,/And raft'ring of my ribs . . ./Though wrought in shop both dark and low'.[103] Prospero's desire to harness the resource of flowing water so that he may take advantage of nature's valuable reproductive potential is voiced by a disgruntled Caliban who protests that it was his own local knowledge of such watery and bountiful spaces which facilitated his master's usurpation of the island: 'When thou cam'st first . . . I loved thee,/And showed thee all the qualities o'th' isle,/The fresh springs, brine-pits, barren place and fertile' (I, ii, 332–8).[104] It is a role which he transfers with ease to the service of Stephano and Trinculo, offering to open nature's hidden rarities to the two shipwrecked strangers:

> I'll show thee every fertile inch o'th' island . . .
> I'll show thee the best springs . . .
> I prithee let me bring thee where crabs grow,
> And I with my long nails will dig thee pig-nuts,
> Show thee a jay's nest, and instruct thee how
> To snare the nimble marmoset. I'll bring thee
> To clust'ring filberts, and sometimes I'll get thee
> Young scamels from the rock. (II, ii, 142–66)

Caliban becomes a connoisseur of nature's curiosities, offering a veritable cabinet of outlandish specimens.[105] The intriguing 'scamels', perhaps a form of crustacean or fish whose natural habitat was thought to be around or under rocks,[106] take their place among a catalogue of exotic names to conjure with, including 'pig-nuts', 'filberts' and marmosets. The 'crabs', of which Caliban has expert knowledge, may not indicate the bitter-tasting 'crab apples' but the crustaceans which were believed, literally, to 'grow' spontaneously from rock-pools and other grotto-like regions, a belief which was frozen for all time, as we have seen, in the earthenware of Bernard Palissy. Caliban's seductive narrative, which dwells upon mysterious grove-like, watery and rocky spaces, the warm and dank cradles of life, replicates the concerns of the first English settlers in the New World. Documents such as the *Strachey Letter* (1610), long recognised as a possible source for Shakespeare's play, reveal that travellers to Virginia and the Bermudas did not only bring with them superstitious beliefs about the wonders they might encounter there, but came armed with geological knowledge which they tested against the alien landscapes in which they lodged:

> When wee came first we digged and found certaine gushings and soft bublings, which . . . sinketh into the earth and vanisheth away . . . without any channell above or upon the superficies of the earth . . . howbeit some low bottoms . . . we found to continue as fishing Ponds, or standing Pooles, continually Summer and Winter, full of fresh water . . . Wee have taken also from under the broken Rockes, Crevises [i.e. crayfish] oftentimes greater then any of our best *English* Lobsters; and likewise abundance of Crabbes, Oysters, and Wilkes [i.e. whelks] . . .

This interest in the properties of moving and static water is not merely incidental but connotes a central aspect of the early modern natural philosophy which was instrumental in shaping the New World encounter. The ethos of subterranean discovery, which turned such reservoirs of generation as 'standing Pooles', 'running Springes of fresh water', and 'broken Rockes' into the readily transposable elements of gardens and grottoes, was part of a general shift in the understanding of the mechanisms which governed the reproduction of living forms.[107] In *The Tempest* these ideas acquire political relevance in the struggle for control over the island. If Caliban offers his knowledge of these natural resources to the bumbling Stephano and Trinculo as a means of circumventing Prospero's rule, Sebastian and Antonio hatch their own conspiratorial plans in terms which resonate closely with the island slave's own natural historical wisdom:

> SEBASTIAN Well? I am *standing water*.
> ANTONIO I'll teach you how to flow.
> SEBASTIAN Do so – to ebb
> Hereditary sloth instructs me.
> ANTONIO . . . ebbing men, indeed,
> Most often do so *near the bottom run*
> By their own fear or sloth.
> SEBASTIAN Prithee, say on.

> The setting of thine eye and cheek proclaim
> A matter from thee, and a birth, indeed,
> Which throes thee much to yield. (II, i, 219–29, my italics)

A recognition of the negative aspects of 'standing water' colours this coded exchange in which the parthenogenic fantasy which underpins the colonial enterprise is symbolically figured forth in the ability to transform a stagnant pool into a flowing river. The fertile qualities of moving water are in turn exemplified in the succeeding childbirth metaphor. However, Sebastian's claim that he can identify Antonio's phantom pregnancy through the 'setting of thine eye and cheek' hints that the 'matter' which he will 'yield' may not be dissimilar to the 'one thing [Sycorax] did' to save her from execution in Algiers, for Prospero describes her as a 'blue-eyed hag [who] was hither brought with child' (I, ii, 266–9). Blue eyelids were popularly believed to be a prognostication of pregnancy.[108] In Sycorax' case this was to result in 'the son that she did litter here,/A freckled whelp, hag-born' (I, ii, 234–5). In early modern embryological and midwifery manuals freckles and birthmarks are described as signs of a surplus of menstrual fluid in the womb during either conception or gestation. Women like Sycorax, who were identified as being 'earthy' in nature (I, ii, 275), were most likely to induce these anomalies in their children. According to the *De Secretis Mulierum* of Albertus Magnus, in 'earthy women, there is so much unconsumed humidity and so much earthy substance that their menses is livid, that is black. Earth is black, and because their menses is very earthy, it follows that it takes on the color of the earth', something which can be passed on to the child in the form of blemishes or a corresponding darkness of skin-tone.[109] Prospero's reference to Caliban as 'earth' (I, ii, 314) and as being 'poisonous' (I, ii, 319) may thus indicate both a darkened appearance and the accumulation of 'poisonous' menstrual matter which predominated during his conception.

That the language appropriated by Sebastian and Antonio is deliberately intended to mirror the peculiarities of Sycorax' maternal condition can be gleaned from such texts as Helkiah Crooke's *A Description of the Body of Man* (1615). This describes the 'Menstruous blood' as a form of 'excrement' which 'by standing periods' is accumulated till it reaches 'a superfluity' before being expelled. In 'waterish women' this process is naturally related to the lunar cycle, with 'that tide of the blood sometimes flowing, again ebbing sometimes' depending on 'the full of the Moon'. Too great a surplus of this 'standing' matter can, however, be harmful and occurs frequently in women because they are 'more sedentary and idle' than men.[110] In his *Child-birth, or The Happy Deliverie of Women*

(1612) Jacques Guillemeau corroborates this, identifying two major factors which threaten the health of the foetus in pregnant mothers:

> First, because they live . . . for the most part in idlenesse, and eate ill meates, which are turned into excrements, and breed many obstructions, the fountaine and beginning of all diseases: the second is, the great suppression and stopping of bloud, whereof they were wont to be purged every Moneth.[111]

Sebastian's 'sloth', which is likened to 'standing water', is 'Hereditary' because in Renaissance anatomical thinking the damaging effects of idleness are seen to proceed from the mother. This has a common cause in nature as well as in the microcosm: the poisonous stagnation which arises from the accumulation of obstructed or motionless matter. John Sadler explains, in *The Sicke Womans Private Looking-Glasse* (1636), that 'In breeding women there is a corrupted matter generated . . . and the stomacke being weake, not able to digest this matter, sometime sends it unto the guts, whereby is caused a flux of the bellie, which greatly stirreth up the faculty of the wombe.'[112] Sebastian's scrutinising of Antonio's 'cheek', which he sees as 'proclaim[ing]' his painful pregnancy, may also allude to the symptoms of a specific type of conception, one engendered by precisely this kind of 'corrupted matter': the Mola. Crooke explains that in order to identify this monstrous birth one must carefully take note of the female complexion, most readily discerned in the colour of the cheeks, for 'the woman which hath conceived a Mola becommeth pale, looseth all her colour, yea and pineth away'.[113] Such a 'vicious conception' writes Sadler, is 'ingendred of the menstruous blood' and occurs 'if the womans seed goes into the wombe and not the mans'.[114] This is echoed by Jacob Rueff in his *De conceptu et generatione hominis* (1554), translated into English in 1637 as *The Expert Midwife*, in which he describes the Mola as 'a piece or lump of mishapen flesh', the cause of which is 'the more copious and abundant seed of the woman . . . [which] by the want of mans seed, the proper worke-man and contriver of it, doth grow together into such a lump'.[115]

The absence of the formative principle with which the male 'seed' is endowed, opens the doors to a nightmare scenario: the horrors of spontaneous female generation. This is dramatically realised in Caliban who is described as the offspring of 'Hag-seed' (I, ii, 364), not the product of a union with a human father but 'got by the devil himself' (I, ii, 319). Guillemeau illustrates that one of the causes of the 'false mola' is its 'waterish' nature, the result of a 'heaping together of waters'. As such it is traditionally associated with the moon and is that 'which we commonly call the Moone-calfe'.[116] Caliban himself is referred to as a 'mooncalf' (II, ii, 102 and 106) and Sycorax is described as a 'mother' who could 'control the moon, make flows and ebbs,/And deal in her command without her power', a capacity which is directly related to the bearing of the 'misshapen knave', her 'bastard' son (V, i, 268–71). In 1600 Moderata Fonte (1555–92) published *The Worth of Women* in which she rehearsed the Renaissance commonplace of the moon's power over the female body:

> The moon is closer to us [women] than any other planet . . . In the air, the moon causes sometimes lightning, thunder, cloud, mists, winds, rain, and storms . . . Nor has it lesser powers over the earth, over fields, crops, and trees . . . And, what's more, with its great humidity, the moon is extremely harmful to our physical health . . . This is why doctors observe the phases of the moon very closely, because one could almost say that the moon disturbs and churns up the human body in the same way that it does the sea.

It is the 'extreme humidity' of the moon which, in particular, poses a threat to the reproductive functions of the female anatomy. Similarly, 'the waxing and waning of the moon' governs the springs and rivers which 'pass through the inner reaches of the earth', the mechanism believed to ensure that 'they are purified and freshened . . . as though they had been distilled'. It is the specific movement of these waters, which radiate from and then 'flow back to the sea by subterranean paths', that accounts for the wondrous 'properties of springs' whose fertile and 'excellent curative' qualities, as Fonte maintains, were discovered by the 'natural historians'.[117]

If the elite owners of grottoes and rooms of wonder used these dramatic spaces as a means of asserting their mastery over the fertile and 'curative' properties of flowing water, thereby reproducing a fundamental propagandist tool of the colonial programme, Sycorax and Caliban are the demonic antitypes to this very endeavour. Sycorax is not controlled by, but governs the moon and in doing so is able to harness the power of water and 'make flows and ebbs' as she pleases. Prospero is in direct competition with Sycorax' memory and with Caliban for dominion over the island's 'brooks, standing lakes, and groves', as well as over the water-nymphs who 'Do chase the ebbing of Neptune, and do fly him/When he comes back' (V, i, 33–6). In ventriloquising his Ovidian prototype, the witch Medea of the *Metamorphoses*, Prospero is brought ever closer to Sycorax whose own power, like that of the island's usurping magus, is based on a terrifying ability to commandeer the processes of birth and procreation. Indeed Sycorax' dangerous mastery over natural reservoirs of flowing and stagnant water is equated with the faculties of her monster-producing womb, made all the more hazardous by its autonomy from the masculine motive principle of generation. As Jane

Sharp maintains, the 'waterish' mole or mooncalf, caused by 'ill purgations coming from the menstruous Veins', can cause 'Monsters of all sorts to be formed in the womb' including 'Worms, Toades, Mice, Serpents'.[118] Just what is at stake in Sycorax' own manipulation of the 'veins o'th' earth' (I, ii, 256), the transmitted knowledge of which Prospero is so keen to wrestle from the island's natives, is revealed by Caliban who has an accurate understanding of the implications of such natural historical wisdom:

> PROSPERO Come forth, I say; there's other business for thee.
> Come, thou tortoise, when?
> *Enter* Ariel, *like a water-nymph* . . .
> CALIBAN As wicked dew as e'er my mother brushed
> With raven's feather from unwholesome fen
> Drop on you both! A south-west blow on ye
> And blister you all o'er! . . . All the charms
> Of Sycorax, toads, beetles, bats, light on you! . . . (I, ii, 315–40)

Ariel's appearance as a '*water-nymph*', that denizen of the grotto-space who represents the life-giving properties of flowing water, is countered by Caliban's evocation of the 'unwholesome fen' and 'south-west' wind, conveyors of the kind of corrupted matter which was thought to facilitate the spontaneous generation of life-forms in stagnant, humid conditions. It is significant that the interchange between master and vassal takes place in the very vicinity of Caliban's cave. The menacing creatures associated here with magical 'charms' are also natural dwellers of such dark and dank places. In *Othello* toads are described as being able to 'live upon the vapour of a dungeon' (III, iii, 275), and are creatures naturally found to 'knot and gender' wherever it is warm and wet as 'a cistern' (IV, ii, 62–3).[119] In *The Duchess of Malfi*, Antonio's exposition of the cardinal's 'temper' (I, i, 46) similarly draws on the myth of the toad's genesis from water, for '[t]he spring in his face is nothing but the engendering of toads . . . for he strews in his way flatterers, panders, intelligencers, atheists, and a thousand such political monsters' (I, i, 150–5).[120]

Caliban's geological and hydrological knowledge, therefore, is characterised by an awareness of the difference between flowing water and the swamps, marshes, stagnant pools and caves which are the potential transmitters of disease, monstrosity and death. It is the inherent properties of these which he seeks to harness against Prospero: 'All the infections that the sun sucks up/From bogs, fens, flats, on Prosper fall, and make him/By inchmeal a disease!' (II, ii, 1–3). Prospero also exploits this knowledge when punishing Caliban's 'confederates' (IV, i, 140), leaving them in the 'filthy-mantled pool . . ./There dancing up to th' chins . . . [in] the foul lake' (IV, i, 182–3). This fate is foreshadowed in the horticultural language which saturates Prospero's stage-managing of Miranda's childbearing potential. Recalling the ocular sign of Sycorax' monstrous birth, Prospero warns Ferdinand that if he should 'break her virgin knot' before marriage 'Sour-eyed disdain, and discord shall bestrew/The union of your bed with weeds', the monstrous effects of which Ferdinand associates with the natural habitat of lustful genii, the 'murkiest den' (IV, i, 15–25).

That Prospero wishes to define Caliban as a product, rather than a knowledgeable surveyor, of these spaces is suggested in his description of him as a 'tortoise'. This may not merely be an allusion to the proverbially slow creature but to its cove-loving relative, the turtle, then termed a tortoise. Indeed, this creature was among the first images of the New World that circulated in England as part of the programme to fashion a taxonomy of natural specimens. In 1585 John White was commissioned as a draftsman for Sir Walter Raleigh's Virginian voyage, to record the most interesting natural features of what is now North Carolina.[121] As well as images of the native Americans of Roanoke he recorded fruit, plants and animals, including a vivid depiction of a Loggerhead turtle (Fig. 2.20)[122] which he clearly found as fascinating as the New-World settlers who, as Strachey documents, found it difficult to classify since they could 'neither absolutely call [it] Fish nor Flesh, keeping most what in the water . . . in the bottome of Coves and Bayes'. What made this water-loving reptile particularly fascinating was its association with the processes of spontaneous generation, since it would leave its eggs 'to the hatching of the Sunne'.[123] That the interest in the role of humidity and the sun in generation concealed an ecologised embryology is traceable in Spenser's account of the birth of Belphoebe in *The Faerie Queene*, who was 'wondrously . . . begot' after her mother Chrysogonee bathed in 'a fresh fountaine . . . the boyling heat t'allay' (III, vi, 6):

> Miraculous may seeme to him, that reades
> So straunge ensample of conception;
> But reason teacheth that the fruitfull seades
> Of all things living, through impression
> Of the sunbeames in moyst complexion,
> Doe life conceive and quickned are by kynd:
> So after *Nilus* inundation,
> Infinite shapes of creatures men do fynd,
> Informed in the mud, on which the Sunne hath shynd. (III, vi, 7–9)

Spenser recapitulates a theory of macrocosmic natural 'generation' which is related to how life is 'fructifide' in the 'pregnant flesh' of the mother. Similarly in Michael Drayton's *Endymion and Phoebe*,[124]

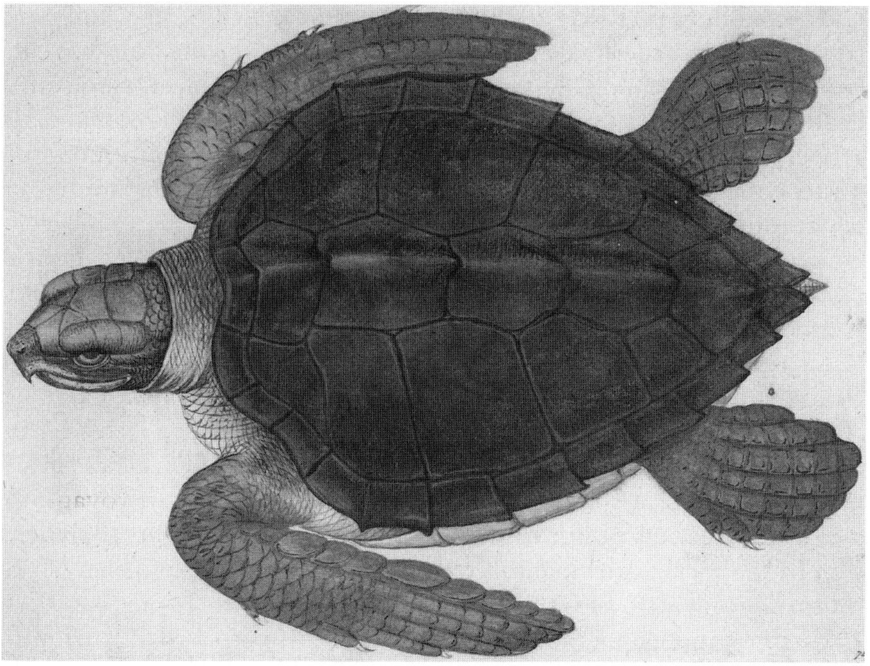

Figure 2.20: John White, Loggerhead Turtle, 1585. British Museum, Department of Prints and Drawings. © The Trustees of the British Museum.

Phoebe is the embodiment of the spontaneously generating powers of rivers acted upon by heat, for she is a 'nymph' of the water, who was 'Begot by Pan on Isis' sacred flood' (181–2). More significantly the dwelling-place of Phoebe is described as a living cabinet of 'curious' artefacts (39), boasting the kind of *naturalia* and *artificialia* so prized by collectors, which 'served for hangings and rich tapestry/To beautify this stately gallery' (37–8). The 'stately grove' (23) which forms the backdrop for these rare commodities also takes on the aspect of a grotto in which there are 'bubbling fountains' with 'straying channels . . . like to a curious maze', whose 'silver sand' glistens like 'orient pearl', the whole sparkling with translucent 'rocks of rarest precious stone' (45–71). It is here that we encounter Phoebe who, encapsulating the nurturing qualities of Iris, is attired in an 'azured mantle . . ./Embossed [with] rainbows' (111–13). A living wonder, Phoebe's visage is inlaid with 'ivory brows', her body adorned with 'rubies set in lozenges of gold,/Trussed up in trammels and in curious pleats' (118–28). That *Endymion and Phoebe* was dedicated to none other than Lucy Harrington of Woburn Abbey, and possible patron of the grotto there, is certainly food for thought. In this poem, perhaps composed as part of the celebrations for

Lucy's wedding in 1594, wonder must be succeeded by the 'fury and conceit' which the female body as cabinet of curiosities foreshadows (877) and 'which doth impart/The thought conceived in the inward heart' (949–50). The neo-Platonic trajectory of such utterances is echoed in Spenser's own poetics of wonder. In the *Amoretti* the admired mistress becomes the locale of all 'wondrous things', the source of 'amaze[ment]' (Sonnet 17), for 'hir lips be Rubies sound . . . hir teeth be pearles . . . her forhead yvory weene'. However such ephemeral wonders must be laid aside in pursuit of the mind's 'vertues manifold' (Sonnet 15).[125] Similarly in *The Faerie Queene* Guyon must destroy the 'pleasant bowres', 'Cabinets' (II, xii, 83) and the glistening fountain 'Of richest substaunce' and 'curious imageree' (II, xii, 60) which make up Acrasia's 'brave' Bower (II, xii, 83), in order to rescue 'the mind of beastly man/That hath so soone forgot the excellence/Of his creation' (II, xii, 87).

This translation from earthly wonder and curiosity to an apprehension of the divine principle follows closely the neo-Platonic bias of the grotto-space which, as we saw in the first part of this chapter, incorporated the same iconographical vocabulary. Prospero's island, with its fantastical automata and '*quaint device[s]*' (stage direction to III, iii), and its wondrous music telling of a 'sea-change' in which bones become coral, eyes turn into pearl, and 'Sea-nymphs' ring knells (I, ii, 398–403) – recalling perhaps the kind of 'rich and strange' mosaics made from marine material which would have adorned a grotto-wall populated with water-gods – seems to undergo a similar apotheosis. Prospero, like the engineers and grotto- and garden-designers who recreated Eden for their powerful patrons, is 'So rare a wondered father . . . [who]/Makes this place paradise' (IV, i, 123). This propensity finds its final dramatic expression in the grand spectacle intended to emblematise the success of his shaping of Miranda's procreative destiny, and echoes the feminine embodiments of wonder which, as we have seen, were so much a part of both grotto-spaces and court masques. The 'marriage-blessing', conducted to ensure the 'continuance, and increasing' of the new royal family, is presided over by Juno, Ceres and Iris who appear as the representatives of an almost gravid *Natura* whose 'goodly burden' serves to secure 'Earth's increase, *foison* plenty' (IV, i, 106–13, my italics).[126] These figures may have appeared on stage in costumes decorated with the natural specimens which grow out of the 'leas' (IV, i, 60), 'broom-groves' (IV, i, 66), and 'watery' (IV, i, 71) spaces they were believed to inhabit. And it is probably no coincidence that one of the favourite abodes of Ceres, goddess of natural generation, seems to be a grotto, the 'sea-marge sterile and rocky-hard' where she 'dost air' (IV, i, 69–70), since the recreational activity of 'taking air' was the functional purpose of these spaces, the design of which deliberately imitated the sea-cove. The very imagery of natural procreation which attends the couple's union is associated throughout the play with the processes of colonial expansionism. Gonzago's utopian fantasy involves harnessing such natural historical knowledge to make 'nature . . . *bring forth*/Of it own kind all *foison*, all abundance' (II, i, 160–1, my italics) and Antonio imagines the infinite reproduction of the island's wealth by 'sowing the kernels of it in the sea, [to] *bring forth* more islands' (II, i, 90–1, my italics).

The play's forcing together of the demands of primogeniture and the mechanisms which undergird the exploitation of natural resources in the New-World encounter are most strongly exemplified by Caliban himself. Caliban is no less aware than his master of the congruity between the value of natural historical knowledge, which affords opportunities for the acquisition of precious materials, and the wondrous reproductive capabilities of the maternal body. Just as Prospero defines Miranda as a 'rich gift' (IV, i, 8), a rare 'acquisition/Worthily purchased' (IV, i, 13–14), Caliban's paean to her rarity makes the mastery over her fertility a necessary adjunct to colonial dominion:

> CALIBAN . . . Burn but his [Prospero's] books.
> He has brave utensils, for so he calls them,
> Which when he has a house, he'll deck withal.
> And that most deeply to consider is
> The beauty of his daughter. He himself
> Calls her a nonpareil. I never saw a woman
> But only Sycorax, my dam, and she;
> But she as far surpasseth Sycorax
> As great'st does least.
> STEPHANO Is it so brave a lass?
> CALIBAN Ay, lord. She will become thy bed, I warrant,
> And *bring thee forth brave brood*. (III, ii, 93–103, my italics)

Though usually described as representing merely magical artefacts,[127] the explicitly domestic setting in which they will be displayed or 'deck[ed]', the tone of admiration, and the apparently exotic nature of these 'brave utensils', are elements remarkably evocative of the cabinet of curiosities. John Tradescant the younger, as we have seen, described the 'utensills' which were an integral part of his father's cabinet of curiosities in his *Musaeum Tradescantianum* (1656).[128] The word 'brave', used three times in the space of ten lines, attaches itself to anything rare and worthy of wonder, whether it be the 'nonpareil' Miranda, or her potential offspring, the 'brave brood'. It is Stephano's ability to determine what this 'brave . . . lass' will 'bring . . . forth' which will secure his usurpation of the island, an endeavour presented as being no different from the collector's acquisition of rare objects.

Prospero, following the masque and grotto traditions, seeks to make the neo-Platonic dissolution of his 'insubstantial pageant' (IV, i, 155) and the rejection of his 'rough magic' (V, i, 50) the necessary precondition of his restored royal privilege. Deploying such rhetoric effectively means securing the panoptic vision of a god on earth, a pattern exemplified in court masques such as *The Vision of Delight* where a personified Wonder appears on stage and poses a series of questions, the elucidation of which will signal her own dissolution:

> Wonder must speak or break: what is this? Grows
> The wealth of nature here, or art? . . .
> Whose breath or beams have *got proud Earth with child*
> Of all the treasure that great Nature's worth,
> And makes her every minute to *bring forth*?
> Whose power is this? what god? (my italics)[129]

The miraculous events inventoried here, including the impregnation of the earth with the natural resources so effectively exploited by the colonial ruler, are not in the final instance caused by Wonder, but *brought forth* by King James I. The meaning of the pageant would have been reinforced by one particular member of the audience known to have been present at this masque: Pocahontas.[130] The epitome of colonised womanhood, her procreative potential is absorbed by the monarch whose ability to control the forces of nature is histrionically bodied forth in his on-stage room of wonders.

Uncovering the spectacle of Miranda and Ferdinand playing chess at the play's close, Prospero gives utterance to the parthenogenic vision which has propelled his directorial management of the island's spectacles, seeking to 'bring forth a wonder' (V, i, 170) which will secure his succeeding lineal power in his 'brave new world' (V, i, 183). The neo-Platonic ethos which animated the propagandist machinery of the evolving discipline of natural history depended upon the early scientist's ability to enslave and control a potentially monstrous and monster-producing maternalised nature. The play unsettles this programme by staging the increasing proximity between the natural historical knowledge demonstrated by Prospero, Caliban and Sycorax, which becomes the locus for the on-going struggle for ownership of the island. By the play's close Prospero has uttered the words which exemplify the logical culmination of this intellectual trajectory: 'This thing of darkess I/Acknowledge mine' (V, i, 275–6). This is the very creed which would become, by the time of Thomas Browne and his intellectual successors, the precondition for the early scientist's engagement with the burgeoning variety of nature.[131] In the age of Shakespeare, however, the very process of establishing an authoritative natural history, which relies on a knowledge of the maternalised productions of creation, brings forth the revelation that dismantles the ideological scaffolding of the colonial enterprise which it was instituted to serve: the natural historian *is* the monster.

Notes

1. I, i, 71–4. Thomas Middleton and William Rowely, *The Changeling*, ed. Joost Daalder (London: A. and C. Black, 1990).
2. Fynes Moryson, *The Itinerary of Fynes Moryson*, vol. 1 (Glasgow: James MacLehouse and Sons Ltd, 1907), pp. 327–8. For more on Fynes Moryson's descriptions of Pratolino see Roy Strong, *The Renaissance Garden in England* (London: Thames and Hudson, 1979), pp. 78–9 and John Dixon Hunt, *Garden and Grove: The Italian Renaissance Garden in the English Imagination 1600–1750* (Philadelphia: University of Pennsylvania Press, 1996), pp. 54–7 and 92–3.
3. For more on the relation between the grotto and the Nymphaeum see Naomi Miller, *Heavenly Caves: Reflections on the Garden Grotto* (Boston, London and Sydney: George Allen and Unwin, 1982), pp. 17–20 and 67–71. For the Pratolino grotto, probably completed some time between 1569 and 1589, see ibid., pp. 47–9.
4. In his article, 'The Mystery of Margate's Shell Temple', which first appeared in *Bygone Kent* (September/October 2006), Mick Twyman provides strong evidence that the grotto was built by the Knights Templar. The article can be seen at the official website of the Margate Shell Grotto: www.shellgrotto.co.uk. I am grateful to Colin Barber for supplying me with images of the grotto.
5. Georgiana Blakiston describes the grotto as 'a charming retreat for conversation and repose on the hottest days of summer', *Woburn and the Russells* (London: Constable, 1980), pp. 54–5.
6. Renaissance works which juxtapose, either textually or schematically, designs for machines, fountains and water-systems with anthropomorphised bodies (incorporating in some instances fountains in the shape of lactating water-nymphs) include Georgius Agricola's *De Re Metallica Libri XII* (1556), BL, 32.g.13; Jacques Besson's *Theatre des instrumens mathematiques et mechaniques* (1579), BL, C.97.f.1; Schopperus Hartmanus' *Omnium illiberalium mechanicarum* (1568), BL, C.27.a.40; and Agostino Ramelli's *Le diverse et artificiose machine* (1588), BL, G.60.55. Christy Anderson makes the point that manuals dedicated to the cultivation of such technologies developed systems of labelling and classification which drew on prototypes associated with anatomical manuals: 'Wild Waters: Hydraulics and the Forces of Nature', in *The Tempest and its Travels*, eds Peter Hulme and William H. Sherman (London: Reaktion Books, 2000), p. 46.

7. In his *Institutio Oratoria* Quintilian defines the emotional and histrionic basis of *admiratio*: 'For when our audience find it a pleasure to listen, their attention and their readiness to believe what they hear are both alike increased, while they are generally filled with delight, and sometimes even transported by admiration' [*plerumque ipsa delectatione capiuntur, nonnunquam admiratione auferuntur*], trans. H. E. Butler, Loeb Classical Library (Cambridge: Harvard University Press, 1921), Book VIII, 3: 5–6, pp. 212–13. For more on the humanist revival of *admiratio* within a specifically neoplatonic framework see T. G. Bishop, *Shakespeare and the Theatre of Wonder* (Cambridge: Cambridge University Press, 1996), pp. 36–41.
8. See also Hazelle Jackson, *Shell Houses and Grottoes* (Buckinghamshire: Shire Publications, 2001), pp. 6–7 and John Anthony, *The Renaissance Garden in Britain* (Buckinghamshire: Shire Garden History, 1991), p. 25.
9. Paula Henderson, *The Tudor House and Garden: Architecture and Landscape in the Sixteenth and Seventeenth Centuries* (New Haven and London: Yale University Press, 2005), p. 166.
10. Strong, *The Renaissance Garden in England*, pp. 73–4 and 87–97 and Hunt, *Garden and Grove*, p. 122.
11. *Les Raisons des forces mouvantes avec diverses machines . . . grotes et fontaines* (Frankfurt: 1615), dedicatory epistle to Book 2, BL, L.40/65.
12. Strong, *The Renaissance Garden in England*, pp. 97–103. Robert Cecil's grotto at Theobalds also contained wild men or 'savages', see Henderson, *The Tudor House and Garden*, p. 165.
13. New hydrographic atlases of the late sixteenth century incorporated this knowledge as part of the ethos of colonial expansionism which sought to exploit the natural contours of the virgin landscape. See Edward Wright's *Hydrographiae Descriptio* (1599), reproduced in Richard Hakluyt's *The Principal Navigations, Voiages, Traffiques and Discoveries of the English Nation*, vol. 1 (London: 1598), BL, 683.h.5; and London: George Bishop, 1599, BL, MAPS 920.(290.). See also Lucas Wagenaer, *The Mariner's Mirrour* (London: 1590), map between pp. 23 and 24, BL, MAPS C.8.b.4. The dedicatory epistle to this work describes the cartographical exploit as being in itself a great wonder since 'the goodlie science of Hidrographie . . . [is] to the publick benefit of the whole body of the common wealth', for 'He that would throughly consider [it], should find matter rather myraculous to wonder at.'
14. *A Declaration of the State of the Colony and Affaires in Virginia* (London: 1622), BL, sigs B–B2, C.32.g.28. See also *A True and Sincere Declaration of the Purpose and Ends of the Plantation Begun in Virginia* (London: 1610), BL, C.32.d.13.
15. Joseph de Acosta, *The Natural and Moral History of the Indies*, ed. Clements R. Markham (London: Hakluyt Society, 1880), p. 81, BL, AC.6172/54. Acosta dedicates a whole section to springs and fountains: pp. 154–6.
16. In his *Civitas Dei* Augustine presented individual wonders as direct demonstrations of divine intervention: 'God decided to create some [monstrous] races in this way, so that we should not suppose that the wisdom with which he fashions the physical being of men has gone astray in the

case of the monsters which are bound to be born among us of human parents': *City of God*, trans. Henry Bettenson (London: Penguin, 1972), Book XVI, pp. 661–4.

17. Acosta, *The Natural and Moral History of the Indies*, p. 104.
18. The date offered by Woburn Abbey for the grotto's construction is broadly estimated between 1619 and 1641: *Woburn Abbey* (Norwich: Woburn Abbey and Jarrold Publishing, 2000), p. 54. The curator of the abbey, Chris Gravett, however has informed me that it probably dates from the early part of this period. Hunt concurs, suggesting that it was completed some time before 1627 (*Garden and Grove*, p. 133), while Jackson gives a more specific date of 1626 (*Shell Houses and Grottoes*, p. 6).
19. The unpublished notes for the abbey's grotto, with which Chris Gravett was kind enough to supply me, identify these nymphs as Neptune and Amphitrite. It is also possible that they represent Tethys and Oceanus, who between them bore the Oceanides or sea-nymphs. See *Dictionary of Mythology* (London: Chancellor Press, 1994), pp. 12 and 161.
20. See also Miller, *Heavenly Caves*, pp. 64–5.
21. Unless otherwise stated the masques referred to are taken from *Court Masques: Jacobean and Caroline Entertainments 1605–1640*, ed. David Lindley (Oxford: Oxford University Press, 1995). The line-numbers are presented in brackets.
22. In *Tethys' Festival*, the rivers actually appear before Tethys in the grotto-like cave, symbolically returning to the sea via underground channels exactly as they were believed to do in early geological theory. For a similar use of river-imagery see Edmund Spenser, *The Faerie Queene*, ed. A. C. Hamilton (London and New York: Longman, 1977), IV, xi.
23. The statue of Bacchus which currently stands in the niche is a later addition. It is not known what would have originally been in its place; perhaps a figure of the type which formed the focal point in the masque, usually a water-nymph or Oceanide. The niches presented both in the grottoes and in the masques formed a central raised platform beneath an arch in the manner of Italian theatres.
24. For more on the Ovidian basis of grotto and garden imagery see Hunt, *Garden and* Grove, pp. 42–58 and 135.
25. This was probably produced around 1623–4. For more on the Whitehall Grotto see Jackson *Shell Houses and Grottoes*, pp. 6–7 and Strong, *The Renaissance Garden in England*, pp. 138–9.
26. For the uncertainty surrounding Lucy Harrington's patronage of the grotto at Moor Park and for the importance of the gardens themselves, see Strong, *The Renaissance Garden in England*, pp. 141–5.
27. Sebastian Fattorini of Skipton Castle has provided me with useful information about the grotto's history and generously supplied me with photographs of its interior. The Skipton grotto has been connected to Lady Anne Clifford: see Gwyn Headley and Wim Meulenkamp, *Follies, Grottoes, and Garden Buildings* (London: Aurum Press, 1986), pp. 563–4.
28. Plato's use of the Cave metaphor in the *Republic* represents, in the words of Val Plumwood, a move from 'the world of Appearance' to 'the

blinding light of Reason' and is figured in a 'journey out of the Cave (which as Plato describes it, remarkably resembles the uterus or matrix)': *Feminism and the Mastery of Nature* (London and New York: Routledge, 1993), p. 93. For the Cave allegory see Plato, *Republic*, trans. Robin Waterfield (Oxford: Oxford University Press, 1993), 514a-18a, pp. 240–5.

29. Francesco Colonna, *Hypnerotomachia Poliphili: The Strife of Love in a Dream*, trans. Joscelyn Godwin (London: Thames and Hudson, 1999), pp. 70–1 and 82–3.
30. Ibid., p. 465.
31. Robert Basset, *Curiosities: or The Cabinet of Nature* (London: 1637), dedicatory epistle to William Lord Craven, Baron of Hamstead, sigs A4v–A6, BL, CUP.407.f.43.
32. Paula Henderson suggests the rock-hewn mount may have contained a grotto inside: *The Tudor House and Garden*, p. 133.
33. Cecil Papers, Bills 58, BHH/282, dated 1611, and BHH/267. I am immensely grateful to Robin Harcourt Williams of Hatfield House for providing me with copies of the accounts for the gardens' construction.
34. Cecil Papers, Bills 58, BHH/284 and BHH/286, dated 1611–12. Other bills dated 30 October 1610 and 25 September 1611 show that Tradescant had been in Flanders and 'other partes beyond, the seas' purchasing more plant-specimens for Cecil: Cecil Papers, BHH/136 and BHH/140.
35. On the influence of the Tradescant family and their collections, see Jennifer Potter, *Strange Blooms: The Curious Lives and Adventures of the John Tradescants* (London: Atlantic Books, 2006). For the gardens at Hatfield see ibid. pp. 53–60.
36. For more on the connection between Shakespeare and Cope, see Mark Thornton Burnett, *Constructing Monsters in Shakespearean Drama and Early Modern Culture* (Houndmills: Palgrave, 2002), p. 23; Peter G. Platt, *Reason Diminished: Shakespeare and the Marvelous* (Lincoln and London: University of Nebraska Press, 1997), pp. 45 and 64–5; and Dennis Kay, 'Who says "Miracles Are Past?": Some Jacobean Marvels and the Margins of the Known', in *Wonders, Marvels, and Monsters in Early Modern Culture*, ed. Peter G. Platt (Newark: University of Delaware Press, 1999), pp. 180–1. Extant records also note Cope's involvement in preparations for the staging of Shakespeare's *Love's Labour's Lost* in 1605 for Queen Anne: *The Oxford Companion to Shakespeare*, eds Michael Dobson and Stanley Wells (Oxford: Oxford University Press, 2001), pp. 88–9.
37. Cecil Papers, Bills 58, BHH/285, dated 1611–12.
38. *Thomas Platter's Travels in England 1599*, trans. Clare Williams (London: Jonathan Cape, 1937), pp. 33–6. Cope's notoriety as a connoisseur of wonders is also indicated by the fact that Edward Grimeston dedicated his English translation of Simon Goulart's *Thrésor d'histoires admirables et memorables de nostre temps* (Paris: 1600) to him, under the title *Admirable and Memorable Histories Containing the Wonders of our Time* (London: 1607), BL, 12356.b.35.
39. John Tradescant, *Musaeum Tradescantianum* (London: 1656), sigs A4 (dedicatory epitaph), and A2, BL, 957.d.34.

40. John Evelyn, *The Diary*, ed. E. S. de Beer (Oxford: Clarendon, 1955), pp. 685–6.
41. Henderson, *The Tudor House and Garden*, pp. 132–3. It is unsurprising that Bacon's servant, the eccentric Thomas Bushell, should have built his own grotto at Enstone in Oxfordshire in the 1620s in which a statue of Neptune lurked among a veritable cabinet of 'many strange forms of Beasts, Fishes and Fowls', according to Robert Plot, *The Natural History of Oxfordshire* (1677). For more on the Bushell grotto, see Hunt, *Garden and Grove*, pp. 137–8; Anthony, *The Renaissance Garden in Britain*, p. 33; and Strong, *The Renaissance Garden in England*, pp. 130–4.
42. *Thomas Aquinas: Selected Writings*, trans. Ralph McInerny (Harmondsworth: Penguin, 1998), 'The Range of Natural Philosophy. Expositions of *Physics* . . .' (1269), pp. 440–3. When Aquinas discourses on 'natural science' this does not indicate what we may today think of as an experimental discipline, but refers to the Aristotelian *scientia*, the acquisition of indisputable knowledge towards the ultimate goal of attaining 'universal truths', as opposed to mere conjecture or opinion: see Lorraine Daston and Katharine Park, *Wonders and the Order of Nature 1150–1750* (New York: Zone Books, 1998), p. 114.
43. *Parasceve*, in *The Works of Francis Bacon*, ed. James Spedding (London: Longmans and Co., 1875), vol. 4, p. 254.
44. Carolyn Merchant, *The Death of Nature: Women, Ecology and the Scientific Revolution* (San Francisco: Harper Collins, 1980), pp. 165; Bacon's *Masculine Birth of Time* is quoted from p. 170.
45. Bacon, *Works*, vol. 4, pp. 168–9.
46. Bacon, *Works*, *Parasceve*, vol. 4, p. 253.
47. *Of the Dignity and Advancement of Learning*, Bacon, *Works*, vol. 4, p. 295.
48. Desiree Hellegers, *Handmaid to Divinity: Natural Philosophy, Poetry, and Gender in Seventeenth-Century England* (Norman: University of Oklahoma Press, 2000), p. 54.
49. Bacon, *Works*, *Parasceve*, vol. 4, p. 253.
50. David Freedberg, *The Eye of the Lynx: Galileo, his Friends, and the Beginnings of Modern Natural History* (Chicago and London: University of Chicago Press, 2002), pp. 57–74. Collecting was an important pastime in the dal Pozzo family. Only recently has evidence come to light which reveals the extent to which Cassiano dal Pozzo's younger brother, Carlo Antonio dal Pozzo, was a central figure in the formation of the early museum. See Donatella L. Sparti, 'Carlo Antonio Dal Pozzo (1606–1689): An Unknown Collector', *Journal of the History of Collections* 2 (1) (1990), pp. 7–19.
51. Evelyn, *The Diary*, ed. E. S. de Beer, p. 277.
52. Freedberg, *Eye of the Lynx*, pp. 75–6. The English prelude to this work was the *Advancement of Learning*, published in 1605. For a further account of the Linceans, see Rea Alexandratos, ' "With the True Eye of the Lynx": The Paper Museum of Cassiano dal Pozzo', in *Amazing Rare Things: The Art of Natural History in the Age of Discovery*, ed. David Attenborough (London: Royal Collection Publications, 2007), pp. 74–105.

53. I would like to thank Rea Alexandratos for all her help and for allowing me complete access to the archive of the Cassiano Project Office, Windsor Castle/Warburg Institute.
54. Windsor Castle Royal Library manuscript numbers (henceforth RL), RL19329/RL19330 (pasted together) and RL19365. See also RL19324, RL19340, RL19355, RL19367.
55. See RL19328 and RL21146 for more 'pregnant' fruit.
56. Govanni Ferrari, *Hesperides, Sive de Malorum Aureorum Cultura et Usu Libri Quartuor* (Rome: 1646), BL, 35.g.2. The *Hesperides* contains a large number of monstrous fruit; one plate for instance clearly identifies a deformed lime as 'MO[N]STROSA', p. 337.
57. RL19341 (deformed chick), Paris Bibliothèque de l'Institut de France, MS 978, f. 357 (hermaphroditic rat) and Paris Bibliothèque de l'Institut de France, MS 978, ff. 360–1 (hydrocephalic child).
58. Paris Bibliothèque de l'Institut de France, MS 976, f. 47. The charming Windsor Castle images are thought to have been largely the work of Vincenzo Leonardi, while the much coarser drawings held in the Paris archives were clearly executed by another artist, or group of artists.
59. Bacon, *Works, Novum Organum*, vol. 4, pp. 171–2.
60. Bacon, *Works*, vol. 8, pp. 334–5.
61. Pliny, *Natural History*, trans. H. Rackham, Loeb Classical Library (Cambridge: Harvard University Press, 1942), Book VII, 2:30, pp. 526–7. For a revealing account of how the *Natural History* came to an English readership, particularly the way in which it was involved in the mercantile aspects of textual exchange, see Lisa Jardine, *Worldly Goods: A New History of the Renaissance* (London: Macmillan, 1996), pp. 143–7.
62. *Palissy the Potter*, trans. Henry Morley (London: Chapman and Hall, 1855, p. 414), BL, 10662.e.1. *Discours Admirables, de la Nature des Eaux et Fonteines* (Paris: 1580), BL, 1171.d.3.
63. I have consulted the 1672 Venice edition, BL, 456.d.16.
64. Quoted in Patrick Mauries, *Cabinets of Curiosities* (London: Thames and Hudson, 2002), p. 155.
65. For the importance of the relation between the cabinet and this concept of *theatri rerum universitatis* see Eva Schulz, 'Notes on the History of Collecting and of Museums: In the Light of Selected Literature of the Sixteenth to the Eighteenth Century', *Journal of the History of Collections* 2 (2) (1990), pp. 205–18. This quotation appears on p. 208. On the connection between the Renaissance garden and grotto and the theatre see Hunt, *Garden and Grove*, pp. 59–72.
66. Quoted in Paula Findlen, 'The Museum: Its Classical Etymology and Renaissance Genealogy', *Journal of the History of Collections* 1 (1) (1989), pp. 59–78. Federico Cesi of the Linceans, following Ferrante Imperato, also described his natural historical project as constituting a 'Theatre of Nature', ibid., p. 64.
67. One of France's most influential patrons, Anne de Montmorency, commissioned Palissy to construct just such a grotto. For more on Palissy and the grotto tradition, see Leonard N. Amico, *Bernard Palissy: In Search of Earthly Paradise* (Paris and New York: Flammarion, 1996), pp. 47–81.

68. Bernard Palissy, *Resources: A Treatise on 'Water and Springs' written by Bernard Palissy in 1557*, trans. E. E. Willett (Brighton: W. J. Smith, 1876), pp. 17 and 1 respectively, BL, 7106.c.1.(13).
69. Ibid., pp. 5–6.
70. Albertus Magnus, *Womens' Secrets: A Translation of Pseudo-Albertus Magnus's De Secretis Mulierum with Commentaries*, trans. Helen Rodnite Lemay (New York: State University of New York Press, 1992), p. 75. On the role that the heat and humidity generated by the sun and planets have in embryological formation see pp. 64 and 84–6. For the dangers of too much heat and humidity on the conception of animals, see Albertus Magnus, *Albertus Magnus On Animals: A Medieval Summa Zoologica*, trans. Kenneth F. Kitchell Jr and Irven Michael Resnick (Baltimore: The John Hopkins University Press, 1999), vol. 2, pp. 1,241–3. Basset also says of places like Africa that 'so many Monsters are there bred' because it is 'a Countrey very hot . . . and heate . . . [is] a friend to nature', *Curiosities: or The Cabinet Of Nature*, pp. 11–12.
71. For more on this, see Martin Kemp, *Visualizations: The Nature Book of Art and Science* (Oxford: Oxford University Press, 2000), p. 19 and, by the same author, *Seen/Unseen: Art, Science, and Intuition from Leonardo to the Hubble Telescope* (Oxford: Oxford University Press, 2006), pp. 96–113.
72. Francis Bacon, *Essays* (1612), 'Of Gardens', in *Francis Bacon: A Critical Edition of the Major Works*, ed. Brian Vickers (Oxford: Oxford University Press, 1996), p. 433.
73. *The Works of Sir Thomas Browne*, ed. Geoffrey Keynes (London: Faber and Faber, 1928), Part 1, s. 39, p. 50.
74. Ibid., Part 1, s. 15, p. 24.
75. Ibid., Part 1, s. 37, pp. 47–8.
76. Ibid., Part 1, s. 55, p. 66. Montaigne makes a similar point about wonders and prodigies: 'Whatever happens against custom we say is against Nature, yet there is nothing whatsoever which is not in harmony with her. May Nature's universal reason chase away that deluded ecstatic amazement which novelty brings to us': Michel de Montaigne, 'On a Monster-Child', *The Complete Essays*, trans. M. A. Screech (Harmondsworth: Penguin, 1991), pp. 807–8.
77. *Sir Thomas Browne: Selected Writings*, ed. Claire Preston (Manchester: Carcanet, 1995), pp. 70–1 (October 1660).
78. All quotations from the play are taken from Shakespeare, *The Tempest*, ed. Stephen Orgel (Oxford: Oxford University Press, 1987).
79. Caliban refers to the cave in which he is 'sty[ed]' (I, ii, 343) as 'this hard rock', suggesting that he may be gesturing towards a physical construction of some kind, perhaps displayed beneath the tiring-house which would have provided a naturally in-set space or niche. Could a grotto-like cave have been suggested to the audience through marine-inspired decoration?
80. Marina Warner, '"The foul witch" and Her "freckled whelp": Circean Mutations in the New World', in Hulme and Sherman, eds, *The Tempest and Its Travels*, p. 99.
81. Hunt, *Garden and Grove*, pp. 123–4.

82. *The Tempest* was probably composed some time between late 1610 and the autumn of 1611, its first recorded performance being at James I's court on 1 November 1611: *The Oxford Companion to Shakespeare*, eds Michael Dobson and Stanley Wells (Oxford: Oxford University Press, 2001), p. 470.
83. The family were the subjects of close scrutiny by natural historians of the age, most notably Ulysses Aldrovandi (1522–1605), professor at the University of Bologna and founder of one of the first public museums, in whose great work, the *Monstrorum Historia* (1642), images of the family were eventually published. Gonsalvus' extraordinary story can be read on the website of the Kunsthistorisches Museum, Vienna: www.khm.at. The portraits of Gonsalvus and his son have been kindly supplied by the museum. Daston and Park also mention Gonsalvus and his children, *Wonders and the Order of Nature*, pp. 412, n. 58 and 416, n. 115.
84. The hermit's 'cell' was often a feature attached to the grotto in Renaissance gardens. The Enstone grotto of Thomas Bushell, for example, contained a monk's cell or 'hermitage' among its many wonders: Miller, *Heavenly Caves*, p. 66. See also pp. 31–4 of the same text for the use of sacred allusions in grotto-spaces. Strong sees the Enstone grotto, with its experimental automata and 'preoccupation with . . . examination of natural phenomena', as evocative of 'the world of the late Renaissance magus', *The Renaissance Garden in England*, p. 130.
85. That this is related to the play's concern with permissible and illicit forms of royal knowledge is suggested in Henry Peacham's *Basilikon Doron* (1610), an emblematised rendering of James I's political tract. The emblem '*Inopportuna Studia*' illustrates the dangers which can beset a kingdom governed by a negligent ruler, recapitulating through the image of a wonder-working magus James' advice to his own heir, in which he insists that the too curious 'studie of . . . liberall artes and sciences . . . cannot but distract you from the pointes of your calling', BL, Royal MS 12 A, LXVI, f. 30. It is pertinent to recall Quintilian's description of *admiratio* in his *Institutio Oratoria*, as an emotion which allows one to be 'transported by admiration' [*admiratione auferuntur*, literally 'carried away'], Loeb Classical Library, pp. 212–13. Augustine warned against that 'curiosity' which is 'a vain inquisitiveness dignified with the title of knowledge and science'. In particular he condemned those who 'study the operations of nature which lie beyond our grasp', such as the magus or astrologer who would use 'the perverted science . . . to achieve things by magical arts': *Confessions*, trans. Henry Chadwick (Oxford: Oxford University Press, 1991), pp. 210–12.
86. Jacob Rueff, *The Expert Midwife* (1637), p. 139, BL, C.112.c.1. See also Jane Sharp, *The Midwives Book, Or the Whole Art of Midwifry Discovered*, ed. Elaine Hobby (Oxford: Oxford University Press, 1999), pp. 84–9.
87. *The Complete English Poems*, ed. A. J. Smith (Harmondsworth: Penguin, 1971), 'First Anniversary', ll. 383–6.
88. Henry Peacham, *The Compleat Gentleman* (London: 1622), pp. 2 and 139, BL, C.124.c.8 (1).
89. Departing from Orgel's text, I follow many previous editors of the play in assigning this speech (I, ii, 350–61) to Prospero rather than Miranda. I have done so because it reproduces a concept of wonder more consistent

with Prospero's treatment of Miranda and the monster Caliban as possessing antithetical value as objects of admiration.

90. On the connection between conception/childbirth and printing, see Margreta de Grazia, 'Imprints: Shakespeare, Gutenberg and Descartes', in *Alternative Shakespeares*, ed. Terence Hawkes (London and New York: Routledge, 1996), vol. 2, pp. 63–94.
91. David Crystal and Ben Crystal, *Shakespeare's Words: A Glossary and Language Companion* (London: Penguin, 2002), p. 337.
92. Edward Fenton, *Certaine Secrete Wonders of Nature, containing a descriptio[n] of sundry strange things, seming Monstrous in our eyes and judgement, bicause we are not privie to the reasons of them* (London: 1569), ff. 48v-9, BL, C.31.d.8.
93. *A Most certain report of a monster borne at Oteringham in Holdernesse, the 9. of Aprill last past. 1595. Also of a most strange and huge fish, which was driven on the sand at outhorn in holdernesse in February . . .* (London: 1595), BL, 1476.b.3.
94. *The forme and shape of a Monstrous Child, borne at Maydstone in Kent, the xxiiii. of October 1568*, BL, Huth .50.38.
95. For telling parallels with the play's monstrous discourse, see Anon., *A Plaine Description of the Auncient Petigree of Dame Slaunder, togither with hir Coheires and fellow members, Lying, Flattering, Backebyting* (London: 1573), sig. G8v, BL, 245.d.4; Nicholas Breton, *A Murmurer* (London: 1607), sigs D3v–D4v, BL, C.27.d.7; and Edmund Spenser's description of Sclaunder (IV, viii, 24–6) and Detraction (V, xii, 33–6), the latter of whom appears as a hybrid serpent-fish, in *The Faerie Queene*, ed. A. C. Hamilton (London and New York: Longman, 1977).
96. Thomas Vaughan, *The Spirit of Detraction . . .* (London: 1611), pp. 85–6, BL, C.122.bb.26. The word 'consopited' from Latin *consopire* carries the subsidiary meaning of 'to compose' (*OED*). 'Embalon' may be a variation of 'embrion', an early version of embryo.
97. Morley, *Palissy the Potter*, pp. 349–50.
98. Ambroise Parè *On Monsters and Marvels*, trans. Janis L. Pallister (Chicago and London: University of Chicago Press, 1982), pp. 53–4.
99. Interestingly Roy Strong identifies the style in which the portrait was executed as indicative of a genre which came to be known as 'curious painting': *Gloriana: Portraits of Queen Elizabeth I* (London: Pimlico, 1987), pp. 135–140.
100. This is the astute conjectural reconstruction of the Ditchley sonnet produced by Louise Schleiner in *Tudor and Stuart Women Writers* (Bloomington and Indianapolis: Indiana University Press, 1994), p. 68. For the purposes of this quotation only I have reproduced her orthographical u/v constructions.
101. See, for example, Georgius Agricola's *De Re Metallica Libri XII* (1556), BL, 32.g.13. For more on mineral deposits, metals and mining and their relation to the concept of earth as 'mother' see Merchant, *The Death of Nature*, pp. 29–41.
102. Thomas Raynalde, *The Birth of Mankynde, otherwyse named the Womans Booke* (London: 1564), ff. 14v–15, BL, 1177.h.1. Compare this to Acosta's description of the precious 'mettalls' retrievable from the new

world in his *Naturall and Morall History of the Indies*: '[T]he fixed veins [of silver] are those which have a continuance in depth and length, like to great branches and armes of trees', p. 195.

103. Randall Martin. (ed.), *Women Writers in Renaissance England* (London and New York: Longman, 1997), p. 332, ll. 43–56.
104. The play's interest in watery spaces as sources of salt and brine also echoes early modern interest in the healing and purifying properties of springs, ideas which go back as far as Jacopo Dondi's *On the Cause of the Saltiness of Waters* (1355). Dondi had analysed the waters of the Monte Grotto as a test-case for the benefits of mineral deposits: see Katherine Park, 'Natural Particulars: Medical Epistemology, Practice, and the Literature of Healing Springs', in *Natural Particulars: Nature and the Disciplines in Renaissance Europe*, eds Anthony Grafton and Nancy Siraisi (Cambridge: MIT Press, 1999), pp. 350–2.
105. Mark Thornton Burnett describes 'Prospero's absorption in natural history' as pointing 'to the proximity of the *wunderkammern* in which, in an anticipation of the "museums" of the eighteenth and nineteenth centuries, natural singularities and "monstrous" aberrations alike vied for prominence': *Constructing 'Monsters'*, pp. 128–9. My reading pushes the play's engagement with natural history back to the contemporary interest in the cultures of geology, hydrology and collecting which exemplified the grotto-space. My focus on Caliban's knowledge of the hidden natural properties of the island is intended to uncover the meaningful inversion the play stages between the monster and the natural historian, an inversion which turns on the fulcrum of early theories of reproduction.
106. Compare the substitution of 'seamews' at II, ii, 164, in the *The Norton Shakespeare*, with the same line in *Mr William Shakespeare's Comedies, Histories, and Tragedies: A Facsimile of the First Folio, 1623* (New York and London: Routledge, 1998), p. 10. See also Stephen Orgel's note to II, ii, 166 of his edition of the play which relates the word to a particular New World variety of fish, the 'fort scameux'. As Helen Hackett has pointed out to me, Milton's reference to 'sea-mews' in Book XI of *Paradise Lost* (l. 835) seems to indicate gulls (see also *OED*).
107. William Strachey, *A true repertory of the wracke, and redemption of Sir Thomas Gates . . . from the Ilands of the Bermudas: his coming to Virginia . . . July 15 1610*, from *Purchas his Pilgrimes* (London: 1624), Part 4, p. 1,740, BL, 679.h.14.
108. See Greenblatt's note to I, ii, 271 in the *Norton* edition of the play.
109. Albertus Magnus, *Womens' Secrets: A Translation of Pseudo-Albertus Magnus's De Secretis Mulierum with Commentaries*, p. 73.
110. Helkiah Crooke, *Microcosmographia: A Description of the Body of Man* (London: 1615), pp. 260–1, BL, 781.k.1. For more on the relation of the moon to the maternal body, see Aristotle, *History of Animals [Historia Animalium]*, trans. D. M. Balme, Loeb Classical Library (Cambridge: Harvard University Press, 1991), Book VII, 582a34–b5.
111. Jacques Guillemeau, *Childbirth, or the Happy Deliverie of Women* (London: 1612), p. 33, BL, 1177.d.40.
112. John Sadler, *The Sicke Womans Private Looking-Glasse* (London: 1636), pp. 188–9. BL, 1175.a.7

113. Crooke, *Microcosmographia*, p. 299.
114. Sadler, *The Sicke Womans Private Looking-Glasse*, p. 124–5.
115. Jacob Rueff, *The Expert Midwife* (London: 1637), p. 139. BL, C.112.c.1.
116. Guillemeau, *Childbirth*, p. 14.
117. Moderata Fonte, *The Worth of Women: Wherein is Clearly Revealed their Nobility and their Superiority to Men*, trans. Virginia Cox (Chicago and London: University of Chicago Press, 1997), pp. 130 and 150–2.
118. Sharpe, *The Midwives Book,* pp. 85–7.
119. *Othello*, ed. E. A. J. Honigmann (Surrey: Arden, 1996).
120. John Webster, *The Duchess of Malfi and Other Plays*, ed. René Weis (Oxford: Oxford University Press, 1996).
121. Raleigh himself did not go to Virginia, but appointed White governor of the second Roanoke Colony in 1587; see Peter Whitfield, *New Found Lands: Maps in the History of Exploration* (London: The British Library, 1998), p. 86. White was, however, accompanied by Thomas Harriot, whose *A Brief and True Report of the New Found Land of Virginia* (1590) contained renderings of White's drawings executed by Theodor de Bry. Harriot was a scientist with, it seems, a particular interest in the properties of water, having conducted experiments on its motion and velocity which enabled him to design a plumbing-system for Petworth House, the country seat of his patron, the Earl of Northumberland. With this skilled mastery over the dynamics of water it is hardly surprising that Harriot was employed to survey accurately the waterways and river-channels of Virginia; see Adam Hart-Davis, *What the Tudors and Stuarts Did for Us* (London: Macmillan, 2002), pp. 102–3.
122. British Museum, Department of Prints and Drawings.
123. Strachey, *Purchas his Pilgrimes*, p. 1,741.
124. All quotations from Drayton's poem are taken from *Silver Poets of the Sixteenth Century*, ed. Douglas Brooks-Davies (London: Everyman, 1992). Line numbers are indicated in brackets.
125. Spenser, *Complete Poetical Works* (Oxford: Oxford University Press, 1970).
126. In Plato's *Theaetetus* wonder has a specific lineage: '[W]onder is the only beginning of philosophy, and he who said that Iris was the child of Thaumas [i.e. meaning wonder or miracle] made a good genealogy', trans. Harold North Fowler, Loeb Classical Library (Cambridge: Harvard University Press, 1921), p. 55.
127. See David Crystal and Ben Crystal, *Shakespeare's Words*, p. 476; and Orgel's note to III, ii, 94.
128. *Musaeum Tradescantianum: or, a Collection of Rarities* (1656), sig. A2.
129. Ben Jonson, *The Complete Masques*, ed. Stephen Orgel (New Haven and London: Yale University Press, 1969), ll. 131–90.
130. Platt, *Reason Diminished*, p. 116.
131. My reading thus moves in the opposite direction to that of Julia Reinhard Lupton, who sees Caliban as struggling to move away from 'a liquid world in which ponds, streams, and fountains teem with the swarming marginalia of mere life' and into a transcendent space 'largely devoid of flora and fauna, of creatures in their extrahuman dimension': 'Creature Caliban', *Shakespeare Quarterly* 51 (1) (2000), p. 22.

Chapter 3

Strange Labours: Maternity and *Maleficium* in the Theatre of Justice

Breaching the Wall: The Archaeologies of Witchcraft and the Maternal Body in Early Modern England

> We are all conceived in close prison; in our mother's wombs, we are close prisoners all; when we are born, we are born but to the liberty of the house; prisoners still, though within larger walls; and then all our life is but a going out to the place of execution . . .
>
> John Donne, *A Sermon preached to the Lords, 28 March 1619*[1]

In 1961 workmen were carrying out structural repairs to the first-floor interior of Lauderdale House, a late-sixteenth-century mansion situated in London's Highgate Hill. As they began to remove bricks near a chimney-breast in what is now the long Tudor gallery they made a grim discovery.[2] They had stumbled upon a hidden compartment which had been blocked up for more than four centuries. One by one the old house gave up its long-held secrets as the workmen began to remove the curious artefacts concealed inside. The extraordinary hoard of carefully-placed objects, which can still be seen at the Museum of London today (Fig. 3.1), consisted of four desiccated chickens, two of which, as forensic evidence suggests, were strangled while the other two may have been, gruesomely, buried alive;[3] a candlestick with a yellow glazed border (Fig. 3.2); a glass drinking goblet; two odd shoes (Fig. 3.3); a cord of plaited rush-matting; and an egg, which may have been laid by one of the chickens while it was trapped inside its stony prison.[4]

Archaeologists have made many such discoveries around the thresholds of Britain's Renaissance houses; above fire-places, beneath doors, and near windows, or on sites where these thresholds are known once to have stood. Used as methods of counter-magic to ward off evil spirits and malevolent witchcraft, or *maleficium*, these objects and their locations tell us something about the way in which ritual and superstition operated within the environs of the domestic sphere. Further archaeological finds include written charms or spells, stone and wooden heads, pots, curiously bent nails, knives etched with

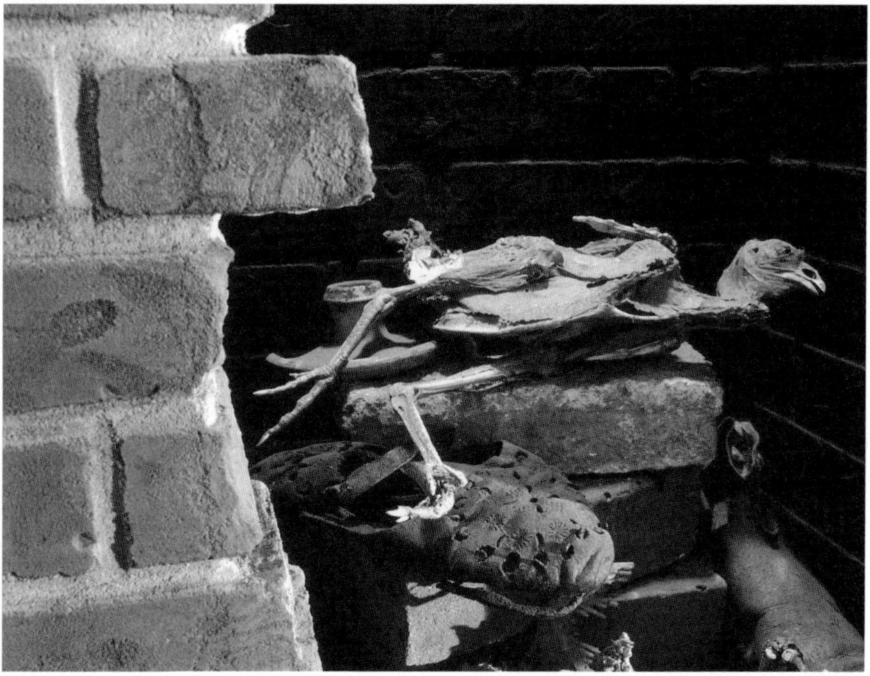

Figure 3.1: Concealed magical artefacts, Lauderdale House, Highgate Hill, London. © Museum of London.

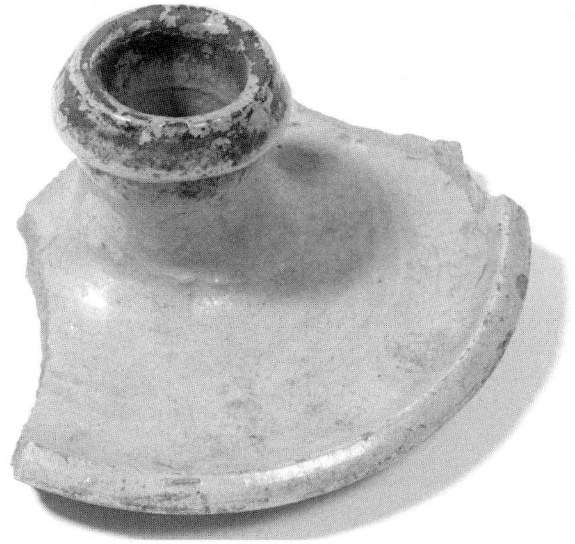

Figure 3.2: Candlestick, late sixteenth or early seventeenth century, part of the cache of concealed magical artefacts found in Lauderdale House, Highgate Hill, London. © Museum of London.

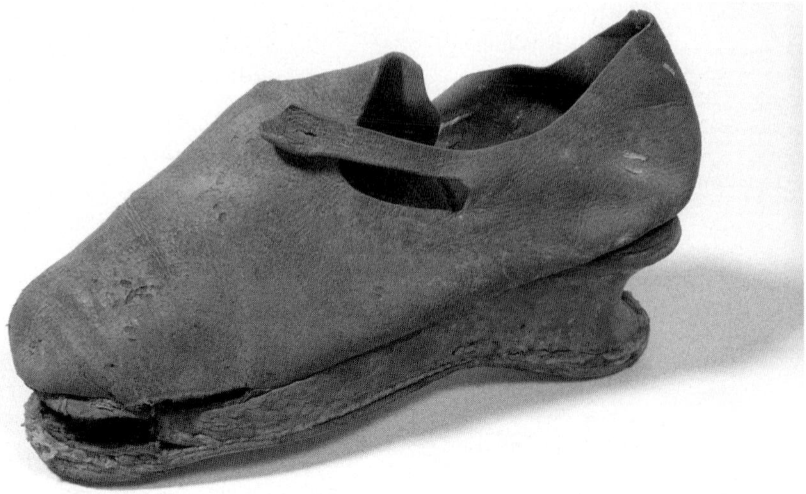

Figure 3.3: Shoe, late sixteenth or early seventeenth century, part of the cache of concealed magical artefacts found in Lauderdale House, Highgate Hill, London. © Museum of London.

occult symbols, magic talismans and stones, dolls and items of clothing, the most common of which are shoes which, in many cultures today, continue to be used as fertility or luck charms.[5] More disturbing still are artefacts of organic origin such as human skulls; the extracted hearts of pigs or bullocks, most often found inserted with pins; and mummified cats, like the early examples which form part of the Norwich Castle Museum collection (Fig. 3.4).[6] By far the most enigmatic archaeological discovery, however, is the so-called witch-bottle; a receptacle containing mysterious magical ingredients which we will go on to consider in more detail. Given the fragmentary nature of the archaeological record, a surprisingly large number of items relating to superstitious practices have survived.[7] That their use was widespread enough in early modern England to be of particular concern to the authorities is suggested by the injunctions against their use which circulated in contemporary legal treatises such as Richard Bernard's *Guide to Grand-Jury Men* which condemned a range of superstitious practices:

> To use a sieve and a paire of sheeres, with certain words: To put something under the threshold, where the suspected [witch] goeth in, or under the stoole where he or she sitteth . . . To burne some cloathes in which the sicke party lyeth, for to torment the Witch; to burne part of the creature in paine; to burne alive one, to save the rest [in cases where cattle and livestock are

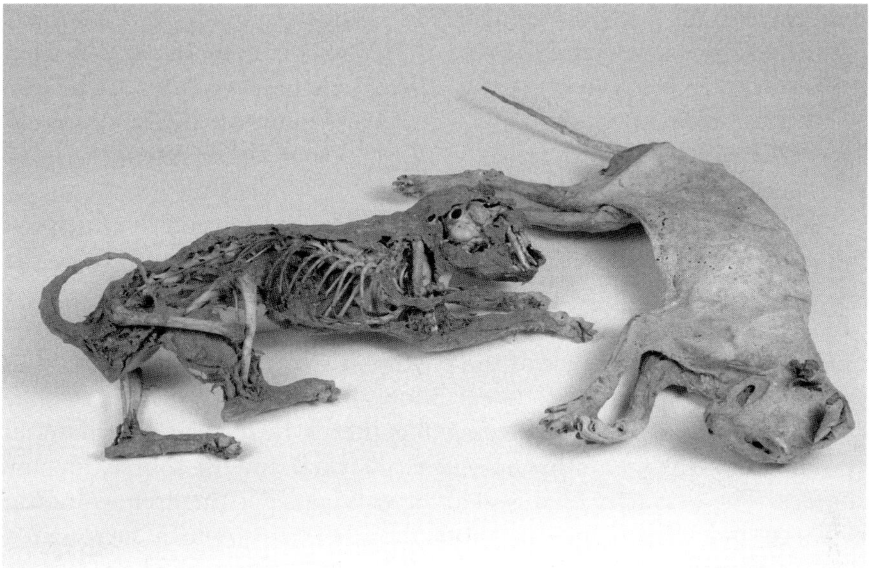

Figure 3.4: Mummified cats. Norwich Castle Museum and Art Gallery. Photo: David Kirkham.

> suspected of being bewitched]; & to make the Witch to come thither [by burning one of her possessions, or the possessions of her victim]: These are execrable sacrifices made to the divell, to be abhorred of all true Christians.[8]

Sieves, shears, stools, clothes, whole animals or parts of animals: Bernard makes reference to a plethora of personal domestic possessions used as a means of attacking the body of the witch and securing the health of the victim. The symmetry of counter-magical measures also suggests the ways in which witchcraft itself was thought to operate, targeting the weakest points of the home, usually its thresholds, as well as sites of domestic production where food is prepared and livestock reared. The burial or blocking up of objects inside walls and under openings in the house was thus thought to stop the flow of maleficent forces into the domestic space. It has been difficult for archaeologists, working with discoveries which enter the formal record as a range of culturally disconnected, site-specific acts, to account for the ways in which these objects functioned as mediating instruments in a far more complex and wide-ranging network of social interactions.[9] Moreover, the rituals of which they formed a part presupposed a direct relation between the agents of malevolent magic and the body of the victim in ways which are now largely lost to us. Equally limiting, however, has been the trajectory of literary-historical research conducted to date, particularly that concerning Renaissance England. While early modern accounts overwhelmingly presented the dark arts, and the methods used to keep them at bay, as being in some way effected through the use and misuse of physical objects, studies of Shakespeare's interest in the maternal aspects of witchcraft have failed to take account of the *material* basis of witchcraft beliefs.[10]

The purpose of this chapter is to begin to suggest ways in which the principles of archaeological enquiry can offer new possibilities for the study of maternity in Shakespeare's plays. This still relatively new facet of interdisciplinary analysis is not, however, merely concerned with the mud-stained, broken relics of the past which we can physically hold in our hands. It seeks rather to unearth long-hidden artefacts from a range of possible *archaeologies*, piecing together a history of the material culture from textual, anthropological, pictorial and, of course, literary sources. The first part of this chapter will consider the archaeological evidence and what it tells us about those anxieties which surrounded domestic nurture and fertility in the early modern family. The materials of magic were often the very stuff of routine labour in the household economy, items of everyday use needed to keep the familial unit and its kinship relations functioning productively. Understanding the ways in which they played a key role in the processes of maternal care-giving, domestic labour and charity will bring us closer to explaining the mystery which has long taxed historians of witchcraft: why it is that most suspected witches in England were women,[11] and why so many accounts of maleficent magic, as we will see, *maternalise* the perpetrators of such crimes. We will then go on, in the second part of this chapter, to apply what we have learnt to our reading of the materials of magic, and their function as the ritualised conduits of malevolent agents, in Shakespeare's *Macbeth*.

In 1582 Bennet Lane, a house-proud woman from Essex, was called upon to give evidence in the trial against her neighbour Annis Herd who, along with other women in St Osyth, had been arraigned for witchcraft. The catalyst for the dispute, which would eventually lead to Bennet's day in court, was a simple dish of milk which she had lent Annis. Only after Bennet had angrily demanded the return of the domestic receptacle did it make its way back to her home. Once in the hands of its rightful owner, however, things began to go badly in the Lane household when Bennet discovered she 'could no lo[n]ger spin nor make a thread to hold'. When all attempts to rectify the problem by conventional means had failed she 'tooke her spindle and put it into the fire, & made it red hot, & then cooled it [a]gaine and went to worke, and then it wrought as well as ever it did at any tyme before'. The next day she experienced further disruptions to her work following a dispute with Annis over two pence promised in exchange for milk. Receiving money from Annis was again the stimulus for her domestic problems:

> [S]he would have fleet her milk bowle, but it wold not abide the fleeting, but would rop & role as it were the white of an egge . . . then shee saith it came into her minde to approove another way, which was, shee tooke a horse shue and made it redde hote, and put it into the milke in the vessals, and so into her creame: and then she saith, she coulde seath her milke, fleete her creame, and make her butter in good sort as she had before.[12]

Faced with a crisis in her ability to nurture her family Bennet falls back on a typical counter-magical measure; the burning of objects believed to be infected with a witch's *maleficium*. In the case of the heated horseshoe, this is added to the bewitched 'vessals' which have become the vehicles of this malevolent power.[13] The suspicions surrounding Annis Herd are fairly typical of the kind of conditions which could trigger an accusation of witchcraft. A disruption to the smooth running of food production and familial nurturing, the illness or death of a child, or even the loss of parental fertility, could be interpreted as a case of demonic intervention by women trying to negotiate the pressures and expectations of their social roles. Indeed, for those participating in a largely female culture of borrowing and exchange while they went about their daily duties as wives and mothers, a bottle of milk, a borrowed pot, a stray dish, or a cup of yeast, could so easily become the pretext for the eruption of social tensions. A particularly striking instance of this appears in a sensational pamphlet, published in 1579, which records the interrogation and execution of three notorious Chelmsford witches. One of the condemned was a Margery Stanton who was accused of craftily exchanging one of her milk bottles for a bottle belonging to the wife of Robert Cornell with the intention of bewitching and then returning the household article:

> [Margery Stanton] came againe, and requested her owne bottle, and restored the other, craving Milke as before[.] [T]he wife of the house alwaies suspectyng her to bee a Witche denied her requeste, and barred the doores against here, whereupon she [Margery Stanton] satte doune uppon her heeles before the doore, and made a Circle uppon the grounde with a knife. After that she digged it full of holes within the compasse . . . [T]he nexte daie the wife commying out at the same doore, was taken sicke, and began to swell . . . as if she had been with child . . . and to this daie is not restored to healthe.[14]

Like many of the magical artefacts discovered in archaeological investigations this more transitory ritual act is attached to one of the domestic thresholds and is accomplished with an ordinary domestic utensil which undergoes a startling process of translation. Stanton's strange behaviour may have reminded the court who heard her case of the necromancer's fashioning of magic circles, such as that recorded in a fifteenth-century manuscript which incorporates talismanic references to the kinds of objects used for ceremonial purposes, including a sword, an oil-vessel, a ring and a royal sceptre (Fig. 3.5).[15] The domestic anxieties for which Stanton's case becomes the fulcrum find expression in the reference to pregnancy which correlates the magical assault on the threshold of the house with an attack on the maternal body itself. Similar concerns surface in Margery's other encounters with her neighbours. Being denied yeast by one Richard Saunder's wife, Margery allegedly bewitched 'her yonge child in the Cradle [who] was taken vehemently sicke'. Taking up the poorly child 'to comforte it', the mother noticed that the cradle began strangely to rock of its own accord 'in [the] presence of one of the Earle of Surreis gentilmen, who seyng it stabbed his dagger three or fower tymes into the Cradle ere it staied: Merily jestyng and saiyng, that he would kill the Devill, if he would bee rocked there'.[16] The act of stabbing the cradle is not necessarily one of mere jocund whimsy, but may have had a magical purpose. In Cade House, West Malling, Kent, archaeologists discovered two knives deliberately hidden behind a wall and similar knives were often concealed beneath thresholds, the occupants of the house believing that they could inflict some harm on the witch.[17]

In this instance the measure used to break the witch's spell occurs at a high point of maternal crisis. It is hardly surprising, therefore, that many suspected cases of bewitchment should revolve around definitions of what constituted legitimate wifely and maternal work as women exchanged physical commodities between them. Elizabeth Francis confessed that, after a visit to one of her female neighbours, 'because she could have no yest (which she required) she caused sathan to destroye the brewing at that tyme' and 'being denyed butter of an other, she caused her to lose the curdes ii. or iii. dayes after'.[18] On another occasion Joan Cunny

> came to one Harry Finches house, to demaund some drink, his wife being busie and a brewing, tolde her she had no leysure to give her any. Then Joane Cunnye went away discontented: and at night Finches wife was greevously taken in her head, and the next day in her side, and so continued in most horrible paine for the space of a week, and then dyed.[19]

If the good wife was expected to be of charitable service to her neighbours as well as her family then an accusation of *maleficium* could exonerate the victim from any incompetence in her role as a bountiful supplier of nourishment and nurture.

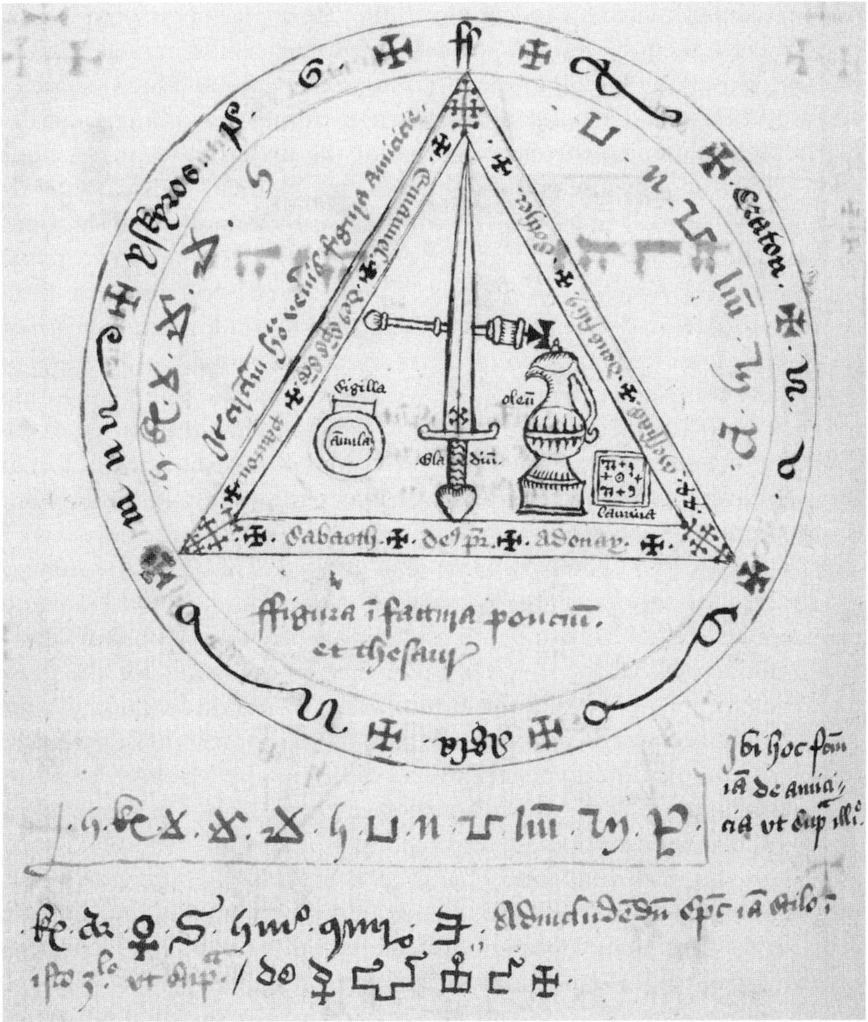

Figure 3.5: Magic circle, fifteenth century, Sloane MS 3853, f. 51v. © British Library Board. All Rights Reserved.

The renowned sceptic Reginald Scot suspected that such motives lay behind allegations of disruptive magic, remarking with no small amount of irony in his *Discoverie of Witchcraft* (1584) that witches 'can also bring to passe, that chearne as long as you list, your butter will not come; especiallie, if either the maids have eaten up the creame; or the goodwife have sold the butter before in the market'.[20] Scot also noticed that many witchcraft accusations were stimulated by some kind of denial of charity.[21] Keith Thomas and Alan Macfarlane have come under recent criticism for the emphasis they have placed on what is now known as the 'charity-refused' model.[22] However, a closer consideration of this topos can, I would argue, illuminate the ways in which women's access to household articles figured in cases of maleficent magic, particularly as it related to the expectations of the maternal ideal. Sermons and conduct manuals which sought to define women's roles as nurturers and providers of charity did so within a larger debate over the extent to which they should have control of domestic production and property.

In *A Lasting Jewell for Religious Women* (1630) William Crompton confidently declared that 'A good woeman was never barren; she cannot but bee a mother of many children, in one sense or other' through her 'workes of pietie and charity'.[23] For William Gouge the wife's obligation to 'be bountifull to the poore' is directly related to her knowledge of the domestic space and its moveable provisions since she knows 'what things are fittest to be given away: for wives commonly know of what things there is greatest store and what may in the house be best spared'.[24] This was echoed by John Downame who insisted in his *Plea of the Poore* (1616) that 'almes deeds are ordinarily done out of houshold store and provision, the administration and disposing wherof doth more properly and immediately belong to the woman then to the man', for she must 'beare children, and guide the house'.[25] A woman's autonomy was, however, limited by the husband's willingness to confer 'the administration of his houshould expences to the discretion of his wife' and this often only applied 'if the almes which shee giveth be but of small value, as bread, drink, cast apparell, and such like', items most closely associated with the nurturing role. This reflects an underlying concern that unrestrained acts of maternal charity could threaten the domestic economy, a fear that 'many undiscreete weomen will abuse it, to the undoing of their husbands and the ruining of their estates'.[26] Women, under enormous moral pressure to conform to the sacred template of maternal charity, particularly when 'the aged and decrepit, the weake widdowes'[27] found themselves at their door-steps, could thus turn to an alternative model of maternity which stressed the woman's role as a protector of the domestic space and its contents. In his *Countrey Contentments* (1623) Gervase Markham appealed to women to limit their expenditure at all times for the 'mother and Mistris of the family' must spend 'according to the competency of her husbands estate & calling . . . for it is a rule if we extend to the uttermost we take away increase . . . [and] enter into consumption'.[28] The diligent housewife should, in the words of Miles Coverdale, guard the family's goods in the same way as a bird 'kepeth the nest, hatcheth the egges, and bryng[eth] forth the frute'.[29]

An accusation of *maleficium*, made by a woman refusing to participate in the exchange of commodities with a neighbour, could allow the housewife to avoid a crisis in her view of herself as capable mother or nurturer if the suspected witch could be grouped among the class of masterless citizens who were deemed to be a threat to the commonwealth, the 'many sturdie beggers, and vagrant rogues, the blemish of our government' not deserving of 'the sacrifice of our almesdeedes' because they 'like idle drones, feede upon the common spoyle'.[30] Indeed, the good wife's status in court, as accuser of a witch, could in part be determined by her ability to demonstrate her awareness of the unstable, and hence demonically translatable, properties of such domestic articles – the material adjuncts of charity and nurture – once they had left her hands. The currency of this knowledge as permissible evidence, however, depended on its mobile nature, on its being equally valuable to the witch as it was to the conscientious wife and mother seeking to protect her home. The Chelmsford community which sentenced Ellen Smith in the April of 1579 were particularly sensitive to the menacingly manipulable nature of household objects. Following her own son's testimony against her, in which he confessed that she had been keeping evil spirits in ordinary domestic receptacles, Ellen's house was searched and two bottles (a 'wicker Bottle' and a 'Leather Bottle') and a 'Wolle Packe' were confiscated by the authorities who used them as evidence against her.[31]

While early representations of witchcraft, like those by Hans Buldung Grien (Figs 3.6 and 3.7), drew on continental models which emphasised the satanic rituals that peppered medieval witchlore,[32] they also began to incorporate elements of the domestic culture which, by the sixteenth century, increasingly provided the immediate context for accusations involving the use of malevolent magic in most parts of Europe. In these images the material relics of feeding and nurture in the home, such as pots, urns, cauldrons, spoons, chalices, plates and serving ewers, practically spill out of each grisly scene. One of Grien's *Weather Witches* is also depicted holding aloft a stopped glass bottle, perhaps containing the spirits which, once released, will execute her murderous intents. This iconographical tradition foreshadows the archival evidence which presents witchcraft as an inverted or corrupted form of maternal nurture. Indeed English accounts of such devilish practices in particular dwell upon the near-maternal relation between a witch and her familiar. In the earliest known witchcraft pamphlet, *The Examination and Confession of certaine Wytches at Chensforde* (1566), Elizabeth Francis confessed that 'she learned this arte of witchcraft at the age of xii yeres of hyr grandmother' who taught her to 'geve of her bloudde to Sathan (as she

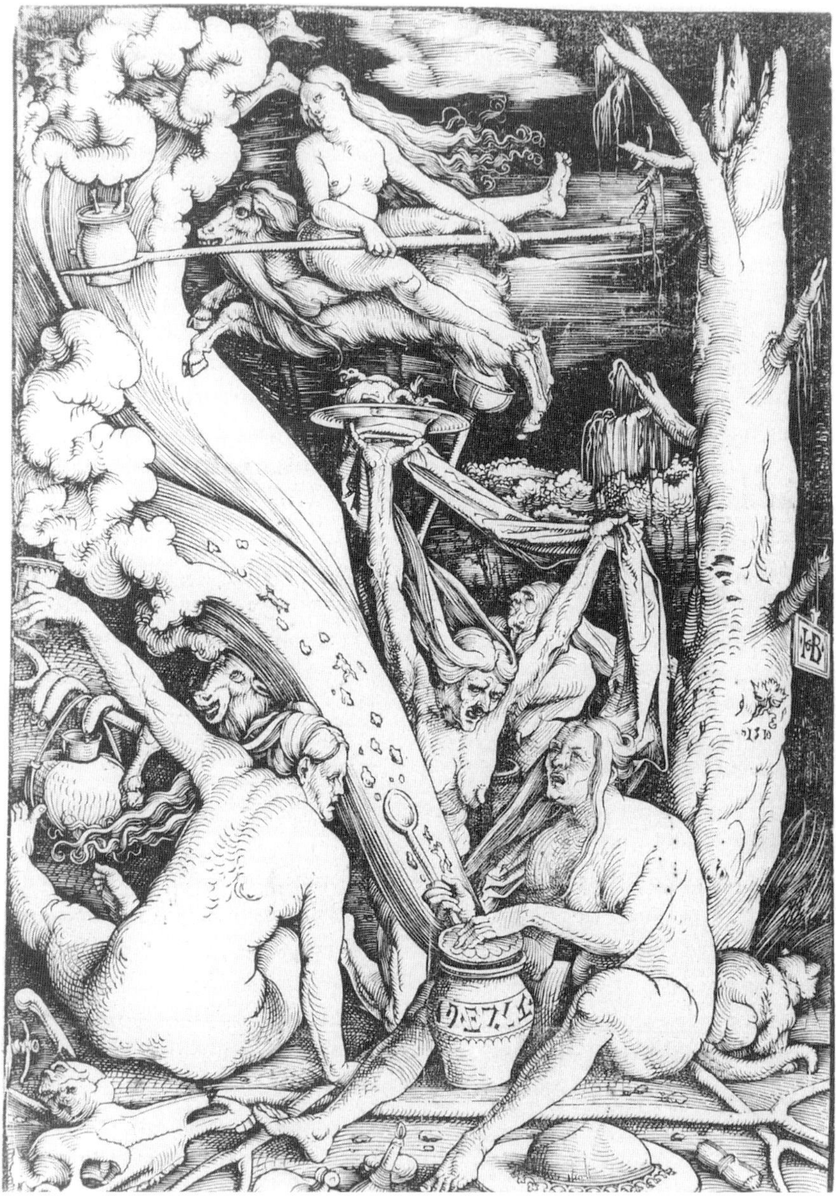

Figure 3.6: Hans Buldung Grien, *The Witches' Sabbath*, 1510. The Warburg Institute, University of London.

termed it) whyche she delyvered her in the lykenesse of a whyte spotted Catte, and taughte her to feede the sayde Catte with breade and mylke'.[33] Likewise, Alison Device claimed to have acquired her occult skills from her grandmother, Elizabeth Sothernes, who succeeded in her

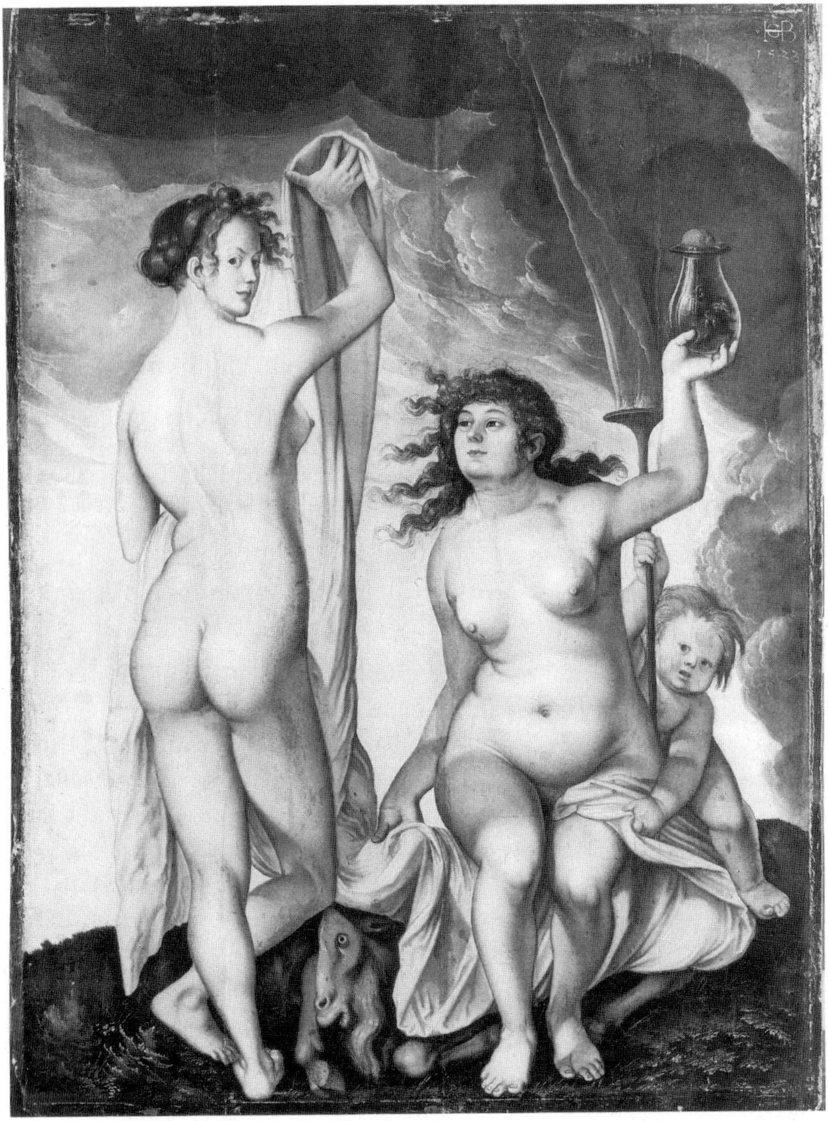

Figure 3.7: Hans Buldung Grien, *Weather Witches*, 1523. Städel Museum, Frankfurt am Main.

attempts to 'perswade and advise this Examinate to let a Divell or a Familiar appeare to her, and . . . suck at some part of her'. A fiend duly appeared in the form of a 'Blacke Dogge' which 'did with his mouth . . . suck at her breast, a little below her paps'.[34] The secrets of witchcraft are passed down from mother to daughter in the same way as legitimate domestic teachings concerning maternal nurture, for as William Perkins writes, 'our witches are wont to communicate their skill to others by tradition, to teach and instruct their children and posteritie, and to initiate them in the grounds and practises of their owne trade'.[35] These witches have learnt through acts of maternal feeding to be good providers in a parody of motherhood which is at once both grotesque and touching. Just how closely this action could be identified with the biological processes of lactation can be seen in Edward Fairfax's manuscript account of the bewitching of his daughters. On one occasion Helen and Elizabeth Fairfax claimed to have been visited in a vision by a witch. The encounter reveals a particular preoccupation with the contaminating effects of a witch's breast-milk even upon human children:

> [A] woman unknown to the children, did appear to th[e]m in trance, & told th[e]m she was daughter to one Umplebie's wife, & that her mother was a Witch, & they saw the woman let a spirit suck upon her breast: to whome Hellen said, th[o]u art a cunning witch indeed, to let thy spirit suck there upon thy Papps head, for noe body can finde any mark upon thee, if th[o]u let thy spirit suck there: hast th[o]u any children? she said noe: the other replyed, it is well: for God help the children th[a]t must suck, where th[a]t spirit sucketh.[36]

Since such close maternal encounters with her familiars, as Helen's testimony indicates, were believed to leave the witch with a visible sign of her damnation, witch-trials came increasingly to focus upon the discovery of the so-called witch's mark. Suspects were assiduously searched by groups of local women or midwives.[37] That this became pivotal to conviction can be ascertained from the second wave of Lancashire witch trials in 1633–4. The charges were brought by Edmund Robinson, a ten-year-old boy who claimed to have been abducted by witches and taken against his will to a secret sabbath.[38] His story, a wild concoction of witch-stereotypes, including accounts of image-magic, shape-changing and riotous bacchic feasting, ensured his status as a local celebrity. A self-styled witch-finder, he was led from church to church and paid to single out clandestine witches from congregations of bemused and terrified female parishioners. One of the accused, Margaret Johnson, confirmed that she had suckled Satan and that 'the devill after hee begins to sucke will make a papp or a dug in a short time & the matter hee sucketh is blood'.[39] Around twenty women were examined for such a mark, including Jannet Hargraves, accused of 'killing a child in the belly of Ellen Robinson' and found with '1 marke in her secrett place', and Mary Aynsworth, indicted 'for killing of Thomas Whittakers an Infant, for killing of Eliz[abeth] Whittakers, and for killing of Georg[e] Crockshawe an Infant', who allegedly had '3 pappes or markes in her secrettes'.[40] When Elizabeth Wright was stripped and searched some sixteen years earlier, the midwives 'found behind her right sholder a thing much like the udder of an ewe that giveth suck with two teates, like unto two great wartes'.[41] Likewise in 1593, after the execution of Alice Samuel, one of the witches of Warboys, her naked body was put to 'open shewe' and a suspected 'teat' near her groin was examined by 'the Jaylors wife' who 'tooke the same teate in her hand, and seeming to straine it, there issued out at the first as if it had been beesenings, (to use the Jaylors worde) which is a mixture of yellow milk and water: at the second time there came out in similitude as cleere milke, and in the ende very bloud it self'.[42]

While the perversely maternalised attributes of the witch have long been recognised by critics and historians, there remains no convincing explanation for the incorporation of this specifically biological dimension in local superstitious customs. This is where the archaeological evidence can offer us new and illuminating insights. Some of the most tantalising artefacts to survive the onslaught of the centuries are witch-bottles. These were receptacles containing ingredients prepared by local wise men or women and were either burned or buried as a means of reversing the bewitchment of people and livestock. The practice has a long chronological history, stretching from the early seventeenth to the early twentieth centuries. During an excavation of a site at Duke's Place in East London the archaeology team of the Museum of London discovered a witch-bottle in an area which once contained domestic dwellings. Its broken base revealed a set of copper alloy pins which had been severely corroded, suggesting the original presence of some other material (Fig. 3.8). This was probably urine, since this often formed an essential ingredient of the witch-bottle.[43] Similar artefacts were found in Stowmarket and Ixworth in Suffolk containing pins and nails.[44] Many such receptacles boasted the characteristic bearded face decoration which was a staple feature of Bellarmine Fretchen-ware bottles imported from Germany from the late sixteenth century onwards.[45] The magical potential of these vessels may have suggested itself to those who used them because of the stereotype of the bearded witch, an image which Shakespeare was to draw upon for his own depiction of the Witches in *Macbeth*.[46] A possibly mid-to-late seventeenth-century witch-bottle which included this decorative motif, discovered in Felmersham, Bedfordshire, had been filled with urine, corroded iron nails and brass pins, each individually bent. Curiously it also included samples of hair from two different individuals. A large coiled lock belonged to a younger person, while strands of grey hair were from someone much older (Figs 3.9a and 3.9b).[47] Another bottle, probably of a similar age, recovered from a mill-stream near Great College Street, Westminster,

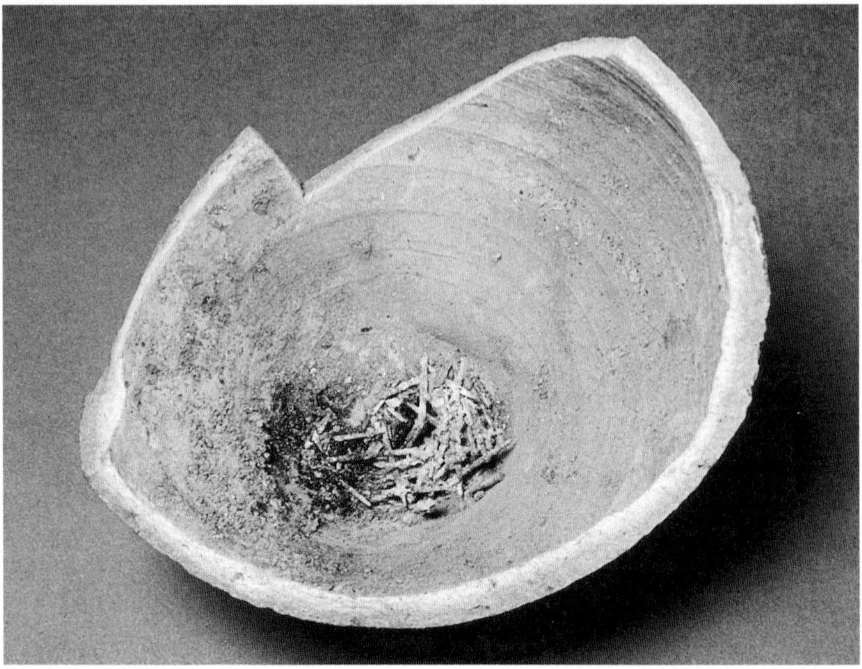

Figure 3.8: Seventeenth-century witch-bottle discovered in Duke's Place, East London, shown with corroded nails. © Museum of London Archaeology Service.

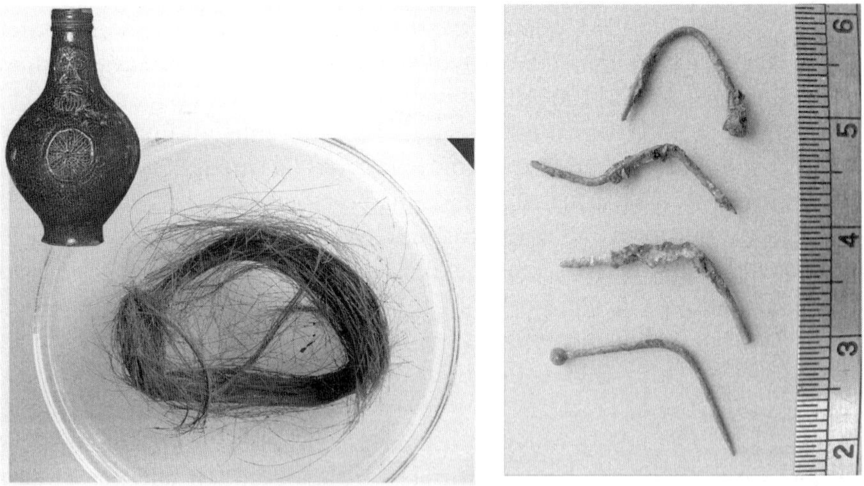

Figures 3.9a and 3.9b: Coil of hair (left) and bent pins (right) from a seventeenth-century witch-bottle (top left) found in Felmersham, Bedfordshire (the lowest brass pin, in a less corroded state, is from another witch-bottle found in Reigate, Surrey). By kind permission of Alan G. Massey and Patrick G. Stone.

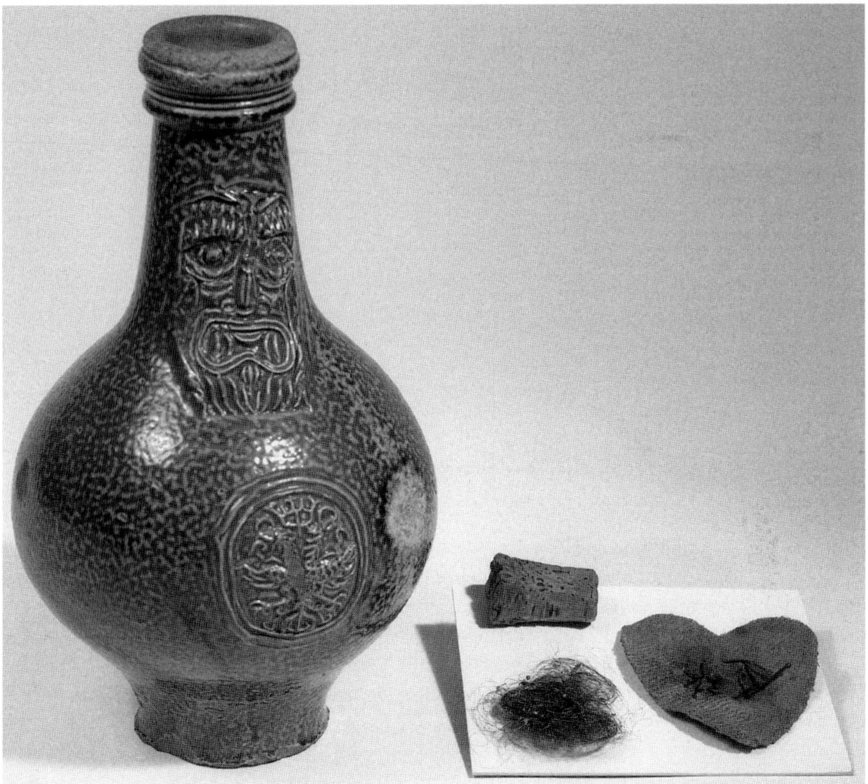

Figure 3.10: Seventeenth-century witch-bottle recovered from a mill-stream near Great College Street, Westminster, containing human hair, nail-clippings and a heart cut out of cloth inserted with pins. Accession number 1910.18.1. Pitt Rivers Museum, University of Oxford.

concealed other enigmatic objects. These were human hair and nail-clippings as well as a heart cut out of cloth (probably made from the victim's own clothing) in which pins had been inserted (Fig. 3.10). An almost identical bottle, fished out of the Thames near St Paul's Wharf, included eleven nails and another heart-shaped piece of cloth with pins.[48] The pierced heart and other related forms of sympathetic magic using pins descends from a long tradition. Among the many instances which survive in the archives is the case of Joanne Harrison whose house was searched by the authorities who discovered a chest packed with a range of bizarre artefacts:

> The Chest being opened, there was first taken out by the Officers all the bones due to the Anatomy of man & woman, and under them haire of all colours that is customarily worne; in the bottome was found a parchment . . . [on which] was coloured (in the purest colours) a heart proportionable to the hart

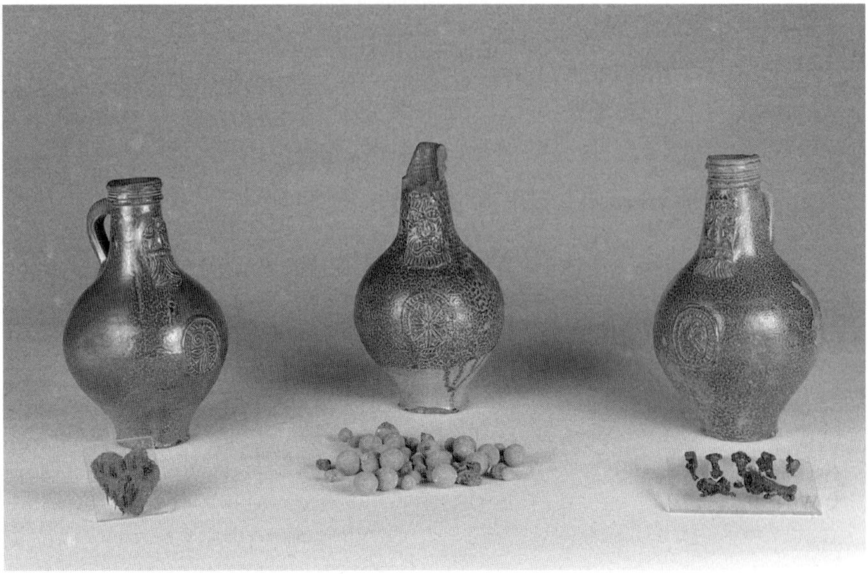

Figure 3.11: Seventeenth-century witch-bottles, displayed with contents of heart-shaped cloth with pins (left) and corroded nails and human hair (right). The central witch-bottle, unusually, contained musket-balls. Norwich Castle Museum and Art Gallery. Photo: David Kirkham.

> of man . . . [and] in briefe the whole joynts and artiers [i.e. arteries] of a man . . . [through which she could inflict pain] by only but pricking the point of a needle in that place of the parchme[n]t, where in his or her body she would have them tortured.[49]

The use of such magical practices may be illuminated by a particularly unusual discovery which has lain hidden among the collections of Norwich Castle Museum. Along with a bottle found in King's Lynn, which contained a heart-shaped piece of cloth inserted with pins, and a bottle retrieved in Norwich in 1950, which had been buried (as most witch-bottles traditionally were) in an inverted position, the castle's holdings produced a bellarmine which concealed a set of musket-balls (Fig. 3.11). It is possible that this was a deliberate use of magical 'artillery' intended to replace that of pins and nails after the civil-war period, from which the bottle may date.[50] What the incorporation of such artefacts suggests is that the idea behind the preparation of a witch-bottle was that the witch's malevolent sorcery could be turned back against its inventor. But how was it thought to work? Among the early accounts of this practice is that by Joseph Blagrave who wrote, in his *Astrological Practice of Physic* (1671), that biological material from the victim was used in witch-bottles:

> because there is part of the vital spirit of the Witch in it, for such is the subtlety of the Devil, that he will not suffer the Witch to infuse any poysonous matter into the body of man or beast, without some of the Witches blood mingled with it.[51]

The witch's magic worked through the infusion of her own corrupted blood and vital spirits in the body of her victim. It was a form of remote poisoning. The extraordinary permeability of the witch's body, with its dangerous excretions, was thus the perceived vehicle of the Devil's power. The fact that the witch-bottle is often found still holding such corporeal remains as urine, hair, nail-clippings and items of clothing, which had an intimate connection to the bewitched party, indicates the sympathetic relation believed to exist between the body of the witch and that of her victim. This makes sense if the natural processes of maternal anatomy were believed to facilitate the dissemination of malevolent magic. Indeed, the witch-bottle was itself perceived as a microcosm of the witch's womb since the use of urine and nails in an upturned vessel was intended to block the witch's own urinary tract, the pain of which would force her to relinquish her magical hold over the innocent party. The witch-bottle therefore symbolically stops up, or obstructs the flow of the 'poysonous matter' thought to proceed from the witch's body. How far this was influenced by the convention of presenting the gravid womb as an upturned flask or bottle in early anatomical tracts is uncertain.[52]

Significantly, blood and vital spirits were, according to the anatomical theorists of the time, the primary agents of the reproductive female body, responsible for the production of breast-milk, menstrual fluid and embryological formation in the womb. Vital spirits in particular mediated the biological connection between mother and child for, as Halkiah Crooke maintains in his *Description of the Body of Man* (1618), the 'Infant . . . draweth not his breath by his mouth, neither doth hee engender any vitall spirits because he draweth them from his Mother'.[53] Similarly, after birth the new-born is fed with the highly 'spiritous' breast-milk which, as John Sadler insists, 'is nothing but the menstrous bloud made whitte in the breasts'.[54] Thomas Raynalde, in *The Birth of Mankynde* (1564), describes how in the process of embryological formation the foetus is fashioned by the mother's 'blood and spirite commixed together' which 'getteth another nature and propertie . . . Even as mettalles and other minerals of the earth'.[55] As we saw in the previous chapter, such anatomical descriptions derive much of their impetus from neo-Platonic readings of the occult workings of nature. For example, in his *Heptaplus*, Pico della Mirandola attempts to uncover the secrets of the 'elemental world' by comparing it to the mechanisms which govern the maternal body:

> [I]f the earth is under the waters and, when irrigated by them, becomes pregnant with what it later brings forth, will not the waters here signify the accidental qualities and affections of matter? By their transient and fluid nature these even have the aspect of waters, moistened by which, as I said, matter becomes pregnant with the form which at the last moment of its time it brings to light . . .[56]

Pico's maternalised anatomy of creation is more than mere analogy. His insistence on the importance of 'accidental qualities' suggests a concept of the autonomousness of maternal 'matter', and the effects which proceed from its 'fluid nature'. Such thinking may explain the persistence of witchcraft beliefs (reflected in the rise of counter-magical practices to which the archaeological record seems to bear witness) well into the seventeenth century, despite increasing scepticism from the likes of Reginald Scot. As the early sciences advanced, such neo-Platonic ideas were given a Paracelsan dimension through the use of alchemical techniques which sought to recreate artificially, in the words of William Newman, 'the materiality of normal female birth'. This was done by combining elements together in glass vials in the belief that, once putrefied, they would behave in the manner of menstrual blood and 'give birth' to a homunculus.[57] Diagrammatic representations of the alchemical union of elements, such as that contained in the fifteenth-century treatise *Opusculum Alchemicum*, gave this process a specifically procreative function (Fig. 3.12). Such ideas provided a naturalised foundation for the powerful remote properties thought to inhere in the primary agents of reproduction. This may explain the peculiar fear of witch's blood which manifested itself in the demonologists' belief that a common ingredient in magical potions was menstrual fluid.[58]

The dramatic destruction in flames, or gradual decomposition in earth of the witch-bottle, filled with matter infected with the witch's own bodily fluids and spirits, was thought to stop up or symbolically obstruct the flow of malevolent agents. It therefore worked in the same way as many of the ritual acts we come across in sixteenth and seventeenth-century accounts, such as the burning or burial of objects belonging to the victim which, when performed by the witch, could cause sterility, physical wasting and finally death, but in the hands of a cunning man or woman could be used to preserve the sufferer by targeting the witch's vital spirits. These ideas were rehearsed dramatically in the space of the court in which women's testimony was mediated by the interpretative demonological machinery which, available to the male legal community who presided over cases of suspected *maleficium*, provided a plausible intellectual rationale for their accusations. A representative example is the trial of Anne Baker of Bottesford, Leicestershire, who was accused

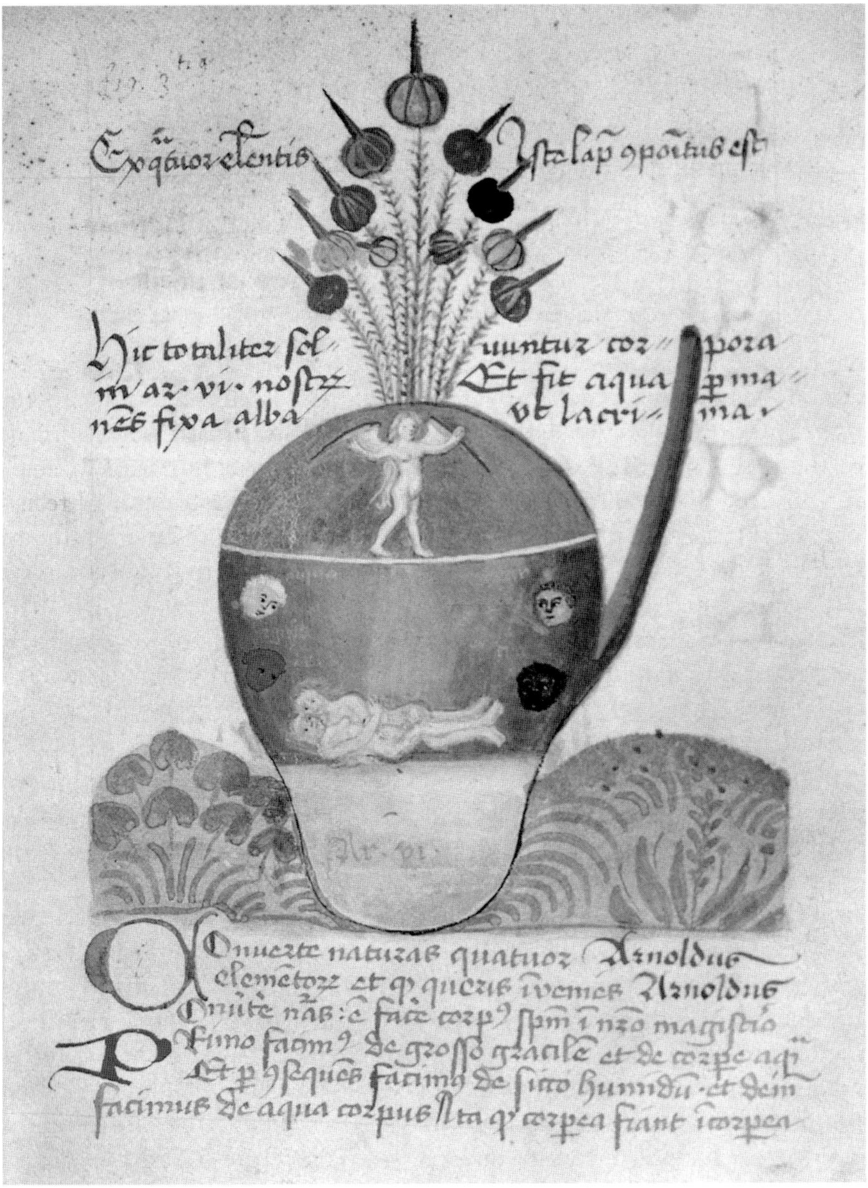

Figure 3.12: Alchemical treatise associated with Arnold of Villanova, *Opusculum Alchemicum*, showing the union of chemical elements, second half of the fifteenth century, Sloane MS 2560, f. 7. © British Library Board. All Rights Reserved.

in 1618 of bewitching a child of Anne Stannidge's to death. Her guilt was proved by her wayward body which had succumbed to exactly the kind of sympathetic magic which underpinned the use of the witch-bottle:

> [B]eing charged by the Mother of the childe, that upon the burning of the haire and the paring of the nailes of the said childe, the said Anne Baker came in and set her downe, and for one houres space could speake nothing; confesseth shee came into the house of the said Anne Stannidge in great paine, but did not know of the burning of the haire and nailes of the said Childe; but said she was so sicke that she did not know whither she went.[59]

That such a means of retaliation was thought possible suggests a common conception that the witch's body possessed the unique ability to extend beyond its own limits, forging an almost corporeal attachment to the recipient of the *maleficium*.[60] The burning or burial of animals functioned in the same way. In 1579 Robert Lathburie of Wimbish blamed Margery Stanton for the demise of twenty of his best hogs, and followed the prescribed magical cure which consisted of burning one 'whereby as he thinketh, he saved the rest'.[61] Likewise in 1593 Robert Throckmorton, a member of an influential family living in Warboys, suspected Alice Samuel of bewitching his livestock. Following the death of 'a very fayre Cowe worth foure markes', he made a 'hole in the ground & buried the same Cowe in it, and threw faggots and fire on her and burnt her: and after that all his cattell did well'.[62] These ideas had their counterpart in the archaeological record too. Just how persistent they were is suggested by an intriguing witch-bottle, probably dating from the mid-seventeen hundreds, which was unearthed in Dorset beneath the remains of the boundary wall which once separated two parishes (Fig. 3.13). It contained an unusual dark-brown glutinous substance which emitted a nauseating smell when opened. Chemical analysis revealed this to be animal fat, probably once belonging to a cow.[63] It is known that during the time in which the bottle was buried cows in the area were stricken with 'distemper of horned cattle', what we might know today as foot-and-mouth disease. It is likely, therefore, that a sample of an infected cow, believed to have been corrupted with a witch's malevolent blood and spirits, was sealed in this bottle and buried under the threshold of the village in the hope that it would protect the remainder of the herd from the same fate.[64]

The relative prevalence of such magical artefacts in the archaeological, as well as textual record, coupled with the chronological duration of the practices they represent, indicate that there was no unproblematic progression from an age of superstition to one of enlightened cynicism. Rather the beliefs that underpinned these ritual acts seemed to

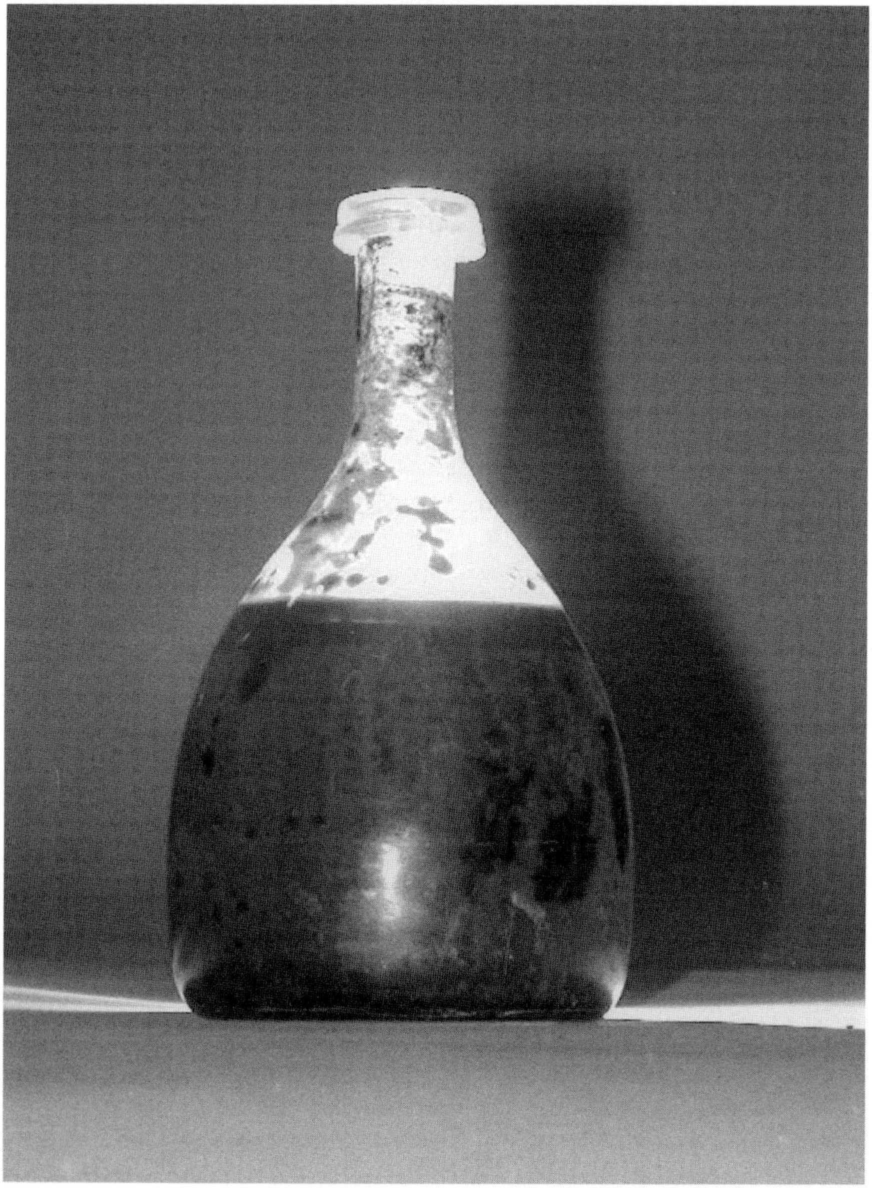

Figure 3.13: Witch-bottle discovered in Dorset, mid-eighteenth century. Courtesy of Alan G. Massey and Patrick G. Stone.

intensify as the seventeenth century progressed, culminating in the bloody reign of Matthew Hopkins.[65] But how could such tragic events have taken place in an age of increasing scientific accomplishment? It was, I would argue, the rise of sceptical attitudes, epitomised in the search for the natural causes of unexplained events, which paradoxically sustained the witch-trial's unique drama of disclosure, a drama in which the laying bare of the female body's maternal products became the necessary precondition for the detection of the witch. While this temporarily energised the search for witches it also laid the foundations for the dismantling of the witch's maternal power altogether.[66] The liminal stage in history which formed the setting for this paradox is bodied forth in Shakespeare's *Macbeth*. Its earliest audiences would have recognised in the magical artefacts which are so much a part of its vocabulary the signature of the demonological discipline which invested these objects with the properties of the witch's maternal body.

Poisoned Chalices: The Reproductive Demonologies of Shakespeare's *Macbeth*

> They say miracles are past; and we have our philosophical persons to make modern and familiar things supernatural and causeless. Hence is it that we make trifles of terrors, ensconcing ourselves into seeming knowledge when we should submit ourselves to an unknown fear.
>
> William Shakespeare, *All's Well That Ends Well*[67]

The paraphernalia of witchcraft, in both its biological and non-organic forms, permeates virtually every scene of Shakespeare's *Macbeth*. Chalices, pots, cauldrons, the accoutrements of alchemy, domestic utensils, the tools of divination, parts of dead animals and human remains are just some of the artefacts presented as posing a potential threat to the integrity of the body and the household through their use as the ritualised conveyors of poisonous substances. The play is carefully structured to make this visibly apparent, staging the circulation of familiar objects in ways which result in their defamiliarisation and mystification. It therefore appropriates the culture which invested material possessions with demonic force, giving dramatic shape to the idea that the same mechanisms which animate the flow of maleficent corporeal agents between the witch and her victim govern the female reproductive anatomy and, in particular, the generation of fluids and vital spirits necessary to procreation and maternal nurture. Characteristic of the play's texture as a whole is Macbeth's own deliberation on the murder of Duncan which encodes the far-reaching, as well as mutually corrupting, influence of such evil acts in maternalised terms:

> We still have judgement here, that we but teach
> Bloody instructions, which being taught, return

To plague th'inventor. This even-handed justice
Commends th'ingredience of our poisoned chalice
To our own lips . . . Besides, this Duncan
Hath borne his faculties so meek . . . that his virtues
Will plead like angels, trumpet-tongued against
The deep damnation of his taking-off;
And pity, like a naked new-born babe . . .
Shall blow the horrid deed in every eye . . . (I, vii, 8–24)[68]

An unsettling reminder of the communion ceremony, Macbeth's 'poisoned chalice' becomes a talismanic object which locates the certainty of his 'deep damnation' in the all-pervasive circulation of plague-infected blood. That its fatal 'ingredience' can be turned ritualistically against – indeed be unwillingly ingested by – the contriver of such 'Bloody' agents is given a corporealised habitation in the ultimate symbol of biological connectivity and dependency; the 'new-born babe'. This imagery amplifies the maternal qualities already attributed to Duncan in the play. Indeed his ability to convey titles and prestige on his subjects is accorded a procreative dimension when he promises he will reward Macbeth for his bravery in battle: 'I have begun to plant thee, and will labour/To make thee full of growing' (I, iv, 29–30). Similarly his desire to 'enfold' Banquo and 'hold thee to my heart', draws the response 'there if I grow/The harvest is your own' (I, iv, 32–4). This ominous echo of the witches' own power to 'look into the seeds of time,/And say which grain will grow, and which will not' (I, iii, 58–9), transforms the crime of regicide that Macbeth will commit in the 'procreant cradle' (I, vi, 8) of his home (against the distinctly maternalised and nurturing body of Duncan), into an extension of the witches' malevolent disruptive influence over the processes of domestic production and fertility.

The witches' mastery over the 'seeds of time', which may in fact indicate the physical manipulation of objects such as leaves, stones or seeds used in the art of divination, is related to their access to domestic objects and organic substances. These include the paraphernalia of food-preparation and charitable distribution, the markers of a fertile and productive home. One of the witches confesses to 'Killing swine' (I, iii, 2), targeting the means of nurture in the family, while another – echoing the charity-refused model of witchcraft – complains that a 'sailor's wife had chestnuts in her lap,/And munched' but refused to share them, believing her to be a 'witch'. This was an affront for which she vowed revenge promising to bewitch her husband, the 'master o'th' *Tiger*', by sabotaging his mercantile vocation and interfering directly in his own bodily functions: 'I'll drain him dry as hay . . ./Weary sev'n-nights, nine times nine,/Shall he dwindle, peak, and pine' (I, iii, 4–23). These are precisely the kind of wasting practices which, as the archaeological evidence suggests, were believed to underpin the use of such objects as witch-bottles and pins, as well as the burial or burning of items of clothing and domestic utensils. The witch boasts that she will use a 'sieve' in order to effect her wicked purpose (I, iii, 8), an apt symbol of the 'drain[ing]' and 'dry[ing]' which may here be indicative of the symptoms of impotence.[69]

As well as condemning the 'use [of] a sieve and a paire of sheeres, with certain words' for magical purposes, Richard Bernard emphasised the need for a thorough investigation, in all cases of alleged *maleficium*, of the closed and secret spaces in which the suspect may have concealed magical paraphernalia: 'search the house diligently, for pictures, or powders, bones, knots, pots, or places where spirits may be kept, oyntments, and for haire cut, books of Witchcraft, or charmes'.[70] It is also perhaps significant that Shakespeare's source for *Macbeth*, Raphael Holdinshed's *Chronicles*, features an account of precisely the kind of domestic demonic magic to which the play tangentially alludes. After 'streict examination' the 'daughter to one of the witches' is made to 'confesse . . . what house in the towne it was where they wrought there mischiefous mysterie'. The authorities, 'breaking into the house, found one of the witches rosting upon a woodden broch an image of wax at the fier, resembling in each feature the kings person' while another 'basted the image with a cereine liquor'.[71] The threat to the patriarchal order which such ritualised objects represent, particularly as they relate to the disruption of sexual potency and fertility, played a central role in the conviction of the suspected perpetrators of such crimes. For example, Margaret and Phillip Flower were granted access to household goods after being 'quickly entertained as Chair-women' under the service of the Earl of Rutland and his wife. Having 'determined to keepe them from having any more children', Margaret, who was responsible for 'looking both to the poultrey abroad and the wash-house within dores', was able to steal a personal possession of the young Lord Henry Rosse in order to bewitch him to death: 'There was a glove of the said Lord buried in the ground; and as that glove did rot and wast, so did the liver of the said Lord rot and wast.'[72]

The sympathetic relation between these acts and the body of the victim they are intended to assault are a particular preoccupation of early modern dramatists. Thomas Dekker's *Whore of Babylon* delineates the motives which underpinned the burial of a rotting piece of 'virgin waxe' and the magical application of pins: 'As this consumes,/So shall shee pine, and after languor die./These pins shall stick like daggers to her heart,/And eating through her breast, turn there to gripings,/. . .

shrinking up her nerves' (II, ii, 207–13).[73] In John Webster's *Duchess of Malfi* the Duchess is confronted with what she thinks are the dead bodies of Antonio and his children and in her despair declares: 'It wastes me more/Than were't my picture, fashioned out of wax,/Stuck with a magical needle, and then buried/In some foul dunghill' (iv, i, 62–5).[74] Similarly in *The Witch*, Thomas Middleton's Hecate alludes to this practice and others of similar ilk: 'Is the heart of wax/Stuck full of magic needles? . . ./And is the farmer's picture and his wife's/Laid down to th'fire yet?' (I, ii, 46–9). As in *Macbeth*, these infernal rites serve as a means of revenge against those women who refuse to share the fruits of their domestic labours:

> Then their marrows are a-melting subtly
> And three months' sickness sucks up life in'em.
> They denied me often flour, barm and milk,
> Goose-grease and tar, when I ne'er hurt their charmings,
> Their brew-locks, nor their batches, nor forspoke
> Any of their breedings. Now I'll meet with'em.
> Seven of their young pigs I have bewitched already . . .
> The dewed-skirted dairy wenches shall stroke
> Dry dugs for this and go home cursing. (I, ii, 51–64)[75]

Like Shakespeare's witches Middleton's Hecate targets human as well as animal reproductiveness, using such enchanted measures as 'skins of serpents', the 'privy gristle of a man', 'needles thrust into their pillows' and 'charmed and retentive knots'. The latter reflects the kind of symapathetic magic that was used in the birthing room to ward off *maleficium* and ease the process of labour: the untying of knots, the loosening of fastenings, the removal of rings and bracelets, and the opening of drawers, the last precaution shown in an Italian childbirth platter of around 1545 (Fig. 3.14).[76] This is reflected in Hecate's use of these bizarre artefacts 'to starve up generation', for once executed 'Neither the man begets nor woman breeds;/No, nor performs the least desires of wedlock' (I, ii, 152–66). Some critics have suggested the possibility that the play alludes to a contemporary scandal involving Robert Devereux, Earl of Essex, who sought a divorce from Frances Howard after accusing her of enlisting the services of Anne Turner, a cunning-woman, in order to inflict him with impotence. When Turner was brought, on 7 November 1615, to the trial which would lead to her execution barely a week later, the evidence deployed to secure a conviction was drawn from suspicious objects removed from her house, including 'certain pictures of a man and a woman in copulation . . . inchanted papers . . . also a figure, in which was written the word Corpus . . . fastened [to] a little piece of the skin of a man'.[77] The court, presented with objects which

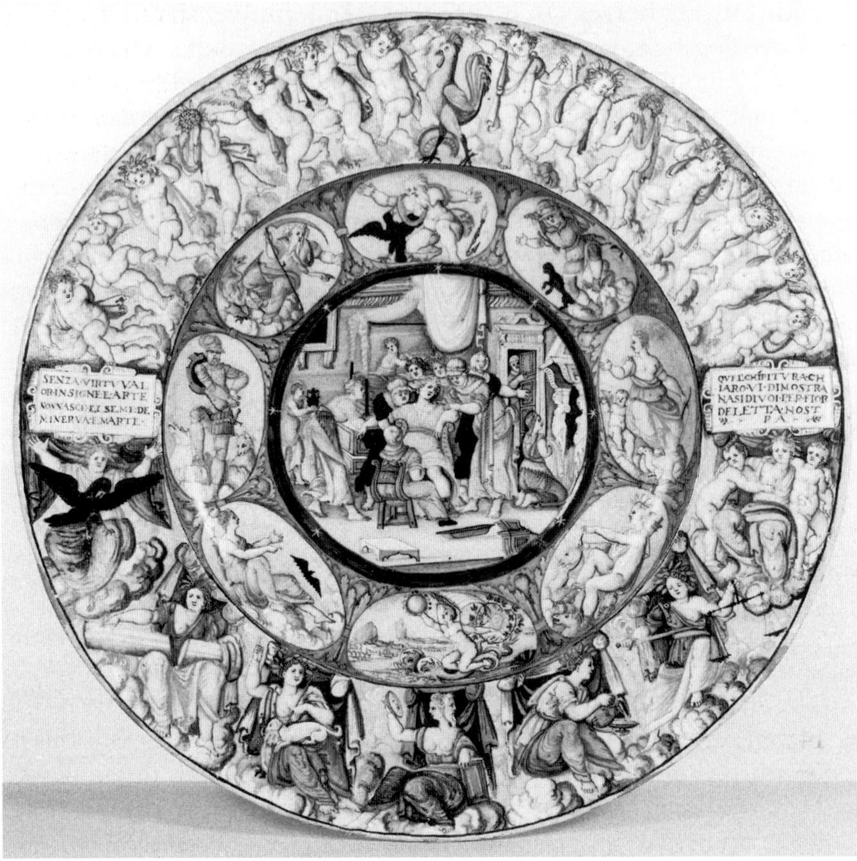

Figure 3.14: Italian childbirth platter, with a central scene in which a woman gives birth, aided by midwives, while another woman opens drawers behind them, c. 1545. © V&A Images/Victoria and Albert Museum, London.

span the erotic and the sacred, is expected to read these enigmatic symbols as confirming the hazardous connection between the objects of witchcraft and the bewitched body, literally the 'Corpus' of the intended victim. With her pernicious arsenal of enchantments, the witch holds the keys to instruments of evil which have the power to emasculate men and drain them of their potency and authority. It is this anxiety which underpins Macbeth's relation to the witches:

> Upon my head they placed a fruitless crown,
> And put a barren sceptre in my gripe,
> Thence to be wrenched with an unlineal hand,
> No son of mine succeeding; if't be so,
> For Banquo's issue have I filed [i.e. defiled] my mind . . .
> Put rancours in the vessel of my peace . . . (III, i, 60–6)

Macbeth's loss of virility, conveyed in unmistakably phallic terms, is associated with the manipulation of talismanic objects which evoke the onset of sterility. The emblems of kingship, materially realised in the 'crown' and 'sceptre', are transmuted into the witches' demonic arsenal. The rituals, therefore, which endow the king with divine authority are made to appear curiously akin to those which invest the witch with her power. The process through which this is effected is presented as being synonymous with the transfer of poisonous fluids ('rancours') into the 'vessel' of Macbeth's mind. This image, taking up Macbeth's earlier reference to the 'poisoned chalice', is not accidental but is intended to accrue demonic significance with the accumulation of the play's many metaphoric references to such domestic receptacles and utensils. Having succeeded in becoming king and queen, the Macbeths lay on a sumptuous banquet which, in its staging, would probably have been accompanied by attendants bearing props such as goblets, ewers and serving dishes; items intended to show the fruitfulness and productivity of the home. Certainly the scene is visibly decked with drinking vessels since Macbeth promises to 'drink a measure / The table round' (III, iv, 11–12), a ritual interrupted by the appearance of Banquo's murderer who is smeared in his victim's blood. Macbeth's witty remark that the blood is 'better thee without than he within' (III, iv, 14), articulates a fantasy of impenetrability – the division of the victim's bodily interior from that of his killer – which is dramatically undermined by the arrival of Banquo's ghost whose haunting presence comes to signify for Macbeth his total immersion in the very substance he thought himself impervious to:

> It will have blood they say: blood will have blood.
> Stones have been known to move, and trees to speak;
> Augures, and understood relations, have
> By maggot-pies, and choughs, and rooks brought forth
> The secret'st man of blood . . . (III, iv, 123–7)

This utterance reflects a governing leitmotif of the play: the idea that the magical relation between the blood or bodily matter of the victim and that of his murderous assailant may be harnessed through the ceremonial use of objects invested with magical properties. As well as enchanted stones and trees, Macbeth refers to a specific ritual of animal sacrifice: the belief that witches or cunning folk are able to divine the future by interpreting the relative positions – what Macbeth calls the 'understood relations' – between the internal organs of eviscerated birds.[78] Whether or not the archaeological instances of sacrificed birds or animals examined in the first part of this chapter, like the Lauderdale chickens (Fig. 3.15), held a similar function, Macbeth's evocation of

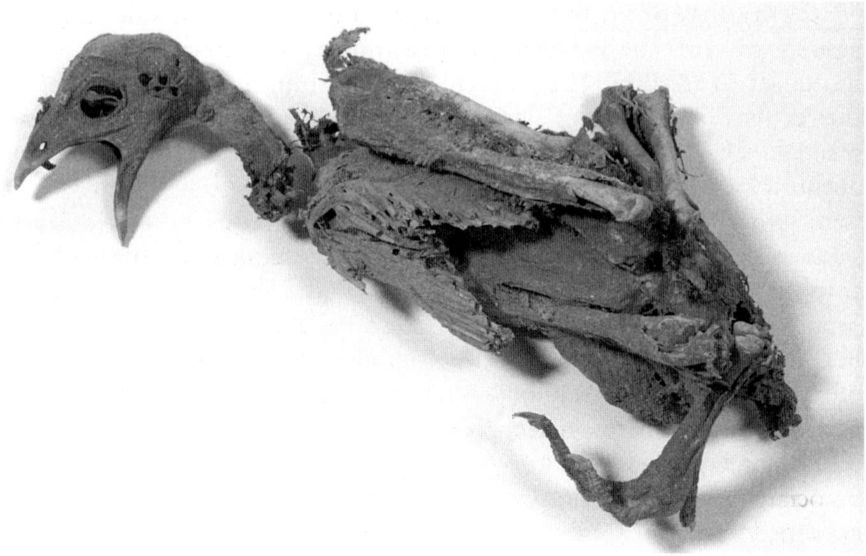

Figure 3.15: Desiccated chicken, late sixteenth or early seventeenth century, part of the cache of concealed magical artefacts found in Lauderdale House, Highgate Hill, London. © Museum of London.

such magical practices ties him to the witches who use animal and human parts for the purposes of divination.

For an audience moving from the banquet's clatter of domestic utensils to Hecate's commanding her attendant witches, just a few lines later, to gather their 'vessels' together (III, v, 18), the juxtaposition would have underscored the notion of witchcraft as a travesty of food production and nurture.[79] The witches go on to mention the 'charmèd pot' into which they throw an assortment of gory ingredients, including animal parts, 'poisoned entrails' (IV, i, 5–9), 'sow's blood, that hath eaten/Her nine farrow' (IV, i, 78–9) and 'three ounces of the red-haired wench' (IV, i, 56). Since red-headed children were believed to have been conceived during a woman's menstrual cycle, the last is particularly indicative of the poisonous matter of the maternal body.[80] That it is through crises in the processes of conception and birth that the witches find fit space to work their 'charm[s]' (IV, i, 38) is suggested by the inclusion of a 'Finger of birth-strangled babe/Ditch-delivered by a drab' (IV, i, 30–1).[81] Macbeth takes up the association between the witches' ritual acts and instances of perverted generation and nurture in his formal invocation: 'I conjure you, by that which you profess,/. . . though the treasure/Of nature's germen [i.e. life-producing seeds] tumble all together' (IV, i, 64–73).

The *conjuring* process which Macbeth hopes will furnish him with knowledge of his dynastic future becomes a type of demonic midwifery as the witches form a magic 'ring' (IV, i, 42) around the cauldron.[82] This is similar to the witches in Ben Jonson's *Masque of Queens* (1609) whose use of 'knots untied' (202), as we have seen the sympathetic precursors to the birthing ritual, heralds their ritualised pouring of 'Both milk and blood' into 'Dame Earth', an act which will make 'her belly . . . ache . . ./Such a birth to make' (232–40).[83] In *Macbeth* the cauldron takes on the symbolic function of the womb, producing a blood-covered infant and tree-bearing child who 'wears upon his baby-brow the round/And top of sovereignty' (IV, i, 102–3). The witches' enchantments once again harness the potency of the paraphernalia of kingship, giving birth to the 'line' of kings who bear the 'two-fold balls, and treble sceptres' which have an almost magical effect upon Macbeth, one which he associates with the paranormally reanimated stopped-up blood-flow of the murdered Banquo whose 'issue [will] ever/Reign' (IV, i, 117–8): 'Thy crown does sear mine eye-balls . . ./For the blood-baltered [i.e. blood-clotted] Banquo smiles upon me' (IV, i, 128–39). The scene forges an unsettling parallel between the witches' ability to cause spontaneous generation and the caesarean birth of Macduff who was 'from his mother's womb/Untimely ripped' (V, vii, 45–6). This also resonates with the witches' slippery rhetoric which gives Macbeth free reign to be 'bloody' since 'none of woman born' can harm him (IV, i, 93–5), an injunction which will result in the spilling of his own blood and the 'crown[ing]' of Malcolm (V, vii, 105). The witches' mastery over the material adjuncts of childbirth (blood and menstrual fluid), becomes indistinguishable from their managed display of the transmitted 'blood' which will guarantee the eventual succession of James I.

The prerequisite for Macbeth's usurpation of power becomes, therefore, the fulfilment of the impossible fantasy of escape from the pernicious influence of the maternal body. Indeed, Stanley J. Kozikowski has argued that Shakespeare may well have been inspired by a contemporary conspiracy, that of the Earl of Gowrie's alleged use of necromancy in order to accomplish the assassination of the then James VI in 1600.[84] In the same year the attempted treason was recorded in *The Earle of Gowries Conspiracie*, a pamphlet which included the testimony of James Weimis which was given on 9 August. Weimis described Gowrie as a 'Nigromancer . . . against the curiositie of nature' who had an interest in the 'Cabbalist of the Jewes', arts which he used in a bid to control the processes of birth and procreation. His desire to eliminate the body of the mother 'that the seed of man and woman, might be brought to perfection otherwise then by the matrix of the woman',[85] is remarkably similar to the alchemical practices which, as we saw in the first part of this chapter, employed the use of incubated vessels for the generation of homunculi from putrefied matter which approximated the properties of menstrual blood. It seems that King James himself, turning crime-scene investigator, was looking for evidence of precisely these kinds of magical props when he searched the earl's pockets and found

> a little close parchment bag, full of Magicall characters, and wordes of inchantment, where in it seemed that hee had put his confidence, thinking himselfe never safe without them, and therefore ever caried them about with him: being also observed, that while they were upon him, his wound whereof he died, bled not, but incontinent after the taking of them away, the blood gushed out in great abundance, to the great admiration of all the beholders.[86]

Gowrie's legally conferred identity as bondman to the Devil in a satanic covenant is sealed by James' disclosing of the material artefacts which act as the guarantors of that blood-pact. The careful scrutiny of the earl's wounds suggests that the corporeal manifestation of the Devil's influence is channelled through the blood and spirits of his earthly vassals, a detail which provides the permissible intellectual framework for the *maleficium* which is now neutralised by the royal presence. Like the magical containers we have been exploring – the witch-bottles with their curious contents – this 'close parchment bag' effected the simultaneous closing or stopping up of the blood and spirits in the body because the physical object was believed to have been infused with these very biological agents. This case may illuminate our reading of *Macbeth* in a number of other ways. There are striking parallels between Gowrie's attempted murder of the king, who was a guest in his own home, and the Macbeths' own rejection of the laws of hospitality. Macbeth expresses his anxiety over this betrayal for he is 'his host/Who should against his murderer shut the door,/Not bear the knife' (I, vii, 14–16).[87] Sermons of thanksgiving, such as John Milwarde's *Jacobs Day of Trouble* (1610), which commemorated James' deliverance from the Gowrie conspiracy, continually resurrected this theme:

> from an enemie? I could then have borne it: But it was thou my *Comes*, my companion and a familiar friend, which did eat at my Table; yea to whom our King . . . enriched, nourished, benefited, honoured them . . . [Y]ea, but to make his Table the snare, and his owne house the slaughter-place, is barbarous and ignoble; and for any man to turne hospitality into hostilitie, is monstrous . . . against the lawes of nature.[88]

Milwarde's obsessive focus on the table and its attendant accoutrements of hospitality illuminates the heavily ritualised nature of domestic paraphernalia in *Macbeth*. In their translated state, as receptacles for the pouring, transferring and stopping up of poisonous fluids and other maleficent ingredients, they represent a breakdown in the idealised political ties which, through the instance of the nurturing King Duncan, come to occupy a space analogous to that of the disrupted maternal function. Indeed, Duncan's body in death seems to recapitulate this very paradigm: 'his gashed stabs looked like a breach in nature/For ruin's wasteful entrance' (II, iii, 115–16).[89] The 'breach in nature', representing the collapse of the social and civic order, results in the birth of 'ruin', an event which is prefigured as a kind of monstrous conception in Lennox's intimation of the 'confused events/New-hatched to th'woeful time' (II, iii, 59–60). Macbeth's belief that he is immune to the crises which any assailant 'of woman born' may visit upon him is undercut by the play's reassertion of the *maternalised* basis of witchcraft in ways which accord with the archaeological evidence we have been discussing. This is better understood if we return briefly to Weimis' account of Gowrie's treason, which presents what may at first seem an odd summation of the earl's necromantic beliefs. As Weimis insists, Gowrie saw his own use of 'Cabbalist' sorcery as being 'no matter of marvel amongst schollers, but that al these things were naturall'.[90] It is precisely this assertion of the ultimately 'naturall' mechanisms which animate the dark arts which works to augment, rather than preclude, the possibility of malevolent sorcery in *Macbeth*.

The witches' ability to drain their victims of their vital, life-sustaining and regenerative bodily essences seems to parallel Lady Macbeth's strange emasculating influence over her husband. And like the witches, Lady Macbeth discloses a desire to determine her destiny through the control of bodily substances; substances associated with the dangerously permeable female reproductive body. Believing Macbeth to be 'too full o'th' milk of human kindness' (I, v, 16), she seeks to contaminate this nurturing material:

> Thou wouldst be great,
> Art not without ambition, but without
> The illness should attend it . . . Hie thee hither,
> That I may pour my spirits in thine ear . . .
> Come, you spirits
> That tend on mortal thoughts, unsex me here,
> And fill me from the crown to the toe, top-full
> Of direst cruelty. Make thick my blood,
> Stop up th'access and passage to remorse,
> That no compunctious visitings of nature
> Shake my fell purpose . . . (I, v, 17–45)

Lady Macbeth imagines herself to be a human vessel filling up with corrupted blood and vital spirits. Her body becomes another of the play's many containers used for the transmission of poisonous matter. As we have seen, for enchanted artefacts to work they must become the conduits for the infusion of the blood and vital 'spirits' of the witch into her victim, and Lady Macbeth proposes nothing less than the pouring of this diseased substance directly into Macbeth. Her relation to the witch is underscored by her invocation to the 'murd'ring ministers' whom she invites, in the recognisable posture of demonic nurturer, to 'Come to my woman's breasts/And take my milk for gall' (I, v, 46–7). As a skilled manipulator of corporeal substances she not only effects the unhindered flow of her polluted matter into those over whom she would have absolute dominion, but also has the power to 'stop up' sympathetically the biological agents most intimately connected with the functions of pregnancy and childbirth.

The proximity of Lady Macbeth's self-translation to the natural causes of the 'illness' to which she alludes is essential to the identification of her malevolent power. As Timothie Bright reveals in his *Treatise of Melancholy* (1586), since the 'purest part' of the blood is responsible for the 'ingendring of spirits' which sustain life, this is most susceptible to corruption and as a result 'that humour which otherwise would yeeld a nutritive juyce, of the best sort, by this occasion is turned into these dregges of melancholie'. He goes on to explain that in sufferers of melancholy this 'aboundance, and *thicknesse* causeth their splene to swell . . . and breedeth *stoppings*, whereby it defileth the whole supply of the humours'. Because the 'melancholicke excrement is . . . drawen of the milte [milk] out of the liver', if produced in 'superfluitie', it can cause an 'obstruction' which 'aboundeth there when it is hindered of such *passage* as nature requireth'.[91] In women this disorder was often directly associated with the various stages which governed the natural life-cycle of the female anatomy during its child-bearing years, particularly in cases when the ordinary course of menstruation was disrupted.

For Reginald Scot accusations of demonic magic could be put down to the 'melancholike imaginations' of middle-aged women, exacerbated by 'the *stopping* of their monethlie melancholike flux or issue of bloud'.[92] It was not only the onset of the menopause which could cause this accumulation of poisonous humours. It also occurred in women afflicted with the melancholy-producing 'greensickness', a disease to which they were not only prone immediately after pregnancy,[93] but from the very earliest stages of sexual maturity. A particularly illuminating instance of this was investigated by Edward Jorden, fellow of the College of Physicians from 1597, who was called upon to provide his learned opinion in the case of one Elizabeth Jenkins who was suspected of bewitching the fourteen-year-old Mary Glover in 1602.[94] Jorden concluded that the young girl was not suffering from the effects of witchcraft but from a medical condition caused by the accumulation of blood, menstruum and corrupted spirits, the so-called 'Suffocation of the Mother':

> Blood is that humor wherewith we are nourished; without which the infant in the mothers wombe could neither grow & increase in bignesse, nor yet live and therefore it was necessarie that those that were fit for generation, should be supplied with sufficient store of this humour . . . [W]here the patients do want those monethly evacuatio[n]s which should discharge theire bodies of this superfluitie . . . [they] have their vaines filled with plenty of blood, which wanting sufficient vent diste[n]deth them in bulck and thicknes, and so contracteth them in their length, whereby the matrix is drawne upwards . . .[95]

The underlying cause of 'the mother' is the same in both young women who have just reached childbearing age, particularly those affected with the greensickness, and in older women who have come to the end of their birthing cycle. An overabundance of blood and spirits which would have ordinarily been voided, or used for the fashioning and nurturing of a growing baby, remain trapped inside the womb, breeding 'corrupt matter', including melancholy, and causing 'the Matrix by consent to impart her offence unto other parts'.[96] While the sceptical attitude to witchcraft espoused by Jorden and Scot depended on the displacement of the witch's demonic agency with the largely autonomous *natural* mechanisms of the reproductive body, it is this widely-accepted belief in the contaminating influence of the womb which, as we will shortly see, came to affirm for demonologists the reality of witchcraft in an age of growing scepticism.[97]

Critics have noted the closeness of Lady Macbeth's invocation to the 'spirits' to contemporary symptomatologies of childbirth and its attendant diseases,[98] but what has not been explored is the relation of these to the play's obsessive engagement with the materials of witchcraft. Lady Macbeth seems to want to hasten the onset of a peculiar moment in the reproductive body's life-stages: when the nutritive maternal function gives way to the corrupted spirits of the enclosed female body.[99] In witchcraft lore this operated in a perverse maternal economy which not only provided the pattern for the witch's relationship with her familiars, but underpinned the actual operation of *maleficium* through the use of enchanted magical artefacts believed to be saturated with these poisonous maternal excrescences. Witches represented a nightmare scenario in which women could control, for their own maleficent purposes, the natural agents of procreation through the mediation of the domestic articles they had most ready access to. Lady Macbeth's ability to temper the very substances which inform the embryological process is akin to that of the witches in that she is able, Macbeth believes, to induce a form of spontaneous birth without the need for the male contribution to conception: 'Bring forth men-children only:/For thy undaunted mettle should compose/Nothing but males' (I, vii, 73–5). The alchemical import of Macbeth's punning reference to the composition of 'metals' resonates with Lady Macbeth's ability to 'stop up' life-giving fluids, or stimulate the flow of poisonous ones, in her foes; a central topos which, in the play's symbolic matrix, is related to Duncan's death which Macbeth reports to Donalbain with the words: 'the fountain of your blood/Is stopped, the very source of it is stopped' (II, iii, 100–1). Donalbain's suggestive response, 'our tears are not yet brewed' (II, iii, 125), picks up on a chain of images inaugurated by Lady Macbeth whose tendency to view herself and others in terms of vessels which can be harnessed through the channelling of fluids, vapours and spirits, is particularly evident in her plan to frame the chamberlains for Duncan's murder:

> his two chamberlains
> Will I with wine and wassail so convince
> That memory, the warder of the brain,
> Shall be a fume, and the receipt of reason
> A limbeck only; when in swinish sleep
> Their drenchèd natures lies as in a death,
> What cannot you and I perform . . . ? (I, vii, 64–70)

The centre of the reasoning faculty in the brains of the chamberlains becomes a 'limbeck'; this is a glass vessel, or alembic, used in alchemy to convey vapours from the heating of chemical substances. Here the article is domesticated through the play's references to the brewing of wine. That Shakespeare associated the limbeck with forms of demonic magic is suggested in Sonnet 119 in which the despairing lover declares: 'What potions have I drunk of siren tears/Distilled from limbecks foul as hell within.'[100] The chamberlains' bodies are thus distilleries for the production of vapours and spirits, and Lady Macbeth's thinking links her directly to Hecate, the witches' ruling deity, whose preparation of ingredients for her own distillery includes 'a vap'rous drop' from the moon which when 'distilled by magic sleights/Shall raise . . . artificial sprites' (III, v, 24–7). That Lady Macbeth's drugging of the chamberlains is reconceived in near-magical terms, as the exchange of contaminated bodily substances, is clear from her insistence that 'That which hath made them drunk, hath made me bold;/What hath quenched them, hath given me fire . . ./. . . I have drugged their/possets' (II, ii, 1–6). The image of the drinking-vessel carrying curdled milk (the traditional recipe for a posset) is particularly indicative of Lady Macbeth's poisoning maternal influence. As with the lover's drinking of the siren's tears in Sonnet 19, the poisoned alchemical substance is remotely shared between victim and assailant. In his poem 'Witchcraft by a Picture' Donne wittily alludes to this process:

> Hadst thou the wicked skill
> By pictures made and marred, to kill,
> How many ways mightst thou perform thy will?
>
> But now I have drunk thy sweet salt tears,
> And though thou pour more I'll depart;
> My picture vanished, vanish fears,
> That I can be endamaged by that art;
> Though thou retain of me
> One picture more, yet that will be,
> Being in thine own heart, from all malice free.[101]

Here Donne refers to such ritual practices as the use of effigies and artificial hearts, as well as the kind of spirit-infused fluids which formed a staple part of love philtres, potions and witch-bottles. By drinking the enchantress' tears he has performed an act of counter-magic, becoming immune to her charms through the ingestion of the vital spirits which contain her feelings of love for him. An ingenious sleight-of-hand turns the lover's body into a bottle in which is contained a magical heart. While this is usually used in witch-bottles as a means of harming the perpetrator of the *maleficium*, it is rendered free of 'malice' because it has been pierced with the speaker's own image. That Shakespeare was aware of the counter-magical properties of bodily fluid is perhaps suggested in *Twelfth Night*:

> SIR TOBY . . . What , man, defy the devil. Consider, he's an enemy to mankind.
> MALVOLIO Do you know what you say?
> MARIA La, you, an you speak ill of the devil, how he takes it at heart. Pray God he be not bewitched.
> FABIAN Carry his water to th' wise woman. (III, iv, 94–9)[102]

While this has almost always been interpreted as a purely medical measure, an opportunity to divine Malvolio's supposed illness through an analysis of his urine, the reference to bewitchment, as well as the archaeological evidence we have amassed, suggests that perhaps what Fabian has in mind is the use of the urine for the fashioning of a counter-magical spell, not unlike that used in witch-bottles. As we will see shortly, such thinking pervades *Macbeth* and is traceable through the play's suggestive imagery of disease which infects on a national scale and seems the horrifying amplification of the contaminated and contaminating body of the 'fiend-like Queen' (V, vii, 99). Lady Macbeth's mental and physical disintegration is met with Macbeth's desire to cure her 'with some sweet oblivious antidote [which will]/Cleanse the stuffed bosom of that perilous stuff/Which weighs upon the heart' (V, iii, 43–4). But the medicalising of Lady Macbeth's condition does not diffuse but rather amplifies the intensity with which the play stages the search for the countermagical measures which will serve as the panacea for the malevolent maternal influence which permeates Macbeth's world.

John Cotta, a physician of Northamptonshire, had it seems a colourful career in the medical profession, one which brought him intimately close to the phenomenon of witchcraft. Writing in 1616 he recalled a particularly memorable patient, 'a right Noble Lady; the cause of whose apparent dangerous estate, divers learned and famous physicions conjoyned with my selfe, could never discover'. The nature of the strange ailment from which she suffered remained concealed until after her death when during 'the dissection of her body . . . her heart was found inclosed with a shining rotten gelly . . . as bigge as a Tenice ball . . . where, in her life, the intolerable paine was seated and fixed'. Had the unfortunate woman been bewitched? Or did her death have a more mundane explanation? Cotta is far from clear as to what he believes could have been the real cause of the fatal affliction, citing the curious episode only as an example of 'the impossibilitie of knowledge unto a Physicion in many and frequent cases'.[103] But rather than signalling the inadequacy of all doubtful accusations of *maleficium* this temporary epistemological crisis becomes the necessary precursor to the disclosure of witchcraft, turning the body and its *natural* biological products into the very wellspring of evidence:

> Many offences also there are, neither manifest to sense, nor evident to reason, against which onely likelihood and presumptions doe arise in judgement; whereby notwithstanding, through narrow search and sifting, strict examination, circumspect and curious view of every circumstance, together with every materiall moment . . . and unto the depth and bottome by subtil disquisition fadomed, the learned, prudent, and discerning judge doth oft detect and bring unto light many hidden, intestine, and secret mischiefes . . .[104]

The malignant forces which are the vehicles of *maleficium* are 'no more inscrutable or hidden from detection in the inquisition thereof . . . then all other intricate or hidden subjects, or objects of the understanding what soever'. This has dramatic, and rather unexpected, implications. The processes which we have come to think of as consonant with the rise of scepticism, the reasoned searching out of material causes, are no less amenable to the exposure of the witch since, as Cotta vehemently maintains, 'Witch-craft is discoverable by sense, and evident by reason.'[105] Such a claim did not spring into the epistemological consciousness in the seventeenth century, however, but was the result of modifications to a much older set of theological paradigms.

In the thirteenth century Thomas Aquinas had made a concerted effort to enumerate the extent of humanity's subjection to the supernatural realm. In his great work of Christian and Aristotelian syncretism, the *Summa Theologiae* (1259–64), he contended that 'God alone can know the thoughts of hearts and the affections of wills', while other spiritual beings merely have access to the operations of the natural world. In the same way as 'physicians can know some affections of the soul from the pulse' both 'angels and the demons' are able to 'examine more subtly the hidden bodily changes' which take place in every corporeal substance.[106] Neither angel nor devil can directly control the human will but, like the physician or anatomist, can influence it indirectly by spying into the secrets of the body. Renaissance demonologists writing after the neo-Platonic school had disseminated its teachings on the occult workings of the *Magicae Naturalis*[107] combined Aquinas' ideas with those of such thinkers as Pico and Ficino; an uneasy marriage which, nevertheless, came to acquire the status of a comprehensive philosophy of witchcraft. Reginald Scot's reputation as arch-sceptic has often obscured the fact that his disquisition on natural magic is dependent upon more orthodox demonological theory, in particular the way in which it can be used as a vehicle for Satan's gradual dominion of the Christian world:

> In this art of naturall magicke, God almightie hath hidden manie secret mysteries; as wherein a man may learne the properties, qualities, and knowledge of all nature. For it teacheth to accomplish maters in such sort and oportunitie, as the common people thinketh the same to be miraculous; and to be compassed none other way, but onelie by witchcraft. And yet in truth, naturall magicke is nothing else, but the worke of nature.[108]

By revealing how these effects of witchcraft 'consist in such experiments and conclusions as are but toies, but neverthelesse lie hid in nature',[109] Scot's forensic disclosures borrow from a contemporary demonological discourse which actually developed in response to a reconceptualisation of the nature of *wonder*. As William Perkins maintained in his *Discourse of the Damned Art of Witchcraft* (1608), although 'Witches may and doe worke wonders', these must be carefully distinguished from a 'true' manifestation of supernatural power:

> A true wonder is a rare worke, done by the power of God simply, either above, or against the power of nature, and it is properly called a *miracle* . . . The second sort of wonders, are lying and deceitfull, which also are extraordinarie workes in regard of man, because they proceed not from the usuall

> and ordinarie course of nature: and yet they be no miracles, because they are done by the vertue of nature, and not above or against nature simply, but above and against the ordinarie course thereof: and these are properly such wonders, as are done by Satan and his instruments.[110]

The 'lying and deceitfull' works of witchcraft are not supernatural at all, but preternatural, deriving from 'hidden causes in nature'.[111] While Scot directly ascribes these acts to the would-be magus or witch, more die-hard demonologists like Henry Holland attributed these 'sathanicall woonders' to the immediate agency of the Devil 'because he excelleth in nature, in swiftnes of motion, and in knowledge'.[112] Perkins agrees that because Satan 'is by nature a spirit' he has 'great understanding, knowledge, & capacitie in all naturall things . . . By reason whereof he can search more deeply & narrowly into the grounds of things, then all corporall creatures that are clothed with flesh and blood'.[113] Although, as Cotta among others insisted, 'the divell is a juggler', the demonologist himself must mimic Satan's role as proto-scientist if he is to defeat his diabolical purpose.[114] The language of demonology thus shared with that of scepticism a concern for recovering the *natural causes* of a witch's apparent power. It is easy therefore to see why bodily fluids and excreta – so often associated with the material artefacts of witchcraft – were given such prominence in the demonological discipline, particularly as they pertained to the legal disclosure of the witch.

In *The Comedy of Errors* Shakespeare gives this a comic twist in Antipholus' insistence that the courtesan is a witch because he finds her desire for a 'chain' to be in keeping with the tendency of 'sorceress[es]' and 'devils' to, in the words of Dromio of Syracuse, 'ask but the parings of one's nail, a rush, a hair, a drop of blood, a pin, a nut, a cherry-stone' (IV, iii, 64–71). Indeed, it is her association with the organic objects – hair, blood, nails – which make up the superstitious rites still in evidence today from witch-bottles and other surviving ceremonial artefacts, that confirm her status as the very epitome of the familiar-nurturing mother-witch, 'the devil's dam' (IV, iii, 49).[115] In *Macbeth* these ideas are subjected to more serious treatment through the forensic scrutiny of Lady Macbeth's body. When the doctor and the waiting-gentlewoman become a secret audience to the sleep-walking queen's 'actual performances' (V, i, 12), 'Stand[ing] close' so that they may better 'Observe her' (V, i, 19), the gentlewoman declines to 'report after her . . . having no witness to confirm my speech' (V, i, 14–17). This is probably not a mere case of modesty on her part but a reference to the strict legal prescriptions which informed the delivery of eye-witness testimony in the judicial process for cases involving witchcraft. William Perkins explained that 'Notorious defamation, is a common report of the greater sort of people, with whome the partie suspected dwelleth, that he or she is a Witch. This yeeldeth a strong suspition.' He does, however, offer a word of caution since 'the Magistrate must be warie in receiving such a report' unless, firstly 'the report be made by men of honestie and credit', and secondly it has, at least, 'the testimonie of two witnesses'.[116] That the doctor takes on an official role as second witness in his capacity as a person of 'credit' is indicated in his readiness to 'set down what comes from her [Lady Macbeth], to satisfy my remembrance the more strongly' (V, i, 31–2). With the correct legal requirements in place he and the gentlewoman are able to begin assessing the corporeal significance of the enigmatic spectacle before them:

> DOCTOR . . . The heart is sorely charged.
> GENTLEWOMAN I would not have such a heart in my
> bosom, for the dignity of the whole body . . .
> DOCTOR This disease is beyond my practice . . .
> Foul whisp'rings are abroad: unnatural deeds
> Do breed unnatural troubles; infected minds
> To their deaf pillows will discharge their secrets:
> More needs she the divine than the physician . . . (V, i, 51–72)

The principles of medical enquiry, which here disclose a 'disease[d]' and 'infected' body responsible for 'breed[ing]' a monstrous and 'unnatural' progeny of 'troubles', do not preclude but actually reinforce the need for 'divine' aid, more befitting cases of suspected bewitchment or demonic possession. Indeed, Timothie Bright laments the 'advantage Satan taketh in this case by the frailtie of the [melancholy-infected] bodies',[117] while George Gifford insists that 'The Divels have power also to infect the humors in mens bodies, and of beasts likewise to bring sores and diseases',[118] for Satan knows the 'naturall causes of tortures and griefe' and all manner of diseases 'in the bodies of men and beastes'.[119] The doctor's diagnosis thus accords with Lady Macbeth's own identification of the 'sightless substances' she had summoned to aid her in her diabolical schemes as agents whose power proceeds from their ability to 'wait on nature's mischief' (I, v, 48–9).

It is this interface between demonological and sceptical attitudes which informs the final realignment of the power structure in *Macbeth*. Symbolically this is bodied forth in a fantasy of decontamination, realised in counter-magical acts which harness the ritualised dissemination of organic fluids and spirits. This is most strongly felt in the play's continuing engagement with the all-pervasive effects of those biological agents most closely connected to Lady Macbeth and the witches: blood, milk, urine and menstruum. Malcolm's nightmare vision of 'Pour[ing] the sweet milk of concord into Hell' (IV, iii, 98) and the thane of Ross' plaintive cry, 'Alas poor country,/. . . It cannot/Be called our mother, but our grave' (IV, iii, 164–6), turn the suffering commonwealth into a maternal body in crisis. The macrocosmic counterpart of the witches' 'charmèd pot', which is at once both hellish womb and receptacle for the fermentation and transmission of maternal matter, the diseased nation is in need of 'the med'cine of the sickly weal' for which Caithness provides the recipe: 'pour we in our country's purge,/Each drop of us' (V, ii, 27–9). The reference to purging evokes again Lady Macbeth's 'stop[ped] up' body, full of contagious contaminants, but deftly suggests a remedy which functions outside the usual parameters of medical prescription. The fact that it is their own blood ('Each drop of *us*') which will form the primary ingredient connotes a sympathetic dimension that resonates closely with those practices we have been exploring, in which the victim's bodily substances formed the basis of potions and spells used to fend off *maleficium*. Similarly, Macbeth's resolution to 'Throw physic to the dogs' (V, iii, 46) is accompanied by his cynical demand that the doctor 'cast/The water of my land, find her disease,/And purge it to a sound and pristine health' (V, iii, 49–51). That this does not merely recapitulate the customary pharmacological application of urine-testing is clear from the play's wider ritualistic vocabulary which locates the antidote for this spread of infected matter – of the 'malady [which] convinces/The great assay of art' (IV, iii, 142–3) – in the 'touch' (IV, iii, 143) of Edward the Confessor. It is he alone who has the power to cure those afflicted with scrofula, 'the disease . . . called the Evil', by employing a potent countermagical measure:

> A most miraculous work in this good King . . .
> . . . strangely visited people,
> All swoll'n and ulcerous, pitiful to the eye,
> The mere despair of surgery, he cures,
> Hanging a golden stamp about their necks
> Put on with holy prayers; and 'tis spoken,
> To the succeeding royalty he leaves
> The healing benediction. With this strange virtue,
> He hath a heavenly gift of prophecy . . . (IV, iii, 146–57)

Drawing on the distinction between a true miracle and a preternatural wonder, the axiom which, as we have seen, formed the first principle of demonology, Malcolm is careful to identify this as a 'miraculous work' in deliberate contrast to the play's other demonstrations of satanic magic. The golden stamp, another of the many ritualised objects which appear in *Macbeth*, is reminiscent of talismans, seals or 'touch-piece' coins

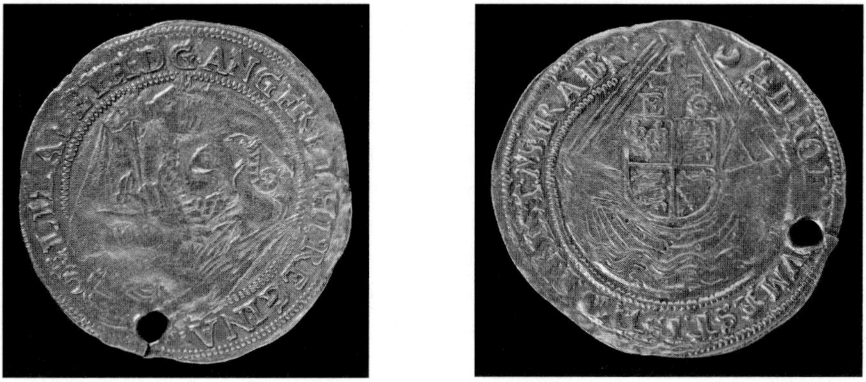

Figure 3.16: Pierced token or 'touch-piece', possibly used in the 'touching' of the King's Evil. Both faces shown. Accession number 1909.60.1. Pitt Rivers Museum, University of Oxford.

invested with magical properties, many of which survive from late antiquity and the medieval period onwards. These artefacts sometimes combined religious iconography, bearing portraits of Christ and the Saints, with a more occult function. They were, in some instances, explicitly translated for ritualistic use, being inscribed with magical characters or pierced, when applied as touch-pieces, probably to allow them to be worn around the neck (as with Fig. 3.16, possibly an Elizabethan gold touch-piece used to cure the King's Evil which shows St George and the dragon on one side and a cross surmounting the Royal Arms on the other).[120] The all-encompassing maternal malevolence of Lady Macbeth and the witches is dissolved by a divinely sanctioned form of counter-magic which, being passed down to 'succeeding royalty' (and, by implication, to James I himself), bespeaks a distinctly masculine parthenogenesis. This is reflected in the precondition that Macduff places upon Malcolm's fitness as ruler: 'the queen that bore thee,/Oft'ner upon her knees than on her feet,/Died every day she lived' (IV, iii, 109–11). Beneath Malcolm's assertion that he is 'yet/Unknown to woman' (IV, iii, 25–6), the self-willed corollary of Macduff's Caesarean birth, lies precisely this implication that the ideal mother of a king is a dead or occluded mother. This is borne out by the play's staging of the transition from the reign of the maternalised Duncan to that of Malcolm, a trajectory which would lead inexorably to the age of James I.

This providentialist unfolding of patriarchal history is, however, disrupted by the proximity we have already identified between the magical materials of witchcraft and those which confer authoritative status on kingship. There is an unsettling symmetry between the Confessor's counter-magical practice and the arts perpetrated by the witches, who have from the play's beginning been associated with the 'gift of prophecy'. The play also implicitly challenges the parthenogenic associations attached to the ritualistic act of 'touching' for the King's Evil by subjecting the magical and 'natural' properties of touch to the scrutiny of one of its most compelling maternal figures, Lady Macduff, who condemns her husband's decision 'to leave his wife, to leave his babes,/. . . He loves us not,/He wants the natural *touch*' (IV, ii, 6–9, my italics). Lady Macduff's complaint restores the maternal to the ideal constitution of both domestic and social order: 'For the poor wren,/The most diminutive of birds, will fight,/Her young ones in her nest, against the owl' (IV, ii, 9–11). Reconfiguring her husband's rejection of the maternal qualities she deems most 'natural' as a political crime, Lady Macduff turns him into a 'traitor' whom she defines as 'one that swears, and lies' (IV, ii, 49–50). This brings him alarmingly close to the type of the equivocator, which in the play is not only associated with the witches, with their doubling pronouncements, but with Satan himself: 'th'equivocation of the fiend/That lies like truth' (V, vi, 43–4). This is given sinister shape in the figure of the 'devil-porter' who, holding the keys to the threshold of the home, turns the domestic space into another of the play's many spectral shadows of the witches' hell-womb:

> [I]f a man were porter of Hell gate, he should have old turning the key . . . Who's there i'th' name of Beelzebub? . . . Faith, here's an equivocator that could swear in both the scales against either scale, who committed treason enough for God's sake, yet could not equivocate to heaven: O come in, equivocator . . . (II, iii, 1–11)

This may be a topical reference to a suspected co-conspirator in the Gun-Powder Plot, Father Henry Garnet, a leader of a Jesuit sect, whose conviction was secured partly on the evidence derived from his book, *A Treatise of Equivocation*, which set out to instruct those professing to the Catholic faith that it is 'lawful to draw words to the sense of thoughts, to cast a mist of error before an eye of single trust' through the use of 'chymical constructions and evasions sophistical' which deceive 'by their distinction of verbal and mental negatives'.[121] But the royalist agenda we would expect such an allusion to fulfil is itself dextrously equivocated. Macduff's status as 'one that swears, and lies' links him to the ultimate traitor, the perpetrator of regicide. But Lady Macduff's critique does not only make him the uncanny doppelgänger of Macbeth. It is Lady Macbeth who mobilises the emotive language of *swearing* in her harrowing vision of infanticide: 'I would, while it was smiling in my face,/Have plucked my nipple from his boneless gums/And dashed the brains out, *had I so sworn*' (I, vii, 55–7, my italics).

There is one particularly disturbing difference between these two swearers, however, and it is in this difference that Shakespeare's ultimate message may inhere. Macduff's professing – his swearing – to the name of father is represented as a lie by Lady Macduff who says of her son, 'Fathered he is, and yet he's fatherless' (IV, ii, 27). Macduff's actions, and by implication the constitution of the lawless and violent patriarchal community he represents, have resulted in the actual deaths of his wife and children. Lady Macbeth's evocation of murderously disrupted maternity, on the other hand, remains a fantasy. It is in fact the worst scenario she can possibly imagine, and its horror lies partly in its being a paradoxical testament to the strength of her maternal instincts and the fidelity of her utterances. In one of Shakespeare's most ingenious dramatic twists Lady Macbeth – the play's most potent vessel for the all-pervasive influence of maternity and its biological functions – becomes a more reliable representative of *truth* than Macduff, the circumstances of whose birth form the symbolic and ideological underpinnings of the new political regime which bases its claim to authority on the rejection of the 'mother's womb' (V, vii, 45).

If Macduff comes to exemplify a parthenogenic mythos which defines itself against a demonised maternity, the measures used to diffuse its poisonous productions reinforce the economy of magical influence that the play has vested in the circulation of the organic materials and ceremonial objects which are the primary props of witchcraft. The play thus deliberately *equivocates* the material adjuncts of *maleficium* with those of kingship, the blood-covered sceptres and crowns, the chalices and talismans, in whose ritualised and 'juggling' manipulation is shown to lie the authority of the king. The ideologically-freighted logic which makes the king's subjects the incorporated members of his divine body is problematised by the demonological epistemology with which it is brought into structural parallel. If the artefacts of witchcraft disclose the remotely-shared contaminating properties of the maternal body's biological agents, the witches expose just how dependent the masculine hegemony is on the analogous 'natural magic' which proceeds from the violent and ritualistic manipulation of the blood, bodily fluids and body-parts of its subjects. The witches are the real archaeologists of the play because they uncover for the audience the buried significance of the materials of kingship. They show us that knowing the witch's maternal body means knowing the fragility of all claims to the authority of political power.

Macbeth was produced within an intellectual framework in which the demonologists' emphasis on the *natural* causes of the witch's diseased body justified the persecution of women but also put under increasing strain the level of corporeal evidence needed to turn suspicion into conviction. James himself, who had during his Scottish reign so virulently persecuted witches, became increasingly interested in the ambiguous sources for the apparent symptoms of *maleficium*.[122] When two young women claimed to have been bewitched in 1604–5, James took a personal interest in their case but rather than pushing for the conviction of the suspected witch he had the women confined and examined by a medical team. That the case had concerned the highest religious authorities is evident in a letter from James Montague to the Archbishop of Canterbury in which he declared that 'the phisitians of Cambridge' have informed 'his Ma[ges]tie that the disease of the maydens is naturall'.[123] A privy seal which tabulates 'the charges of [the] two maydes suspected to be bewitched, and kept . . . at Cambridge for their triall' lists, among other costs incurred, payments made for 'the Appothecaries byll' and 'chardges of phisicke'. An additional sum was also recorded as 'his ma[ges]ties reward to the Phisisians', totalling twenty-two shillings.[124] The dichotomous nature of seventeenth-century attitudes towards witchcraft can be gleaned in a letter which James I penned to Viscount Cranborne, whom the king addresses affectionately as 'My littel beagill'.[125] In it he apologises for having 'bene out of privie intelligence' with him, since he has

> bene ever kept so bussie with hunting of witches, prophetis, puritanes, deade cattis, & haires, yett will I not suffer this bearare, youre fellow secretarie to goe, unaccumpanied with this present, quho shoulde have carried the witches with him as ye desyred, hadde it not bene that he rydes poste, & witches rydes never poste but to the devill, he hath conjured all the devills heir with his welshe tounge, for the devill him self I trow darre not speake welshe . . .[126]

The jocund tone, laden with witty quips and comical stereotypes, is evocative of the kind of sceptical language used by James' old arch-rival, Reginald Scot. This should not, however, prevent us from acknowledging the seriousness with which these issues were taken. James' pursuit of 'puritanes' and witches clearly demands the expenditure of both time and money, comprising a significant portion of his royal duties. We may never be able to recover a context for James' quest after 'dead cattis, & haires', tanstalising though it may be to speculate, but we do know that during this period he was much preoccupied with the supposed bewitchment of one Anne Gunter. Not only did he question her himself, he also enlisted the help of both Jorden and the sceptic Samuel Harsnett who exposed the girl as a fraud after numerous medical experiments.[127]

Though the law officially retained its uncompromising attitude towards witchcraft, harsher penalties having been enforced for the crime upon James' accession to the English throne, this did not reflect the actual rate of prosecutions. Cases continued to find their way into the courts but, as we have seen, what was in effect a new theology of demoniacal agency actually served to increase the burden of proof necessary to secure convictions. As this demonology insisted upon the ever more corporeal nature of the Devil's intervention, the female body – and the materials which were used to harness and disseminate its powers – came under greater scrutiny. The possibility of *maleficium* which the maternal function disclosed thus went hand-in-hand with the gradual dismantling of the epistemologies which sustained witchcraft beliefs. It is no wonder then that Dr William Harvey's intervention in the Lancashire witch trials served to undermine the validity of the witch's mark;[128] that Margaret Russell probably evaded conviction because her alleged victim, Elizabeth Jennings, was rediagnosed by Dr Richard Napier with 'the disease Epileptica Matricis, and Morbus Matricis';[129] that when Joane Harvye tried to break the *maleficium* of Mother Francis by employing the counter-magical measure of scratching, it was she who found herself in court before a group of witnesses, some of whom claimed that 'the mayde counterfeted' while others insisted that 'it was as they thought, some naturall diseaze'.[130]

The suspected witch was not therefore entirely at the mercy of the legal, demonological and sceptical discourses, at the intersection of which she would have stood as she faced her accusers in the court room. Her maternalised body was a potential site of disruption and resistance. Although the horrifying durability of the early modern witch-hunt was due in part to the unique conjunction of demonology and scepticism we have been tracing in this chapter, the centrality of the female reproductive anatomy as the locus of legal *truth*, which found its way into the court room through the materials of *maleficium*, was to prove the catalyst for the eventual dissolution of the intellectual machinery which had sustained its terrible enterprise for so long.

Notes

1. *John Donne: A Critical Edition of the Major Works*, ed. John Carey (Oxford: Oxford University Press, 1990), p. 280.
2. I am grateful to Katherine Ives, general manager at Lauderdale House, for opening the house for me and allowing me to examine the still extant Tudor fireplace above which the items were discovered. Lauderdale House was originally built in 1582 and probably occupied by Richard Martin the younger (d. 1616) who followed his father's profession as master-worker of the Royal Mint. See Peter Barber, Oliver Cox and

Michael Curwen, *Lauderdale Revealed: A History of Lauderdale House, Highgate. The Building, its Owners and Occupiers: 1582–1993* (London: The Lauderdale House Society, 1993), pp. 19–20.

3. Jane Liddle of the London Archaeological Archive Research Centre (LAARC) has discussed with me the prevalence of objects found sealed behind walls for magical purposes and I am grateful to her for her expert forensic input on the Lauderdale chickens. Ralph Merrifield deals with the Lauderdale discovery in *The Archaeology of Ritual and Magic* (London: Guild Publishing, 1987), pp. 129–30. I am especially indebted to Jacqui Pearce of LAARC for her much-valued assistance and our numerous discussions on the subject of witchcraft and archaeology.
4. The Museum of London (MoL) ID number for these finds is L21/1–9. The objects have been broadly dated from the late sixteenth to the early seventeenth centuries and are itemised in the museum's own finds records which Nikola Burdon (MoL specialist services) was kind enough to supply me with. I owe my knowledge of the Lauderdale House artefacts to Hazel Forsyth, curator of the Tudor/Stuart galleries (MoL). June Swann notes that the discovery of another concealed hoard of chicken-parts which included an egg may indicate that the Lauderdale chickens were not buried alive, see 'Shoes Concealed in Buildings', *Costume* 30 (1996), pp. 56–9. The article can be accessed at the website produced by Brian Hoggard, devoted to the archaeology of magical ritual, www.apotropaios.co.uk.
5. As well as listing the superstitious connotations of shoes, Swann records that around twenty deliberately concealed shoes are extant from the sixteenth century and 154 from the seventeenth century: 'Shoes Concealed in Buildings'. See also the Deliberately Concealed Garments Project, run in collaboration with the AHRC and the Textile Conservation Centre of the University of Southampton by Brian Hoggard: www.concealedgarments.org. I am also grateful to Professor Ivor Noel Hume, former archaeologist at the Guildhall Museum, and David Jones of the Ipswich Museum for their input on the significance of concealed shoes.
6. I am indebted to Tim Pestell, Curator of Archaeology at the Norwich Castle Museum, for arranging for the photography of these ritual artefacts as part of a National Trust project to catalogue finds in the castle's collection. He informs me that the cat with the exposed skeleton was discovered in a building (formerly Greene's Bakery) in Upper Olland Street, Bungay, while the other was removed from a building in Norwich. It is not possible to date these finds accurately, but they are likely to be early deliberately-concealed examples as they mirror closely the state of other 400-year-old specimens identified by Alan Massey in 'Spooky or What?', *Period House Magazine* (November 2003), p. 95. Further examples of archaeological finds related to magic and superstition are tabulated in the Dorset Survey compiled by Jeremy Harte. This is available for viewing at www.apotropaios.co.uk.
7. Around 200 early English witch-bottles have been identified, though it is almost impossible to give a precise estimation since a great number of these discoveries remain unrecorded or even unrecognised. See Massey, 'Spooky or What?', pp. 92–5.

8. Richard Bernard, *A Guide to Grand-Jury Men* (London: 1627), p. 213, BL, 518.a.4.
9. Indicative of this is the tendency to define such discoveries as the Lauderdale hoard as merely part of the routine practice of the 'builder's sacrifice' (MoL description for the find). A witchcraft case involving the *maleficium* of Anne Kerke against a child was presided over by one Sir Richard Martin, who had himself indulged in the kinds of ritual counter-magic investigated in this chapter, ordering the cutting of the witch's hair which he attempted to burn (a measure believed to cause pain to the witch thus exposing her guilt). Could this be the same Sir Richard Martin (1534–1617) who originally built Lauderdale House? Martin was Lord Mayor in 1589 and in 1594, just five years before this incident, and his position of influence may well have led to his serving as a 'justice' in important trials. This, if confirmed, along with the findings presented in this study, would suggest that ritual acts, like that reflected by the Lauderdale hoard, constitute more than a 'builder's sacrifice', representing a richer and more complicated social and legal dynamic between victim and witch than has hitherto been understood. For a summary of Kerke's trial, which is recorded in *The Triall of Maist[er] Dorell* (1599), see C. L'Estrange Ewen, *Witchcraft and Demonianism* (London: Heath Cranton, 1933), pp. 189–90.
10. For readings which rely heavily on maternity as a means of interpreting witchcraft, though without extended reference to the material basis of ritual and superstition, see Frances E. Dolan, *Dangerous Familiars: Representations of Domestic Crime in England 1550–1700* (Ithaca: Cornell University Press, 1994); Janet Adelman, '"Born of Woman": Fantasies of Maternal Power in Macbeth', in *Shakespearean Tragedy and Gender*, eds Shirley Nelson Garner and Madelon Sprengnether (Bloomington and Indianapolis: Indiana University Press, 1996), pp. 105–31; Deborah Willis, 'Shakespeare and the English Witch-Hunts: Enclosing the Maternal Body', in *Enclosure Acts: Sexuality, Property, and Culture in Early Modern England*, eds Richard Burt and John Michael Archer (Ithaca and London: Cornell University Press, 1994), pp. 96–120; and Deborah Willis, *Malevolent Nurture: Witch-Hunting and Maternal Power in Early Modern England* (Ithaca and London: Cornell University Press, 1995). One exception to this is Diane Purkiss' *The Witch in History: Early Modern and Twentieth-Century Representations* (New York and London: Routledge, 1996), which incorporates a greater sensitivity to the ritual artefacts of *maleficium*.
11. This question has recently been at the forefront of gender studies. See J. A. Sharpe, 'Witchcraft and Women in Seventeenth-Century England: Some Northern Evidence', *Continuity and Change* 6 (2) (1991), pp. 179–99.
12. W. W., *A true and just Recorde of the Information, Examination and Confession of all the Witches, taken at S. Oses in the countie of Essex . . .* (London: 1582), sigs E8–E8v, BL, C.27.a.2.
13. In his *Astrological Practice of Physick* (London: 1671), Joseph Blagrave explained that a 'way [to reverse *maleficium*] is to get two new horse-shooes, heat one of them red hot, and quench him [i.e. it] in the patients

urine, taken immediately nail him on the inside of the threshold of the door with three nailes', p. 154, BL, 1034.b.23. A related instance of the application of heat can be seen in the use of shoes in the case of Alice Gooderige. Following the demonic possession of their thirteen-year-old son Thomas, the Darling family of Stafford agreed to employ the services of a 'Cunning man' who forced a witch to confess her crimes by 'put[ting] a paire of new shooes on her feet, [and] 'setting her close to the fire, till the shooes being extreame hot, might constrayne her thorough increase of the paine to confesse'. Although the bizarre ritual is defined by the cynical author as a merely practical means of inducing pain, it is probable that the cunning man may have attached some magical significance to shoes when exposed to the heat of a fire, believing, like the many families who had concealed shoes and other items of clothing behind walls or near to fire-places during this period, that they had some special power over the witch, *The most wonderfull and true storie, of a certaine Witch named Al[i]se Gooderige of Stapen hill* . . . (London: 1597), pp. 24–5, Lambeth Palace Library, (zz)1597.15.

14. *A Detection of Damnable Driftes, practized by three Witches arraigned at Chelmisforde in Essex* . . . (London: 1579), sigs A8–A8v, BL, C.27.a.8.
15. BL, Sloane MS 3853, f. 51v. For more on this manuscript and on the use of necromancy, see Richard Kieckhefer, *Magic in the Middle Ages* (Cambridge: Cambridge University Press, 1989), pp. 151–75.
16. *A Detection of Damnable Driftes*, sig. A7v.
17. The Cade House knives date from the late sixteenth to the early seventeenth centuries. Merrifield, *The Archaeology of Ritual and Magic*, p. 162.
18. *The Examination and Confession of certaine Wytches at Chensforde in the Countie of Essex* (London: 1566), sig. B1v, Lambeth Palace Library, (zz)1587.12.03.
19. *The Apprehension and confession of three notorious Witches. Arreigned and by Justice condemned and executed at Chelmes-forde, in the Countye of Essex* . . . (London: 1589), sig. A4, Lambeth Palace Library, (zz)1597.15.03.
20. Reginald Scot, *The Discoverie of Witchcraft* (London: 1584), pp. 7–8, BL, G.19129.
21. Ibid., Epistle to Sir Thomas Scot, sig. A6v.
22. Keith Thomas, *Religion and the Decline of Magic: Studies in Popular Beliefs in Sixteenth- and Seventeenth-Century England* (Harmondsworth: Penguin, 1971), pp. 660–7, and Alan MacFarlane, *Witchcraft in Tudor and Stuart England: A Regional and Comparative Study* (New York and London: Routledge, 1970), pp. 105, 196–7 and 206. For a summary of the 'Macfarlane-Thomas paradigm' as well as some of the challenges to it, see James Sharpe, *Witchcraft in Early Modern England* (London: Longman, 2001), pp. 12 and 36–42, and Stuart Clark's introduction to *Languages of Witchcraft: Narrative, Ideology and Meaning in Early Modern Culture* (London: Macmillan Press, 2001), pp. 5–6.
23. William Crompton, *A Lasting Jewell for Religious Women* . . . (London: 1630), p. 9, BL, 4903.cc.46. See also Thomas Tusser, *A Hundreth Good Points of Husbandrie, Lately Maried unto a Hundrethe Good Points of Huswifry* . . . (London: 1571), p. 28, BL, G.11233. For more sermons

dealing with issues of charity, see *Three Sermons or Homelies, To Move Compassion towards the Poor and Needie in these Times* (London: 1596), BL, 4479.bb.37; Henry Bedel, *A Sermon Exhortyng to Pitie the Poore . . .* (London: 1572), BL, C.142.cc.4; and Robert Allen, *The Odifferous Garden of Charitie* (London: 1603), BL, Huth 53.

24. William Gouge, *Of Domesticall Duties* (London: 1622), pp. 264–5, BL, 722.i.23.
25. John Downame, *The Plea of the Poore. Or a Treatise of Beneficence and Almes-Deeds* (London: 1616), p. 118, BL, 873.h.3.
26. Ibid., pp. 103 and 125.
27. Ibid., p. 39.
28. Gervase Markham, *Countrey Contentments, or the English Huswife . . .* (London: 1623), pp. 2–3, BL, 7074.c.31.
29. Miles Coverdale, *The Christian State of Matrimony* (1543), quoted in Natasha Korda, *Shakespeare's Domestic Economies: Gender and Property in Early Modern England* (Philadelphia: University of Pennsylvania Press, 2002), p. 28. Korda discusses the idea propounded in Renaissance conduct manuals that a woman should 'mother' the household goods, pp. 28–38.
30. Downame, *The Plea of the Poore,* p. 38.
31. *A Detection of Damnable Driftes*, sig. A6v.
32. The earliest manuscript accounts and iconographical renderings of witchcraft focus upon the heretical dimensions of the crime rather than its potential to harm the family. See, for example, the *Chroniques de France ou de Saint Denis*, composed some time in the second quarter of the fourteenth century, BL, Royal MS 16 G. VI. The popular image of witchcraft circulated by Dürer and Grien derives largely from texts like Johannes Nider's *Formicarius* (c. 1435–7), a work which influenced the composition of what was to become the standard sourcebook of witch-beliefs on the continent: the *Malleus Maleficarum*, which was published in 1487. In the same year Ulrich Molitor crystallised the teachings of the *Malleus* in pictorial form in the first printed book to contain illustrations of witches, the *Des Sorcerieres et des devineresses*. For a detailed study of the changing iconography of the witch see Jane P. Davidson, *The Witch in Northern European Art, 1470–1750* , Science and Research, vol. 2, (Freren: Luca Verlag, 1987).
33. *The Examination and Confession of certaine Wytches at Chensforde*, sigs A5–A5v.
34. Thomas Potts, *The Wonderfull Discoverie of Witches in the Countie of Lancaster* (London: 1613), sig. R3v, BL, C.27.b.37. For a similar account of the maternalised feeding of witch-familiars in a domestic setting see *A Rehearsall both straung and true, of hainous and horrible actes committed by Elizabeth Stile, Alias Rockingham, Mother Dutten, Mother Devell, Mother Margaret, Fower notorious Witches, apprehended at Winsore . . .* (London: 1579), sig. Av, BL, C.27.a.11.
35. Perkins, *A Discourse of the Damned Art of Witchcraft . . .* (Cambridge: 1608) p. 193, BL, 1607/788.(1).
36. Edward Fairfax, *A Discourse of Witchcraft as it was Acted in the Family of M[aste]r Edward Fairfax*, 1621–3, BL, additional MS 32496, f. 21v.
37. See Clive Holmes, 'Women: Witnesses and Witches', *Past and Present* 140 (August 1993), pp. 45–78. Also see David Harley's, 'Historians as

Demonologists: The Myth of the Midwife-Witch', *Social History of Medicine* 3 (1990), pp. 1–26, which counters Thomas R. Forbes' identification of the midwife as witch in his 'Midwifery and Witchcraft', *Journal of the History of Medicine* 17 (1962), pp. 264–83.

38. *The examinac[i]on of Edmund Robinson . . . of Pendle Forrest*, 10 Feb. 1633, BL, additional MS 36674, ff. 193–3v.
39. *The Examinac[i]on & voluntary confession of Margret Johnson of Marsden*, 9 March 1633, BL, additional MS 36674, f. 196.
40. *The offenders condemned & accused for witch craft w[i]th their markes at their Attainder*, 1633, a list of the so-called Lancaster Witches, BL, additional MS 36674, f. 199.
41. *The most wonderfull and true storie, of a certaine Witch named Al[i]se Gooderige*, sigs B2v–B3.
42. *The most strange and admirable discourse of the three Witches of Warboys . . .* (London: 1593), sig. O3v, BL, G.2393.
43. The cite code for the bottle is Duk 77 Context 2. I have inspected the bottle (which probably dates from the second half or last quarter of the seventeenth century) and its contents myself and noted that, among the smaller remains which were cleared out and stored separately after its discovery, there appeared to be fragments of bone. But whether these were part of its original contents or merely accidental additions is impossible to ascertain. For more on this particular discovery see Catherine Maloney, 'A Witch-Bottle from Dukes Place, Aldgate', *Transactions of the London & Middlesex Archaeological Society* 31 (1980), pp. 157–8. Jacqui Pearce and Lyn Blackmore of LAARC have kindly given me their own unpublished research notes, from J. Schofield and R. Lear, *Holy Trinity Priory, Aldgate, City of London: An Archaeological Reconstruction and History*, MoLAS Monogr Ser, forthcoming.
44. For more on Suffolk witch-bottles see Ralph Merrifield and Norman Smedley, 'Two Witch-Bottles from Suffolk', *Proceedings of the Suffolk Institute of Archaeology* 28 (1958–60), pp. 97–101 and Norman Smedley and Elizabeth Owles, 'More Suffolk Witch-Bottles', *Proceedings of the Suffolk Institute of Archaeology* 30 (1964–6), pp. 84–93.
45. For more on Fretchen-ware and its use in England, see David Gaimster, *German Stoneware 1200–1900* (London: British Museum Press, 1997).
46. On the significance of this bearded-face decoration and its relation to the witch, see Ralph Merrifield, 'Folk-Lore in London Archaeology, Part 2: The Post-Roman Period', *London Archaeologist* 2 (1969), p. 102.
47. The presence of urine in the bottle was indicated by infrared spectroscopic examination which disclosed traces of sulphate, nitrate, chloride, carbonate and phosphate anions. Dr Alan Massey, honorary fellow of the Department of Chemistry, Loughborough University, has kindly provided me with his own unpublished reports on the discovery, and the results of the chemical analyses conducted on its contents, including Alan Massey, *The Bedfordshire Witch Bottle: A Preliminary Report*, and Alan Massey, Brian Hoggard, Patrick Stone, Andrew Wilson, *The Felmersham Witch Bottle* (the latter text has since been published in *Bedfordshire County Life Magazine* (2004), pp. 7–8).

48. The ID number for the St Paul's Wharf bottle is 18013. The MoL finds records, supplied by Meriel Jeater, Assistant Curator in Early Finds, give a broad date of 1550–1700. This is because some of the contents may have an earlier date, while the bottle itself could date from around the mid-to-late seventeenth century. Many of the bottles found in East Anglia were located in thresholds, under doors in particular. Professor Ivor Noel Hume has informed me that he has a witch-bottle in his personal collection which he discovered in a cottage in Stratford St Mary, Suffolk, beneath the kitchen hearth, the very heart of early modern domestic production. See also Merrifield's extensive analysis of witch-bottles in *The Archaeology of Ritual and Magic*, pp. 163–75.
49. *The most cruell and bloody murther committed by an Inkeepers Wife, called Annis Dell . . . With the severall Witchcrafts, and most damnable practises of one Johane Harrison and her Daughter* (London: 1606), sigs C2v–C3, BL, C.27.c.28.
50. The accession number for the bottle found in King's Lynn (beneath the threshold of the Plough Inn, Kings Street) is 1932.19, while that for the Norwich bottle is 1950.98. The bottle with the musket balls has no recorded accession number (thanks are again due to Tim Pestell for supplying me with photographs of, and historical information about, these bottles). Another interesting instance is a witch-bottle found in a pit in High Street, Guildford, for which Jacqui Pearce has provided me with copies of the preliminary conclusions of the scientific analysis conducted by Lisa Gray (MoL Specialist Services). The bottle contained a pin and fragments of cloth and printed paper (once comprising a magical charm?) as well as some mysterious 'charred remains', *Assessment of Bottle Contents from a pit, High Street, Guildford, TVAS, HSG 01/08 TS, SU 99600 49490*, unpublished.
51. *Blagraves Astrological Practice of Physick*, p. 155.
52. See, for example, Wellcome Library, Western MS 49 *Apocalypse*, c. 1420, f. 37v, which includes an image showing a row of flasks containing foetuses and a diagrammatic figure of the matrix in which the base of the womb is presented as a fluid-filled upturned glass bottle.
53. *A Description of the Body of Man* (London: 1618), p. 267, BL, 781.k.1.
54. *The Sicke Womans Private Looking-Glasse* (London: 1636), p. 8, BL, 1175.a.7.
55. *The Birth of Mankynde, otherwyse named the Womans Booke* (London: 1564), f. 15, BL, 1177.h.1.
56. Pico della Mirandola, *On the Dignity of Man, On Being and the One, Heptaplus*, trans. Charles Glenn Wallis, Paul J. W. Miller and Douglas Carmichael (Indianapolis: Hackett Publishing Company, 1965), pp. 87–8.
57. William Newman, 'The Homunculus and his Forebears: Wonders of Art and Nature', in *Natural Particulars: Nature and the Disciplines in Renaissance Europe*, eds Anthony Grafton and Nancy Siraisi (Cambridge and London: MIT Press, 1999), p. 336.
58. For more on the association between menstruum and *maleficium*, see Christina Larner, *Enemies of God: The Witch-Hunt in Scotland* (Edinburgh: John Donald, 1981), p. 93.

59. *The wonderful discoverie of the Witchcrafts of Margaret and Phillip Flower* . . . (London: 1619), sigs D4v–E, BL, C.27.b.35.
60. For instances of the use of counter-magic or 'unwitching' in the birthing room see W. W., A true and just . . . *Confession of all the Witches, taken at S. Oses*, sig. A2, and the case of Barbara Napier, one of the accused North Berwick witches, who was found 'culpable and convi[c]tt[ed] of the seeking of consulta[io]n fr[o]m Annie Sampson ane wit[c]h for the help of Dame Jeane Lyon lady angus to keep her fr[o]m vomiet[in]g quhen sche was in br[ee]ding of bairne [i.e. when she was pregnant]': Court minutes (dittays) of the examination and confession of Barbara Napier, National Archives of Scotland, JC2/2, *Book of Adjournal*, 8–10 May 1591, f. 213. Agnes Sampson, herself a cunning woman, helped another suspected witch, Euphame MacCalzean, at the time of her birth by allegedly placing graveyard earth beneath her bed as a magical means of minimising labour pains. For the latter, see also Lawrence Normand and Gareth Roberts, *Witchcraft in Early Modern Scotland: James VI's Demonology and the North Berwick Witches* (Exeter: University of Exeter Press, 2000), p. 241. In his case-study of the practice-notes of Dr Richard Napier, Michael MacDonald estimates that more than 500 of the Renaissance physician's patients believed themselves to have been bewitched. This included a large number of women, some of whom thought they had been affected by *maleficium* after failing to invite a female neighbour to a childbirth or lying-in, Bodleian Library MSS: Ash. 224, ff. 124v, 171 (Bower); Ash. 198, ff. 53, 76, 83 (Baneberry); Ash. 227, f. 119 (Whitting); Ash. 230, f. 26 (Boddington); Ash. 414, f. 200v (Cock). Joan Brytton suspected that her barrenness was caused by witchcraft and asked Napier for a magical amulet as a form of protection (Ash. 238, f. 159), *Mystical Bedlam* (Cambridge: Cambridge University Press, 1981), pp. 107–9.
61. *A Detection of Damnable Driftes*, sig. B1.
62. *The most strange and admirable discourse of the three Witches of Warboys*, sig. O2.
63. The substance comprised a series of long-chain fatty acids, characteristic of animal fat, and this was confirmed by a nuclear magnetic resonance (NMR) study. See Alan Massey, Roger M. Smith, and Tim A. D. Smith, 'A Witch Bottle from Dorset', *Education in Chemistry* (July 2003), pp. 97–100. I am immensely grateful to Alan Massey for providing me with photographs and scientific data on the many witch-bottles he has investigated.
64. I am also grateful to Brian Hoggard for supplying me with information about a similar seventeenth-century bottle discovered below a hearth in Exton, Rutland, which contained traces of animal and human hair, plant extractives and animal fat. I further owe to Brian knowledge of witch-bottles discovered in Reigate, Surrey (a bellarmine dated to c. 1600) and Stratford St Mary (dated to c. 1620). The latter was discovered beneath the hearth of a cottage in Goose Acre and contained sprigs of blackthorn, nails and urine. Details of this can be found in I. A. W. Bunn, ' "A Devil's Shield": Notes on Suffolk Witch-Bottles', *Lantern* 39 (Autumn 1982), pp. 3–7.
65. On Matthew Hopkins, see Malcolm Gaskill, *Witchfinders: A Seventeenth-Century English Tragedy* (London: John Murray, 2005).

66. This was accelerated by the gradual replacement of neo-Platonic and humoral theories, which had provided the intellectual scaffolding for the belief in the efficacy of the witch's biological agents, with the discoveries of Harveian science. Harvey published his theory of the circulation of the blood in his *Exercitatio Anatomica De Mortu Cordis et Sanguinis in Animalibus* in 1628, but it was not until the late seventeenth century that his ideas became widely disseminated enough to have a decisive impact on witch-lore. Harvey discovered the female ovum in 1651 and Robert Boyle's *Memoirs for the Natural History of Humane Blood* presented an alternative to the humoral theory of blood in 1684. See Gail Kern Paster, *The Body Embarrassed: Drama and the Disciplines of Shame in Early Modern England* (Ithaca and London: Cornell University Press, 1993), pp. 17 and 66–7.
67. II, iii, 1–5. *The Norton Shakespeare*, eds Stephen Greenblatt et al. (New York and London: W. W. Norton and Company, 1997).
68. All quotations from the play are taken from Shakespeare, *Macbeth*, ed. Nicholas Brooke (Oxford: Oxford University Press, 1990).
69. It is possible that Shakespeare was familiar with the notorious North Berwick witch-hunts and incorporated elements of them into *Macbeth*. A pamphlet which reported the scandalous trial reveals the attempted murder of James VI of Scotland by the witches who, it was claimed, had caused a storm in order to wreck his sailing ship. In another echo of *Macbeth*, the witches are described as travelling 'by Sea each one in a Riddle or Cive [sieve]'. The witches' ability to pervert the traditional practices of birth, fertility and legitimacy are underscored by their use of magical paraphernalia, since they 'tooke a Cat and christened it, and afterward bound to each parte of that Cat, the cheefest partes of a dead man, and severall joynts of his bodie': *Newes from Scotland, Declaring the damnable life and death of Doctor Fian* (London: 1591–2), sigs A3–A4v-C, Lambeth Palace Library, (zz)1597.15.04. For more on the case, see the court minutes (dittays) of the examination and confession of Doctor John Fian, alias Cunningham, JC2/2, *Book of Adjournal*, 26 December 1590, National Archives of Scotland, Edinburgh.
70. *A Guide to Grand-Jury Men*, pp. 213 and 234, BL, 518.a.4.
71. *Narrative and Dramatic Sources of Shakespeare*, vol. 7, ed. Geoffrey Bullough (London: Routledge and Kegan Paul, 1973), pp. 479–80.
72. *The wonderful discoverie of the Witchcrafts of Margaret and Phillip Flower . . .*, sigs D2, C2v, C3v and Ev.
73. Thomas Dekker, *The Whore of Babylon: A Critical Edition*, ed. Marianne Gateson Riely (New York and London: Garland Publishing, 1980).
74. John Webster, *The Duchess of Malfi and Other Plays*, ed. René Weis (Oxford: Oxford University Press, 1996).
75. *Three Jacobean Witchcraft Plays: The Tragedy of Sophonisba; The Witch; The Witch of Edmonton*, eds Peter Corbin and Douglas Sedge (Manchester and New York: Manchester University Press, 1986).
76. Victoria and Albert Museum, Mus. no. C2223-1910.
77. 'The Trial of Anne Turner, Widow, at the King's-Bench, the 7th of November, for the Murder of Sir Thomas Overbury . . . 1615', in *Cobbett's Complete Collection of State Trials and Proceedings for High*

Treason and other Crimes 1603–1627, ed. T. B. Howell (London: 1809), vol. 2 pp. 932–3. See also 'The Trial of the Lady Frances Countess of Somerset, the 24th of May, for the Murder of Sir Thomas Overbury . . . 1616', ibid., pp. 951–66. For more on this case see Purkiss, *The Witch in History*, pp. 215–22.

78. See corresponding footnote in Brooke's Oxford edition of the play.
79. This would have gained a special visual impetus if the same props that graced the banquet table were also used to supply the witches with their own demonic paraphernalia.
80. The effects of menstrual blood on the development of the foetus are discussed in more detail in relation to Caliban in the second chapter of this study.
81. For an instance in which a crisis in the birthing room triggers the use of a 'charme', see the example of Agnes Bowker who allegedly gave birth to a monstrous cat: BL, Lansdowne MS 101, f. 22. The case is also described in David Cressy's *Travesties and Transgressions in Tudor and Stuart England* (Oxford: Oxford University Press, 2000).
82. For a masterly account of the relationship between midwifery and witchcraft which incorporates *Macbeth*, see Caroline Bicks, *Midwiving Subjects in Shakespeare's England* (Aldershot: Ashgage, 2003), pp. 126–60.
83. *Court Masques*, ed. David Lindley (Oxford: Oxford University Press, 1995).
84. Stanley J. Kozikowski, 'The Gowrie Conspiracy against James VI: A New Source for Shakespeare's *Macbeth*', *Shakespeare Studies* 13 (1980), pp. 197–212. Shakespeare's familiarity with the attempted treason seems likely as its events were dramatised in a (now lost) play in December 1604, staged by the King's Players.
85. *The Earle of Gowries Conspiracie against the Kings Majestie of Scotland* (London: 1600), sigs C3v–C4, BL, G.5126.
86. Ibid., sig. C2v.
87. For the importance of the early modern conception of hospitality, see Felicity Heal, 'The Idea of Hospitality in Early Modern England', *Past and Present* 102 (February 1984), pp. 66–93.
88. John Milwarde, *Jacobs Day of Trouble, and Deliverance. A Sermon preached at Pauls Crosse, the fifth of August 1607. upon his Majesties Deliverance from the Earle of Gowries Treason and Conspiracie* (London: 1610), sigs F2v–F3v, BL, 4479.bb.33.
89. Like Spenser's allegorical description of the house of Alma in *The Faerie Queene* whose 'fowle and wast' matter is ejected from the body by being 'close convaid, and to the back-gate brought' (ed. A. C. Hamilton (London and New York: Longman, 1977), II, ix, 32), Duncan's blood, the 'life o'th' building' (II, iii, 71), runs through a 'wasteful entrance', an image which is at once scatological and gynaecological. Alice Fox associates the passage's repetition of breach/breeched with a network of imagery connoting the 'bloody circumstance' of a breech birth, 'Obstetrics and Gynecology in Macbeth', *Shakespeare Studies* 12 (1979), p. 135.
90. *Gowries Conspiracie*, sig. C3v.
91. Timothie Bright, *A Treatise of Melancholy* . . . (London: 1586), pp. 25, 31–2 and 181 (my italics), BL, C.95.b.30.

92. Reginald Scot, *The Discoverie of Witchcraft*, pp. 54–8 (my italics).
93. In the Renaissance a woman who had just given birth and been sequestered during her lying-in was known as a 'green woman'. This was because the period before her churching would have been seen as a time when she was most susceptible to the 'greensickness', before the normal resumption of the menstrual cycle. See David Cressy, *Birth, Marriage and Death: Ritual, Religion, and the Life-Cycle in Tudor and Stuart England* (Oxford: Oxford University Press, 1999), p. 203, and by the same author, 'Purification, Thanksgiving and the Churching of Women in Post-Reformation England', *Past and Present* 141 (1993), pp. 106–46. On the relation between melancholy and 'the green-sickness' which 'often happeneth to young women' see Robert Burton, *The Anatomy of Melancholy*, ed. Holbrook Jackson (New York: New York Review Books, 2001), Part 3, p. 133.
94. Michael MacDonald, *Witchcraft and Hysteria in Elizabethan London: Edward Jorden and the Mary Glover Case* (London and New York: Tavistock/Routledge, 1991), p. viii.
95. Edward Jorden, *A Briefe discourse of a Disease called the Suffocation of the Mother* (London: 1603), ff. 16v–19v, BL, 1177.c.1.(1).
96. Ibid., ff. 5v, 19v and 8v–9.
97. For more on the subject of scepticism in *Macbeth*, see 'Macbeth's Deeds', in Millicent Bell's, *Shakespeare's Tragic Skepticism* (New Haven and London: Yale University Press, 2002), pp. 191–240.
98. Alice Fox, 'Obstetrics and Gynecology in *Macbeth*', *Shakespeare Studies* 12 (1979), pp. 127–41 and Jenijoy La Belle, ' "A Strange Infirmity": Lady Macbeth's Amenorrhea', *Shakespeare Quarterly* 31 (1980), pp. 381–6.
99. This would carry added resonance if Lady Macbeth had indeed been a mother or had only recently given birth. She herself passionately exclaims: 'I have given suck, and know/How tender 'tis to love the babe that milks me' (I, vii, 54–5). Her evocation of murderously disrupted post-partum feeding acts as a reminder of the nurturing biological materials produced by the recently-delivered mother which, without their intended recipient, would be left 'stop[ped] up' in her body.
100. *Shakespeare's Sonnets*, ed. Katharine Duncan-Jones (London: Arden, 1997).
101. John Donne, *The Complete English Poems*, ed. A. J. Smith (Harmondsworth: Penguin, 1996), p. 91.
102. *Twelfth Night*, eds Roger Warren and Stanley Wells (Oxford: Oxford University Press, 1994).
103. Cotta, *The Triall of Witch-craft, shewing the true and right methode of the discovery with a confutation of erroneous wayes* (London: 1616), p. 100, BL, 1608/727.
104. Ibid., p. 18.
105. Ibid., p. 100–1.
106. Thomas Aquinas, *Thomas Aquinas: Selected Writings*, trans. Ralph McInerny (Harmondsworth: Penguin, 1998), p. 395.
107. The phrase is from the title of Giambattista della Porta's influential treatise on the art of natural magic, the *Magicae Naturalis* (1558).
108. Scot, *Discoverie of Witchcraft*, p. 290.

109. Ibid., pp. 290–1.
110. William Perkins, *A Discourse of the Damned Art of Witchcraft; so farre forth as it is revealed in the Scriptures, and manifest by true experience* (Cambridge: 1608), pp. 6 and 13–18, BL 1607/788.
111. Ibid., p. 6. For more on the distinction between supernatural, preternatural and natural, see Lorraine Daston's 'Marvelous Facts and Miraculous Evidence in Early Modern Europe', in *Wonders, Marvels, and Monsters in Early Modern Culture*, ed. Peter G. Platt (Newark: University of Delaware Press, 1999), pp. 76–104.
112. *A Treatise against Witchcraft* (Cambridge: 1590), sigs F3 and C2v, BL 1608/2297.
113. Perkins, *A Discourse of the Damned Art of Witchcraft*, p. 19.
114. Cotta, *The Triall of Witch-craft,* p. 33.
115. *The Comedy of Errors*, ed. R. A. Foakes (London: Arden, 1962).
116. Perkins, *A Discourse of the Damned Art of Witchcraft*, pp. 201 and 213. On the requirement of the minimum number of witnesses in witchcraft cases, see MacFarlane, *Witchcraft in Tudor and Stuart England*, p. 17.
117. Bright, *Treatise of Melancholy*, p. 183.
118. George Gifford, *A Discourse of the Subtill Practises of Devills by Witches and Sorcerers* (London: 1587), sig. D4v, BL 8630.e.19.
119. Gifford, *A Dialogue Concerning Witches and Witchcrafts* (London: 1603), sigs C2 and I, BL, 1395.b.5.
120. I would like to thank Tabitha Cadbury, for providing me with information on navigating the archaeological archives of Cambridge University's Museum of Archaeology and Anthropology, and Jeremy Coote, Joint Head of Collections at the Pitt Rivers Museum, University of Oxford, for his valuable input on artefacts with ritualistic or magical associations in the Pitt Rivers' collections.
121. From the speech of the Earl of Northampton in 'The Trial of Henry Garnet, Superior of the Jesuits in England, at the Guildhall of London, for High Treason, being a Conspirator in the Gunpowder Plot . . .', *Cobbett's Complete Collection of State Trials*, ed. T. B. Howell, vol. 2, pp. 286–7. For more on this specific case in relation to the politics of equivocation, see Steven Mullaney, 'Lying like Truth: Riddle, Representation and Treason in Renaissance England', *English Literary History* 47 (1980), pp. 32–47; and Gary Wills, *Witches and Jesuits: Shakespeare's Macbeth* (Oxford: Oxford University Press, 1995).
122. For more on James' persecution of witches during the Scottish witch-hunts, see Christina Larner, *Enemies of God*, and *The Scottish Witch-Hunt in Context*, ed. Julian Goodare (Manchester and New York: Manchester University Press, 2002).
123. Letter from James Montague, Dean of the Chapel, to the Archbishop of Canterbury, 23 Feb. 1604–5, Hatfield MS 104.39.
124. A copy of a privy seal dealing with witchcraft, 27 May 1605, Hatfield MS 111.11–13.
125. Most of the documents relating to witchcraft prosecutions in the Cecil papers, held at Hatfield House, involve Cranborne in some way. He appears to have been charged with the responsibility of handling most of the cases that came to James' attention. That he is referred to as a 'beagill'

may hint at his role of master-spy, since a beagle was thought particularly adept at hunting hares.

126. Letter from King James to Viscount Cranborne, c. March 1605[?], Hatfield MS 134.71.
127. MacDonald, *Witchcraft and Hysteria*, p. xlviii.
128. Harvey reported, after examining the accused witches, that he found no signs of 'any hollowness or issue for any blood or juice' in any of the suspected marks. *State Papers* (Dom.), 1634–5, pp. 78–9, in Ewen, *Witchcraft and Demonianism*, p. 250.
129. Examinations and Confessions of Margaret Russell, 30 July 1622, BL, additional MS 36674, f. 137.
130. *Circumstances to be considered in the cawse of the mayde of Hockh[a]m, for scratching of an old witch there, nowe deade . . .*, undated, but probably mid- to late seventeenth century, BL, additional MS 28223, f. 15.

Chapter 4

Speaking Stones: Memory and Maternity in the Theatre of Death

Voce Pia Mater: Memorialising Mothers and the Death-Ritual in Early Modern England

Mothers and sculptors work
By small rehearsed caresses in the block
Each to redeeming ends,
By shame or kisses print
Good citizens, good lovers and good friends.

Lawrence Durrell, 'Notebook'[1]

In a gloomy corner of St Edmund's Chapel in Westminster Abbey stands the monument of Elizabeth Russell who died in 1600 at the untimely age of twenty-five (Fig. 4.1). The first seated effigy of its type to be erected in an English church, it was commissioned by Elizabeth's sister Anne and as such offers a visible testimony of the enduring bond between two women. Garnished with a simple yet poignant epitaph which reads 'She is not dead but sleepeth', Russell's stony doppelgänger adopts what one eighteenth-century commentator described as a 'very melancholy posture'.[2] Countless visitors file past this arresting figure on a daily basis, stopping perhaps to admire the quality of the carving or the richness of the age-coloured marble, entirely unaware that it remains at the heart of an enduring mystery.

It has not yet been explained why this tomb, dedicated to an unmarried woman,[3] became the template for a number of similar memorials in the early years of the seventeenth century, all of which were, intriguingly, devoted to mothers who had fatally succumbed to the rigours of childbirth. The earliest of these can be seen in All Saints' Church in Fulham and is dedicated to Lady Margaret Legh who passed away in 1603, a mother to nine children, three of whom died in infancy (Fig. 4.2). With her hand pressed against her chest in the attitude of grief, Legh's carved alter ego sits beside a swaddled infant while clutching a second baby in a loving embrace.[4] Just one year after its completion a similar tomb was erected to the memory of Lady Elizabeth South

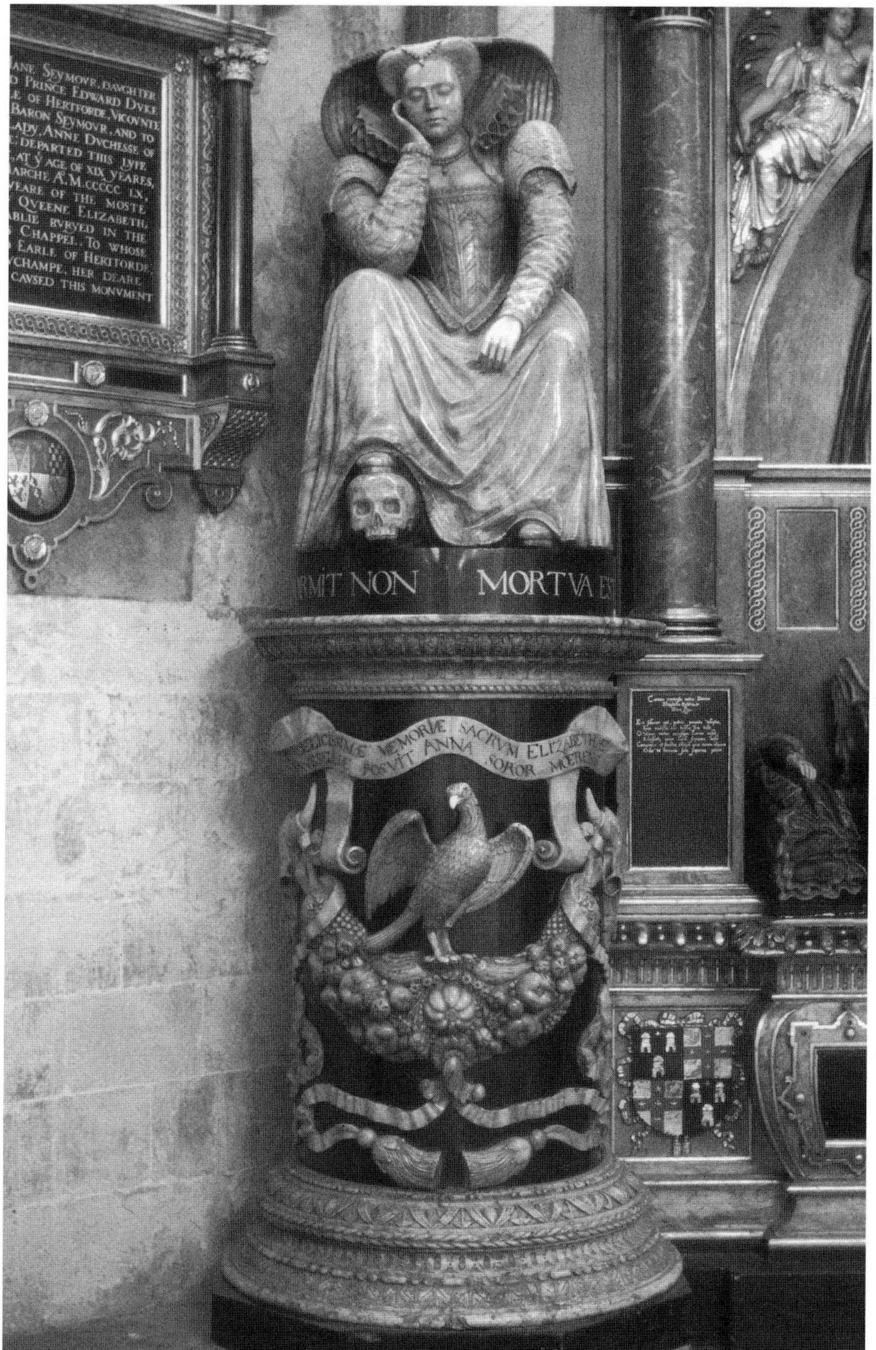

Figure 4.1: Monument of Elizabeth Russell, d. 1600, Westminster Abbey. By kind permission of the Dean and Chapter of Westminster.

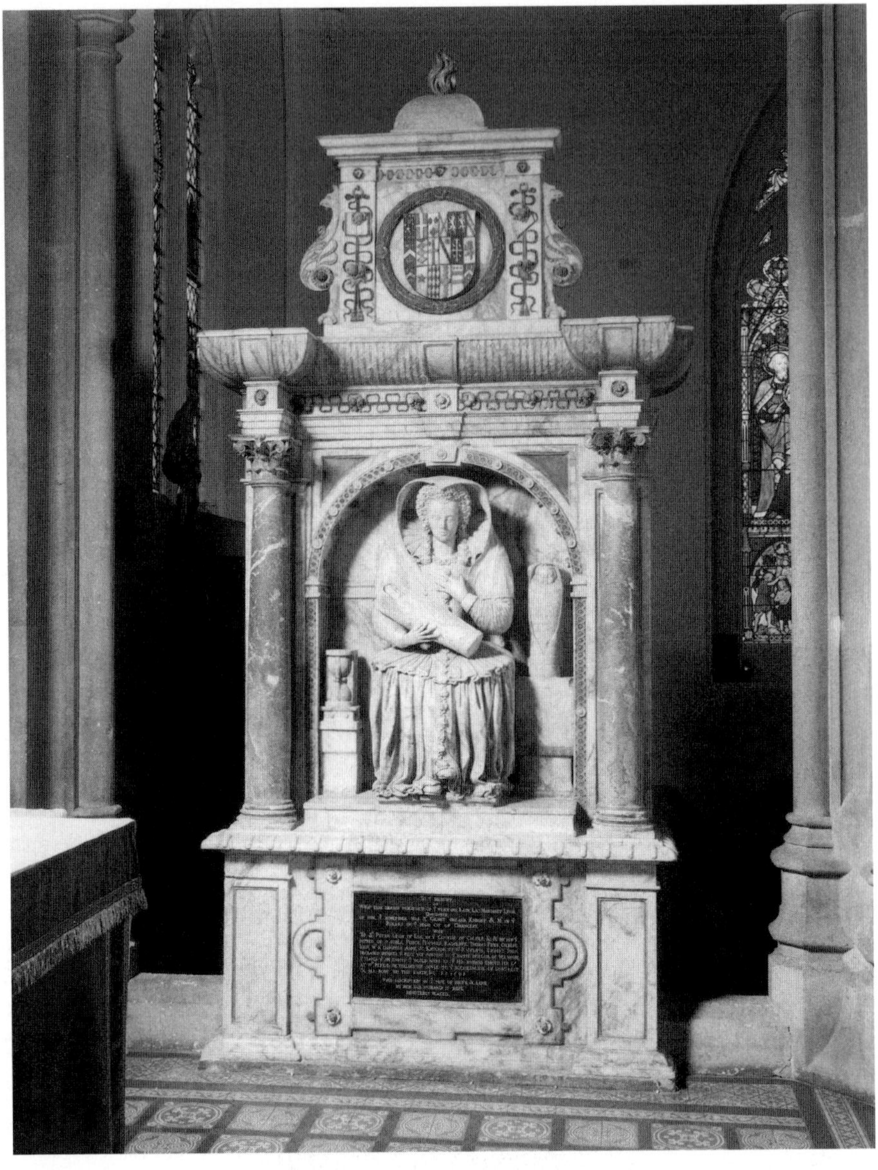

Figure 4.2: Monument of Lady Margaret Legh, d. 1603, All Saints' Church, Fulham. Conway Library, The Courtauld Institute of Art, London.

in Kelstern, Lincolnshire (Fig. 4.3). It presents two contrasting images of infancy. At the base of the monument, just beneath the skirts of its seated mother, a tiny baby is nestled in contemporary bedding clothes. It seems small and frail, in need of its mother's protection, unlike the two robust classical putti who stand on either side of the central figure

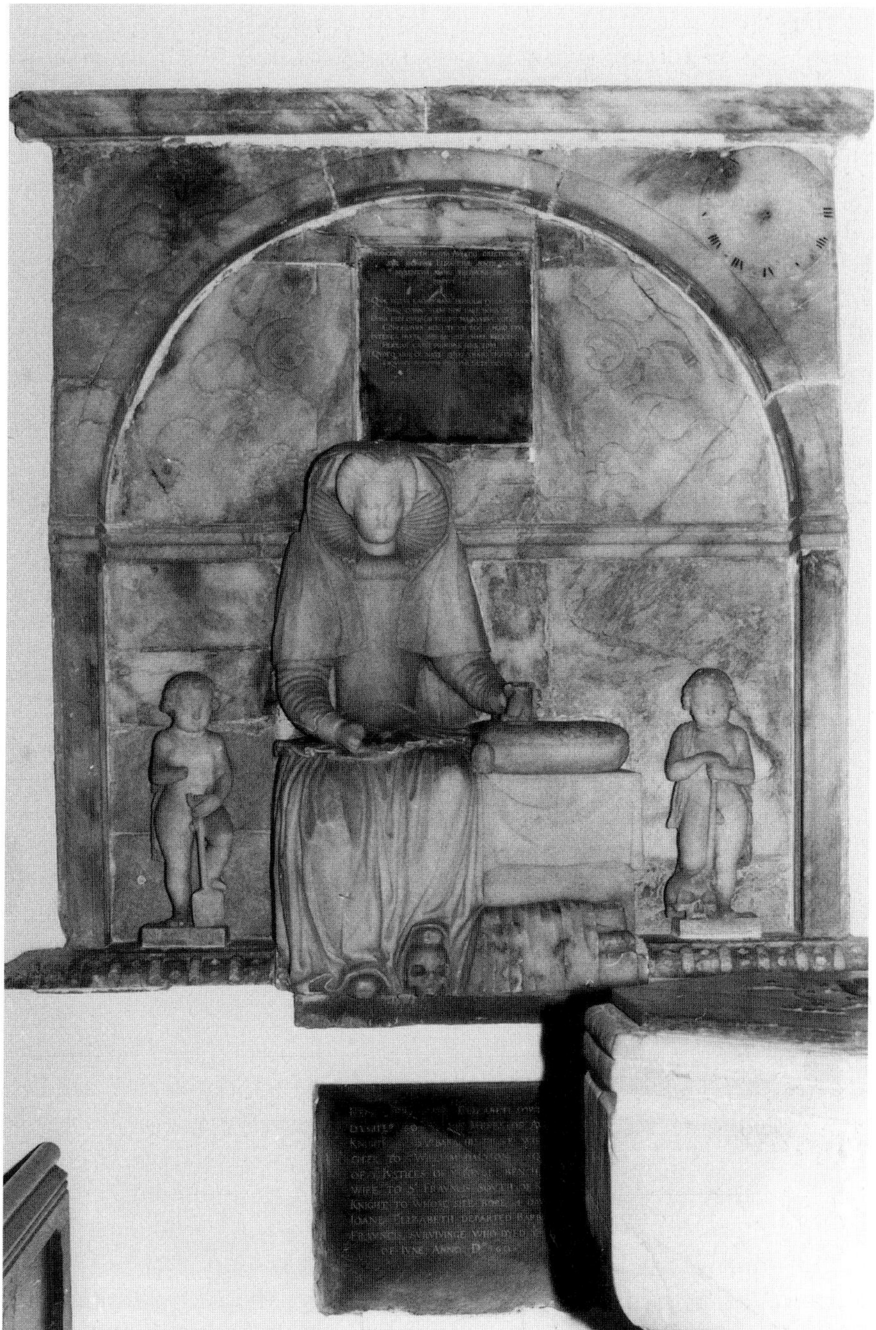

Figure 4.3: Monument of Lady Elizabeth South, 1604, Kelstern, Lincolnshire. Conway Library, The Courtauld Institute of Art, London.

bearing the traditional emblems of death; a shovel and a skull.[5] Lady South's expression conveys a mixture of melancholy and self-restraint, her lips pursed closely together. In St Lawrence's Church, in Hertfordshire, stands the memorial of Mary Plomer who died in 1605 after giving birth to her eleventh child (Fig. 4.4). Her moving epitaph describes her as 'bewties flower/Cropt of in untymly hower' and the onlooker is told that even 't[h]e stone it self doth weepe/To thinck on her w[hi]ch it doth keepe'. The mother seems to gaze out at the world, while cradling her newly-born child in her arms. Below her the carver of the tomb has incorporated a vignette of Plomer's family in mourning, adopting the traditional postures of prayerful devotion. This motif, which emphasises the role of the good mother who raises her children in the Christian faith, came to be particularly prominent on wall monuments like that of Katherine Hart, who died in the same year (Fig. 4.5). Katherine is described as having 'lived vertuouslie & died Godlie' and her deep maternal affection is suggested by the touching way in which she caresses her son's head, a gesture which carries echoes of the Renaissance ritual of the mother's blessing. As onlookers we feel that we have stumbled upon an intensely private moment, captured forever in stone. Margaret Hobbes, who died around 1608–9, was laid to rest in the church of St John the Baptist, West Wickham, in Kent (Fig. 4.6). Her effigy points to a swaddled child while clutching a bible, emphasising the link between piety and maternity. But the figure which most closely imitates the posture of the Russell monument is that commissioned for Elizabeth Marshall, who died in 1613 (Fig. 4.7). In St Lawrence's Church, East Donyland, Essex, the tomb's dedicatee rests her right foot upon a skull, while supporting her right cheek with her hand. Her stare is intense and engaging. The frieze below her contains a relief depicting two swaddled children who appear alongside their eldest sister as she kneels piously in prayer.

These monuments are very different from the two-dimensional funerary brasses which showed the dead wrapped in their burial shrouds, like those belonging to the Fayrey family who were commemorated in Bedfordshire around 1520 (Fig. 4.8), and from the recumbent effigies which, characterised by their stiffness and lack of animation, adorned many a church from the medieval period onwards. A particularly splendid example of the latter is the early sixteenth-century tomb of Henry VII and Elizabeth of York in Westminster Abbey (Fig. 4.9). But why did these extraordinary stylistic innovations take place and could the unique vocabulary of memory which they came to exemplify have informed Shakespeare's representation of Cleopatra's own maternal postures of death? In the first part of this chapter we will take the first tentative

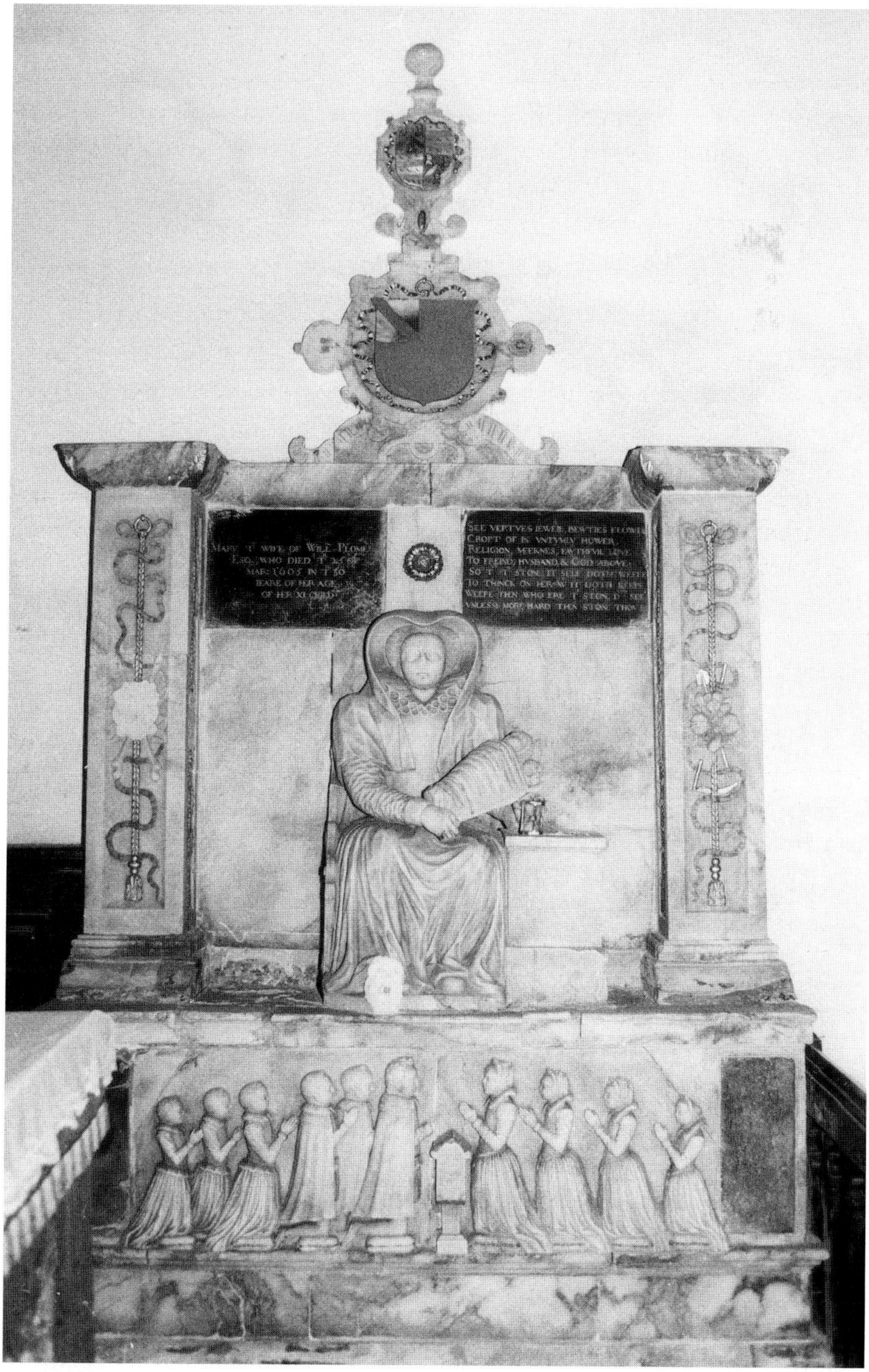
WHO DIED
IEARE OF HER AGE
OF HER XI CHILD
CROPT OF IN VNTYMLY HOWER
RELIGION, MEEKNES, FAYTHFVL
TO FREIND, HVSBAND & GOD ABOVE
VNLESS MORE HARD THA STON

Figure 4.4: Monument of Mary Plomer, d. 1605, St Lawrence's Church, Radwell, Hertfordshire. Conway Library, The Courtauld Institute of Art, London.

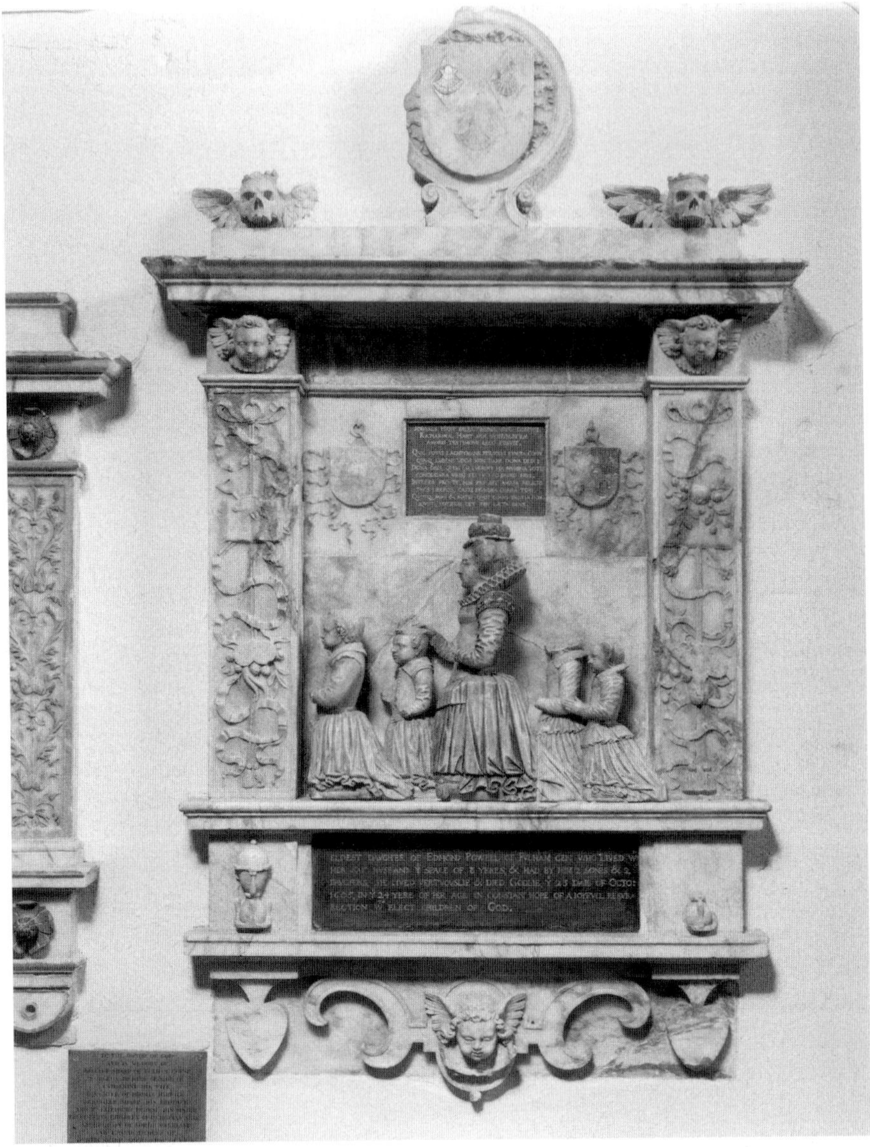

Figure 4.5: Wall monument of Katherine Hart, d. 1605, All Saints' Church, Fulham. Conway Library, The Courtauld Institute of Art, London.

steps towards elucidating the enigma of the specifically maternalised cast of the memorials which followed the appearance of the Russell monument. This will shortly take us to the small parish of Bisham in Berkshire, to a beautiful church which stands on the banks of the Thames river there, and to the nearby Bisham Abbey where, as legend

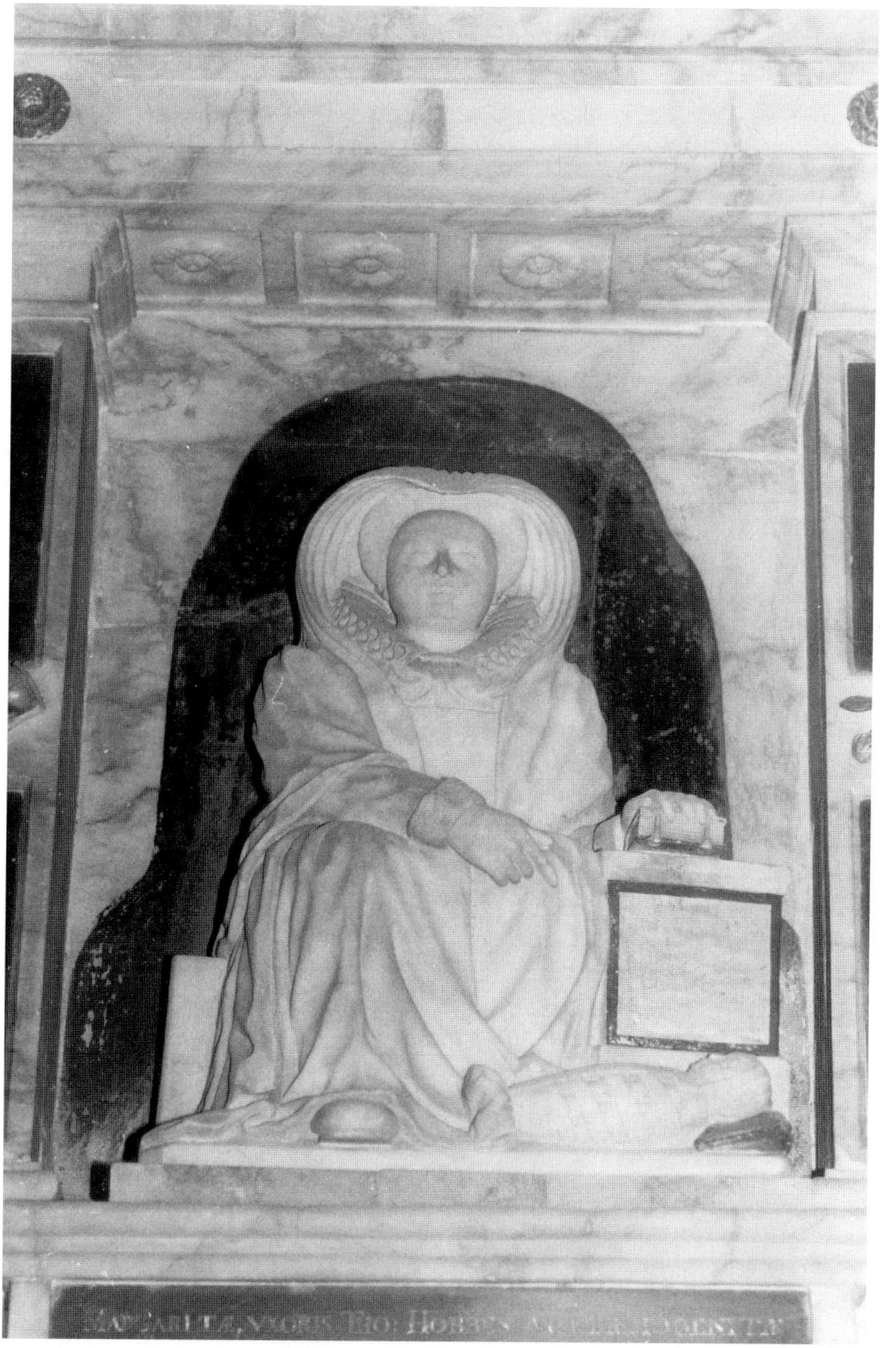

Figure 4.6: Monument of Margaret Hobbes, d. 1608–9, Church of St John the Baptist, West Wickham, Kent. Conway Library, The Courtauld Institute of Art, London.

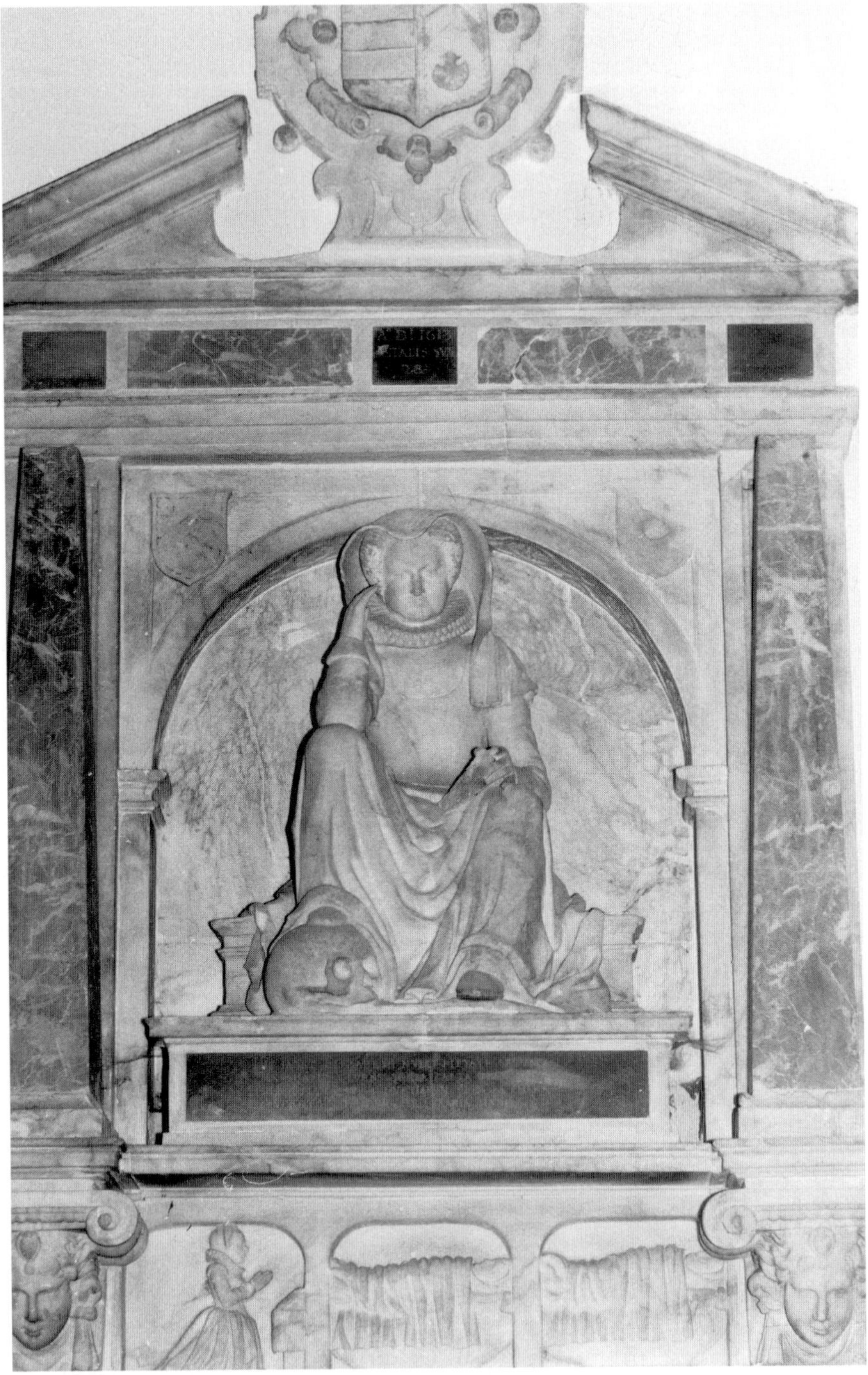

Figure 4.7: Monument of Elizabeth Marshall, d. 1613, St Lawrence's Church, East Donyland, Essex. Conway Library, The Courtauld Institute of Art, London.

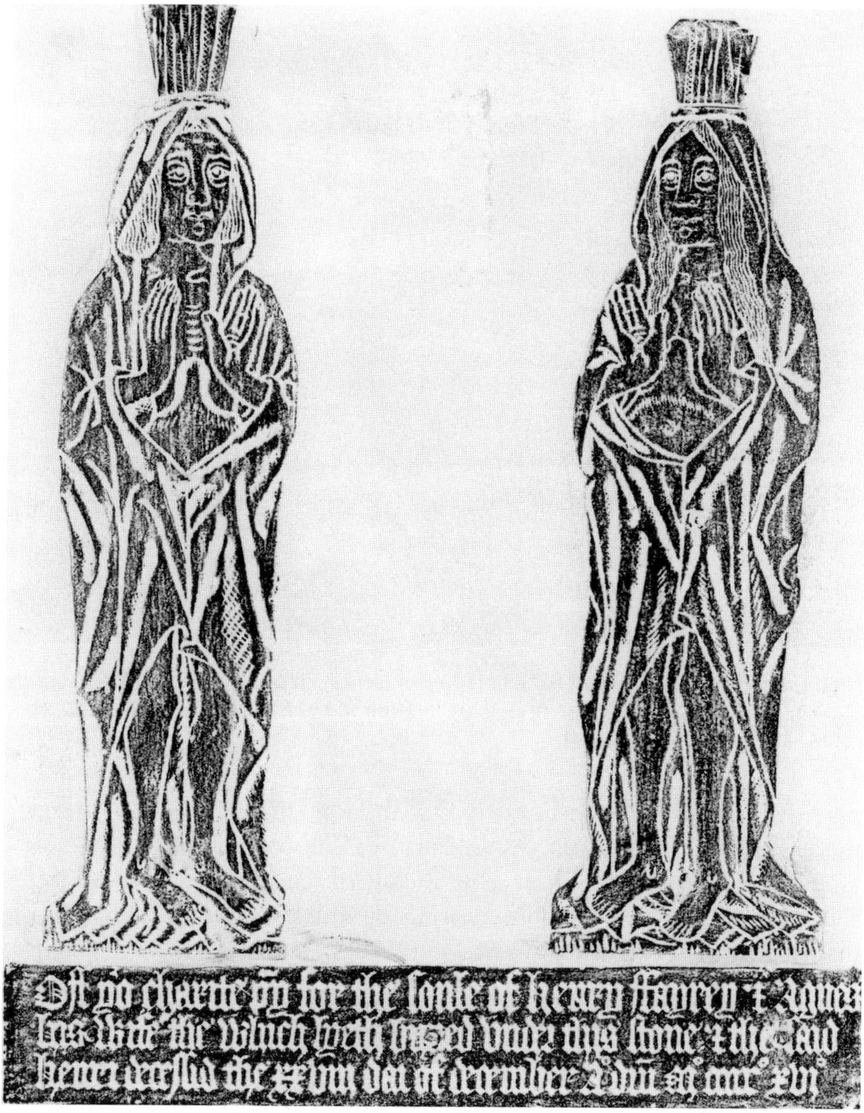

Figure 4.8: Funerary brasses of the Fayrey family, c. 1520, Bedfordshire. © V&A Images/Victoria and Albert Museum, London.

has it, and as residents of the village have informed me, a ghost is said to walk the corridors; the apparition of a mournful mother. It is a journey which will enable us to explore the role of women as both the objects of, and catalysts for changes to, the commemorative practices which accompanied the death-ritual. I will then go on, in the second part of this chapter, to demonstrate the way in which Shakespeare's

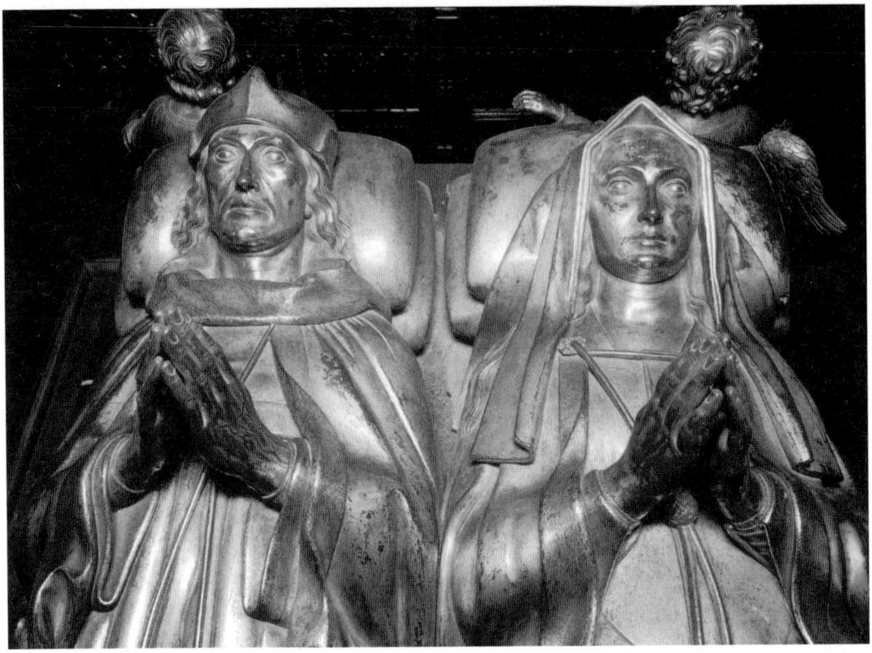

Figure 4.9: Recumbent monumental effigies of Henry VII and Elizabeth of York, early sixteenth century, Westminster Abbey. By kind permission of the Dean and Chapter of Westminster.

play dramatises this conflict between already entrenched and emergent modes of memorialisation. As we will see, Cleopatra manipulates a new language of maternal memory, her means of resistance against an imperialist programme of commemoration which becomes the defining instrument of Octavius' power.

In Renaissance England formalised ceremonial functions, particularly those which involved the upper echelons of society, often fell under the auspices of the College of Arms. Among their powers, the principal officers, the 'Kinges of Armes', claimed jurisdiction over 'the disposing and ordering of all combates . . . [and the] bearing of banners . . . in all Justes, Triumphes, & Turnamentes'. The college also managed the allocation of 'grauntes of new Armes' and 'creastes', and stipulated their use in all pivotal rites of passage for which they acted as mediators, including that of death.[6] Conducted with pomp and histrionic flair, the ideological impetus of the heraldic funeral was to emphasise the continuity of the familial line through the inter-generational transmission of wealth, property and titles. This was symbolically enacted in the ceremony of the 'offertory', a ritualised foreshadowing of legal succession

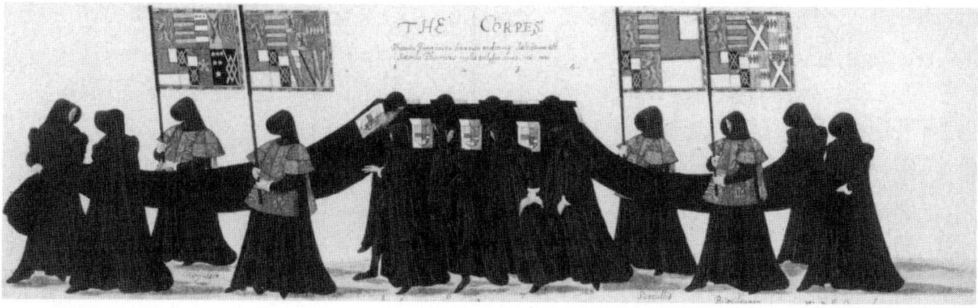

Figure 4.10: Funeral procession of Lady Lumley, 1578, Additional MS 35324, f. 20. © British Library Board. All Rights Reserved.

which involved the offering of the 'hatchments' to the surviving heir; potent emblems of valour and public service which included the defunct's sword, helmet, target or shield, and coat of arms.[7] Where the deceased was a woman, palls of black cloth or money were exchanged in place of the hatchments,[8] though these funereal pageants were no less saturated with the traditional insignia of heraldry. The procedures stipulated by the heralds for the funeral of a woman usually included an order for her body 'to be [disem]boweled[,] trameled and well wrapped in cerecloth and . . . conveyd with a pall of blacke velvet garneshed with Escucheons', to be accompanied in procession by a 'Banner of Armes borne by the Garter principall Kinge of Armes'.[9] What this may have looked like can be seen in a manuscript illustration of the funeral of Lady Lumley, solemnised in 1578, which shows the heralds in their emblazoned gowns, carrying heraldic banners beside a coffin embellished with the family's coats of arms (Fig. 4.10).[10]

Because the heraldic funeral constituted an explicit endorsement of primogeniture, this meant that the passing of mothers was not accorded equal ritual significance with that of fathers.[11] Strict protocols were enforced regarding not only the gender and rank of the principal mourners, but also the way in which they were permitted to *perform* their grief in public. A husband or wife could not be a chief mourner for their spouse and women, segregated from men in the funerary ceremony, were expected to adhere more closely to the formalised gestures of female mourning.[12] There was therefore no room in the heraldic funeral for an open display of familial affection, nor for a laudatory summation of the deceased's maternal qualities. Instead emphasis was placed on one's position in the hierarchical economy.[13] In the funeral of Lady Lennox in 1606, the crucial moment of transition in which the corpse entered the sacred confines of the House of God for the offertory was not to be mediated by the family of the deceased, but by professional members of the church and college of Westminster with all 'the Mynisters, Clearkes, and Schollers . . . me[e]t[ing] the corpes, att the West door, and the Mynister to saye, or singe I am the resurrection . . . as is appoynted in the Book of service for the buriall of the deade'.[14] The family did not really have a chance to commune directly until after the funeral when it was customary for a dinner to be held, as was the case following the burial of the Countess of Exeter in 1609. The records of Westminster Abbey show, however, that the formalities and rituals of the heraldic funeral were taken into the home, where the heralds continued to exercise control over the proceedings. Expenses for the funeral included an

> Allowance of Blackes to officers w[i]thin the house, the dinner beinge kept there: w[i]th composition for blackes to be hunge up w[i]thin the house. And somethinge to be distributed to the poore of the parishe of St Margarettes as allowences in the like occation hath binne donne.[15]

The dinner was a time for the family to make a public demonstration of their hospitality and largesse. Charitable offerings to the poor were a common feature of these events. In some cases, however, women and men remained separated even in these social occasions. The heralds' prescriptions insisted that 'the Lady cheife mourner and the other ladies mourners at the funerall of a Countesse, keep state in the great chamber at dinner, and no men with them at that table'.[16] These dinners offered the opportunity for the relatives of the deceased to cement their ties with other members of their own social milieu, and while more private condolences may have been exchanged (after all, the trauma of personal loss is just as keenly felt by a simple yeoman as it is by a king), these did not form a conspicuous part of the approved heraldic programme. With its finger on the pulse of the body-politic, the College of Arms employed its full heraldic arsenal – crests, coats, escutcheons, banners, processions and triumphs – in its role as the official guarantor of social distinction.

It is easy to see how this kind of ostentation could become a double-edged sword. As the seventeenth century got under way the College of Arms began to lose its control over the English death-ritual.[17] Other styles of burial were fast becoming fashionable, most notably the nocturnal ceremony which allowed the unmediated participation of family and loved ones in a setting that was altogether more intimate.[18] This should not, however, be seen as representing a sudden thrust towards individualism, nor as exemplifying a simple binary opposition between public and private modes of mourning.[19] The absence of a heraldic service could make just as strong a statement as the lavish spectacle it displaced and the College of Arms saw this as a significant enough threat to warrant the issuing of a petition to the Archbishop of Canterbury, enlisting the co-operation of the Church in the obliteration of the newer burial rituals:

> It hath wrought greate confusion amonge the gentrie of the kingdom for that the officers of Armes can take noe notice of the times of theire deathes nor of theire posteritie. And manie in the darke doe presume without warant or right to bury the dead; eaither with new invented ensignes of gentry or with such as justly belonge to other men: or with theire owne unduely marshalled & ordered.[20]

The dark of nightfall becomes a metaphor for the social confusion wrought by the decline of the heraldic funeral. The unregulated ceremony is a microcosm of a world in which hierarchical degree is no longer observed and in which power may even be usurped by those of meaner station. What emerging trends in the death-ritual, and ironically in commemorative art, made strikingly apparent to the disgruntled guardians of the social order was that the dynastic destiny of society's elite was no longer set in stone. Indeed, by visibly challenging the primacy of more traditional recumbent monuments the new tomb-styles which began to take up more floor-space in churches and cathedrals, of which the Russell memorial is a notable example, actually undermined the most histrionic elements of the heraldic funeral. The monumental display of the supine figure recapitulated the wooden and wax effigies that adorned the hearse as it was presented in the heraldic funeral and was therefore intended, in the words of Nigel Llewellyn, to be 'mourned in perpetuity and remind us continually of the body in the grave'.[21] A manuscript held by the still extant College of Arms, the *Book of Monuments* (1619), constitutes an aborted attempt at curbing such innovations in monumental design, those which were not in keeping with its ideological programme, by pictorially recording all officially-sanctioned memorials. The vibrant depiction of Queen Anne of Denmark's funerary catafalque and effigy, with all its conspicuous blazonry, serves as the template for the tombs of the elite which echo the decorative and architectural principles of heraldic funerary display (Fig. 4.11). That this cataloguing programme was an unsuccessful enterprise indicates the speed with which newer monumental models were being implemented, models which were no longer solely mediated by the iconographical language of the funerary service itself.[22] Monuments which recorded living postures, like the maternal memorials which took their cue from Elizabeth Russell's effigy, effectively erased the visible markers that were intended to enshrine for all time the ceremonial gestures of the heraldic funeral.

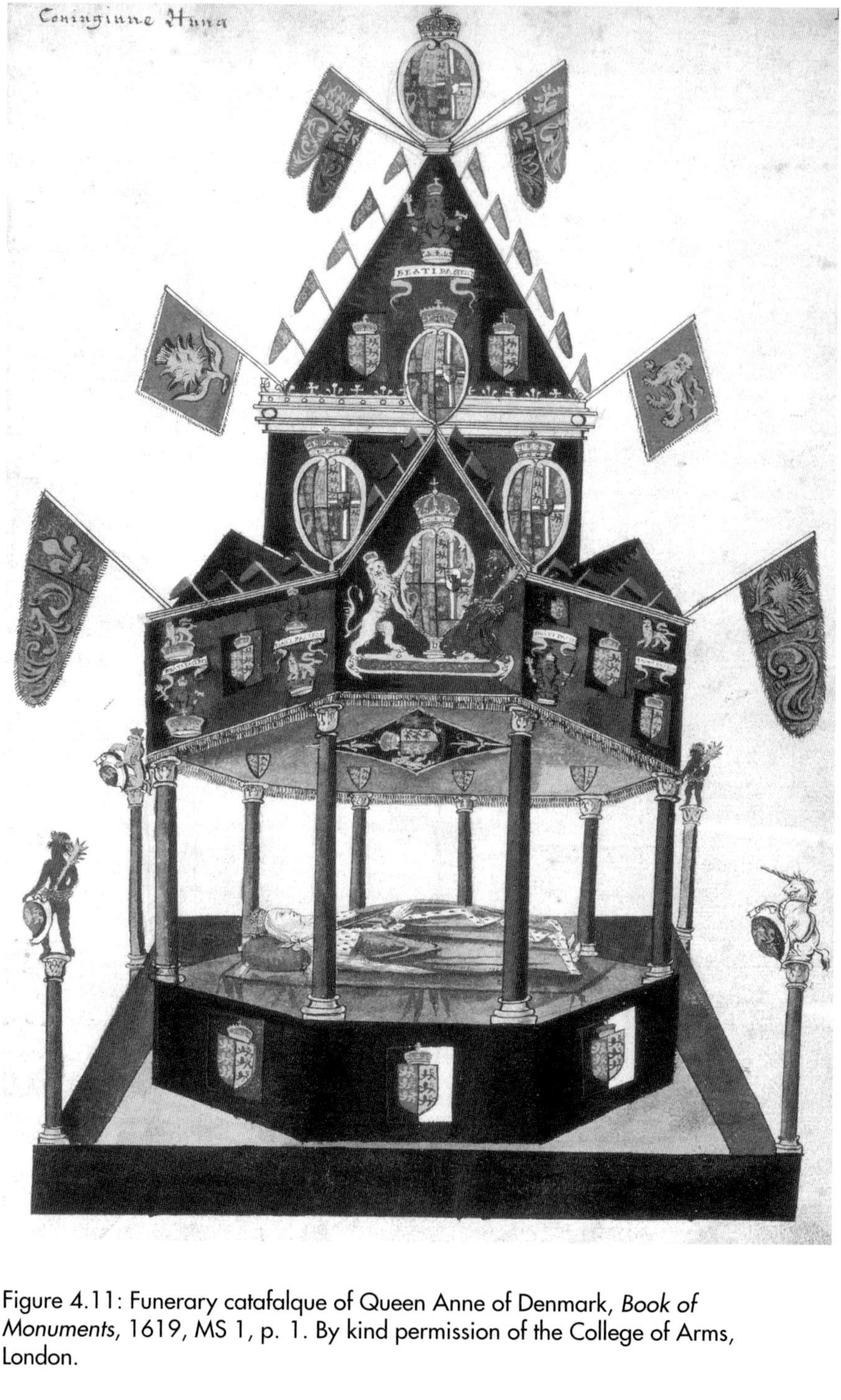

Figure 4.11: Funerary catafalque of Queen Anne of Denmark, *Book of Monuments*, 1619, MS 1, p. 1. By kind permission of the College of Arms, London.

There was, however, no sudden or dramatic break with heraldic custom, rather the accoutrements of memory were negotiated by women as well as men over an extended period. One woman was especially interested in the practices of the College of Arms, and more specifically, in the possibilities open to her with regard to her own and her family's commemoration. This was Lady Elizabeth Hoby Russell, none other than the mother of the young Elizabeth Russell whose commemoration proved so influential.[23] It was she who, in the latter part of her life, wrote a letter to William Dethick, Garter King of Arms, asking for particulars regarding the manner of proceeding at her own funeral, including 'the number of mourners due to my calling . . . with their charge of blacks . . . the charges of the hearse, heralds, and church'.[24] Despite her deference to the heralds, Hoby Russell was not content to take a back-seat when it came to the ordering of such solemnities, nor would she allow the college to delimit her public role as chief mourner following the deaths of her loved ones. From the late sixteenth century she became one of the Renaissance's most prolific memorialisers, somewhat of an aficionado of death, commissioning and erecting tombs, composing epitaphs and elegies in Latin, Greek and English. And it was her manipulation of such arts of memory which allowed her to fashion for herself a lasting identity as an exemplum of maternity.

In the parish church of Bisham stands the impressive monument of Elizabeth Hoby Russell, the design for which she finalised herself (Fig. 4.12).[25] She is presented as an ideal mother schooling her children in their religious devotions. Before her lies the effigy of her son Francis, from her second marriage, while her three daughters from her first marriage, all of whom suffered early deaths, kneel behind her, their hands clasped in prayer. The two youngest Hoby daughters, Elizabeth and Anne (not to be confused with their namesakes from the Russell marriage), died within a week of each other in 1571 and are commemorated in a moving Latin epitaph composed by their mother.[26] It begins with the heart-rending exclamation '*eheu mea viscera*', an interjection of maternal anguish which repeats the throes of childbirth.[27] This emotional timbre is extended in Hoby Russell's explicit self-identification as the orchestrator of her children's memory, for she had 'determined for [them] to share one burial' as they had once been 'in one womb . . . borne'.[28] Elizabeth Hoby Russell also uses the occasion of her husband's death to emphasise her maternal role. The Bisham monument of Sir Thomas Hoby (d. 1566) is thus the very setting for her elegiac self-dramatisation as an 'unhappy mother' (*infaelix mater*) who, in a posture of mourning, holds her surviving 'children's languid limbs' (*prolis languida membra*), while her husband's future heir, with

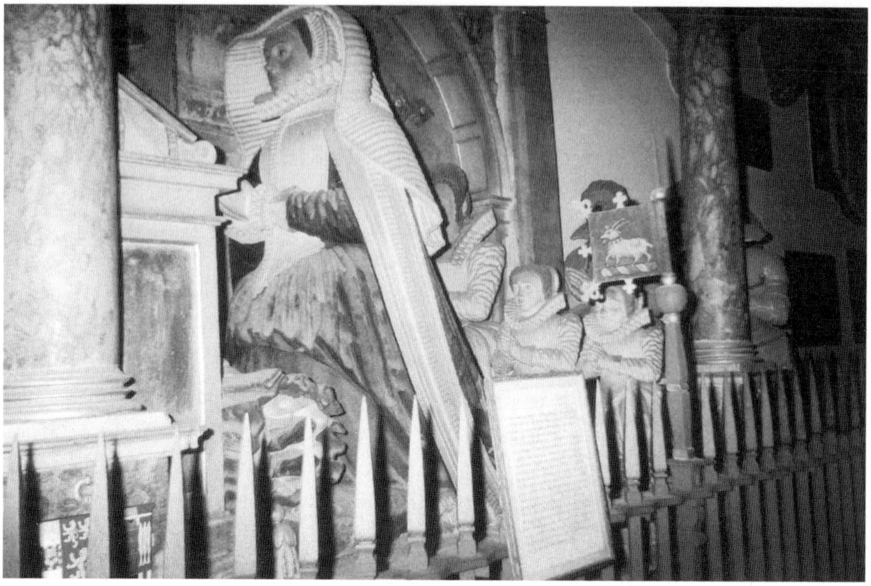

Figure 4.12: Monument of Elizabeth Hoby Russell, d. 1609, All Saints' Church, Bisham, Berkshire. By kind permission of the Church Warden. Photo: author.

whom she was still pregnant after his death and whom she would fittingly name Posthumus, grows within her 'flourishing womb' (*uterum gestans*).

Bisham was not the only public space which provided Elizabeth Hoby Russell with a stage for her performances of memory for, after the death of her first husband, she married Lord John Russell (d. 1584), the son of the second Earl of Bedford.[29] This meant that the programme of familial commemoration she was so eager to initiate would be displayed in one of England's largest and most influential repositories of funerary art, Westminster Abbey. And it was there that the seated memorial of her daughter, Elizabeth Russell, would stand, surrounded by the epitaphs and elegies which were composed by her mother (Fig. 4.1). Among them is the epitaph of Francis Russell in which Elizabeth Hoby Russell describes herself as a 'lamenting mother' (*aerumnosae matris*), forced to take an unwilling command over her son's death-ritual: 'O I wish your mother lay dead/That you had discharged my last rites first.'[30] The fact that Anne Russell chose to present herself as her sister's official memorialiser, by commissioning her tomb, indicates that she wanted to be seen as her mother's protégée, following in her footsteps as a choreographer of memory. That the two women, participating in a specifically feminised discourse of mourning, were engaged in a subtle reshaping of the death-ritual can be surmised from Elizabeth Hoby Russell's epitaphic utterance on her husband's tomb: 'All that is lawful I have performed, I would more were lawful.'[31] It is hard not to see in this simple phrase the anxiety which surrounds any kind of female-authored commemorative practice. While it acknowledges the limits placed upon women by official heraldic decorums, it also implies an earnest desire to stretch those boundaries. It was Elizabeth Hoby Russell's willingness to dwell upon the sorrows and cares of maternity, even in such public contexts, that allowed her to gesture towards a more liberating mode of commemoration, something which is echoed elsewhere in her writings. It was only when she began to sense the approach of death, in 1605, that she felt able to publish her early translation of John Ponet's *A Way of Reconciliation of a Good and Learned Man*, in which she composed a poignant dedicatory epistle to Anne:

> Most vertuous and woorthilie beloved daughter, Even as from your first birth and cradle I ever was most careful, above any worldly thing, to have you sucke the perfect milke of sincere Religion: So willing to ende as I beganne, I have left to you, as my last Legacie, this Booke. A most precious Jewell to the comfort of your Soule . . .

That it is the imminence of her death which authorises her maternal voice is suggested by the Latin *mother's blessing* with which she closes her dedication, asking the Lord to take heed of the prayers and supplications of 'a tender mother' (*Voce Pia Mater, Suplice Mente Precor*).[32] The lactating body's aptness as a natural vehicle for this type of divinely sanctioned matrilineal transmission is most succinctly expressed in *The Countesse of Lincolnes Nurserie* (1622), in which mothers are urged to

> thinke againe how your Babe crying for your breast, sucking hartily the milke out of it, and growing by it, is the *Lords owne instruction*, every houre, and every day, that you are suckling it, instructing you to shew that you are his *New borne Babes*, by your earnest desire after his word.[33]

One of the first texts to identify itself explicitly as a mother's 'last Legacie', Hoby Russell's *Reconciliation* both engages in, and in some sense initiates a tradition of maternal legacies which grew in popularity from the early seventeenth century.[34] Dorothy Leigh's *The Mothers Blessing*, presented as a 'Legacy' in its subtitle, appeared in no fewer than twenty-three editions between 1616 and 1674, making it arguably the most popular work by a female author of that century.[35] In terms remarkably similar to those used by Hoby Russell, Leigh's text paradoxically reconstitutes the nurturing powers of the maternal body whose anticipated extinction provides the very occasion for the work's conception:

> Is it possible, that shee which hath carried her child within her, so neere her heart, and brought it forth into this world with so much bitter pain, so many grones and cryes, can forget it? Nay rather, will she not labour now till Christ bee formed in it? . . . Will she not blesse it every time it sucks on her brests, when shee feeleth the bloud come from her heart to nourish it? Will shee not instruct it in the youth . . .?[36]

Leigh's meditation on the interchangeability of lactation and instruction actually reconceptualises death as an implicitly creative, even nutritive act. The imperatives of female biology, of 'Motherly affection', are therefore placed in critical opposition to a different type of inheritance. Exposing the limitations of the very medium from which the text borrows its own discursive paradigms, the ancient patriarchal machinery of primogeniture, Leigh condemns those who 'labour . . . to inrich their children[,] . . . many hazzarding their soules, some by bribery, some by simony, others by perjury and a multitude by usury[,] . . . not caring if the whole Common-wealth be impoverished, so their children be inriched'.[37] The posthumous transference of worldly goods and titles, the very mainstay of the patrilineal system, becomes not the bulwark of the social order, but a corrosive element which threatens its integrity. These sentiments may well have influenced Elizabeth Joceline, who composed *The Mothers Legacie to her unborne Childe* (1624) in expectation of what she believed, all too prophetically, would be her death-in-childbed:

> [I]t had been a weake request to desire thee onely for an heire to my fortune. No, I never aimed at so poore an inheritance for thee, as the whole world: Neither would I have begged of God so much paine, as I know I must endure, to have only possest thee with earthly riches, of which to day thou maist be a great man, tomorrow a poore begger.[38]

The specifically feminine kind of death-bed legacy Joceline advocates is entirely unmediated by official structures and takes its impetus from the pains of the suffering maternal body. Even the cultivation of an honourable reputation, the culminating endeavour of the death-ritual itself, is to be achieved not by adhering to the strict protocols which govern female commemorative acts, but through the apparently spontaneous outpouring of 'motherly zeale';[39] as Joceline maintains, 'neither the true knowledge of mine owne weaknesse, nor the feare this may come to the worlds eye, & bring scorne upon my grave, can stay my hand from expressing how much I covet thy salvation'.[40] Such textual legacies allowed their female authors to secure a posthumous voice – a lasting memory – by subordinating the masculine machinery of inheritance to the biological and spiritual imperatives of the maternal bond.

What, I would argue, underpins this newly emerging vocabulary of maternal commemoration, in both its textual and monumental forms, is a more orthodox notion of the art of dying well. As the Reformation wore away at the machinery of intercession, the death-bed became the focus of increased attention. Friends and family scrutinised the dying for signs of Christ's imminent saving grace. Final speeches in particular were seen as an important indicator of one's elect status. Many women were thus listened to with a diligence not afforded them during healthier years. In extant sermons from the period, death-bed speeches and mothers' blessings are often presented as natural extensions of the maternal or nurturing role. In Stephen Denison's *The Monument or Tomb-stone* (1620), Elizabeth Juxon is singled out for praise because she would not 'put forth her children to be nursed abroad, according to the practise of the proud women . . . but tooke paines to nurse them with her own breasts'. The preacher noted that as death approached 'she was able both to speak divinely, to instruct her servants and children, and to write letters in the very language of Canaan with great sufficiency'.[41] Significantly, Canaan is the proverbial land of milk and honey, the archetypal symbol of abundant and unending nurture. This is just one of many such documents which identified themselves as 'monuments' and which claimed to provide eye-witness evidence of the deceased's virtuous ending. The same year saw the publication of *The Honour of Vertue. Or The Monument erected . . . to the immortall memory of . . . Mrs Elizabeth Crashawe. Who dyed in child-birth*. In an elegy by one G. Williams for the deceased mother, her death itself becomes a legacy which circumvents the strictures of 'Covert Baron':[42]

> This rare blest wife. Her Infant Birthright gave
> And (loving mother) digged her selfe a grave.
> A Phaenix sure she was. if vertuouse, merit
> [M]ay what she's heire to without wronge inherit.[43]

Likewise Hanniball Gamon in his sermon *The Praise of a Godly Woman* (1627), commends 'Ladie Francis Roberts' for wishing to leave a legacy of instruction to her children and cites as textual evidence her letters to a 'learned professor' of Oxford University, which he writes are 'worthy to be kept as a monument of her truly Noble spirit and godly desire . . . to have the fruit of her Body become the fruit of the Spirit'. In her final moments 'being summoned by Sicknesse', he continues, 'she spake to the Hearts of Her Children, Friends, and Servants that were then about Her (like Jacob) by putting them in remembrance of Her Departure and their Duties'.[44] In justification of her own mother's legacy, which she began in 1606, Elizabeth Richardson also imitates the prerogative exercised by Jacob, the first biblical will-writer,[45] exclaiming that 'God established a testimony in Jacob, & ordeined a Law in Israell, w[hi]ch he com[m]aunded th[a]t thei should teach th[ei]r children, that the posteritie might know it . . . I have written . . . for the direction of my children . . . th[a]t they may . . . injoye after death, a blessed inheritance.'[46] In her *Ladies Legacy to her Daughters*, written in 1625 but published some twenty years later, this endeavour is set against her own husband's failure to supply an adequate inheritance for his children following his death:

> I have long and much grieved for your misfortunes, and want of preferments in the world: but now I have learned in what estate soever I am, therewith to be content, and to account these vile and transitorie things to be but vaine and losse . . . But though I am so unhappy as to be left destitute, not able to raise you portions of wealth, yet shall I joy as much to adde unto the portion of Grace, which I trust, and pray, that God will give to each of you . . . And here I send you a motherly remembrance, and commend this my labour into your loving acceptance . . .

This 'labour' through which she will 'still travell in care for the new birth of your soules' constitutes the nativity of the text itself as the 'greatest treasure', in value exceeding that of any worldly inheritance.[47] Most importantly, the legacy becomes a 'motherly remembrance', a permanent reminder of the mother-daughter bond. That this is the affective rhetoric which underpins the type of textualised memorial Richardson wished to bequeath is most clearly demonstrated through a correction made to the presentation copy of the first published edition for Richardson's brother, Henry Beaumont, in which the original title, *A Ladies Legacie to her Daughters*, has been amended by hand to read *A Mothers Legacie to her Sixe Daughters*.[48] The change is a testament to the growing popularity of this maternal genre and to the textually-legitimising potential of the fecund reproductive body. Writing mothers could thus draw on two traditions: a rich biblical heritage which defined a spiritualised form of will-making as a parental duty, and a Protestant conception of the 'good death' which both valorised the transmission of death-bed speech and, in the case of women, reconstituted that speech as particularly fruitful.

The transitional nature of the period we have been discussing is encapsulated in a painting by the English artist John Souch, which commemorates Sir Thomas Aston's wife, Magdelene, who died in childbirth in 1635 (Fig. 4.13).[49] Here the most heraldic of emblems, the coat of arms, is encircled by a half-withered laurel garland. Moreover, the pose adopted by Thomas and his son, which closely adheres to the pattern of dynastic portraits,[50] is challenged not only by young Thomas' unbreeched state, which ties him more closely to the world of the mother, but also by the demeanour of the mysterious woman who sits at the foot of the empty cradle.[51] The intensity of her gaze, the crumpled handkerchief in her hand, her melancholic carriage, confront us with a

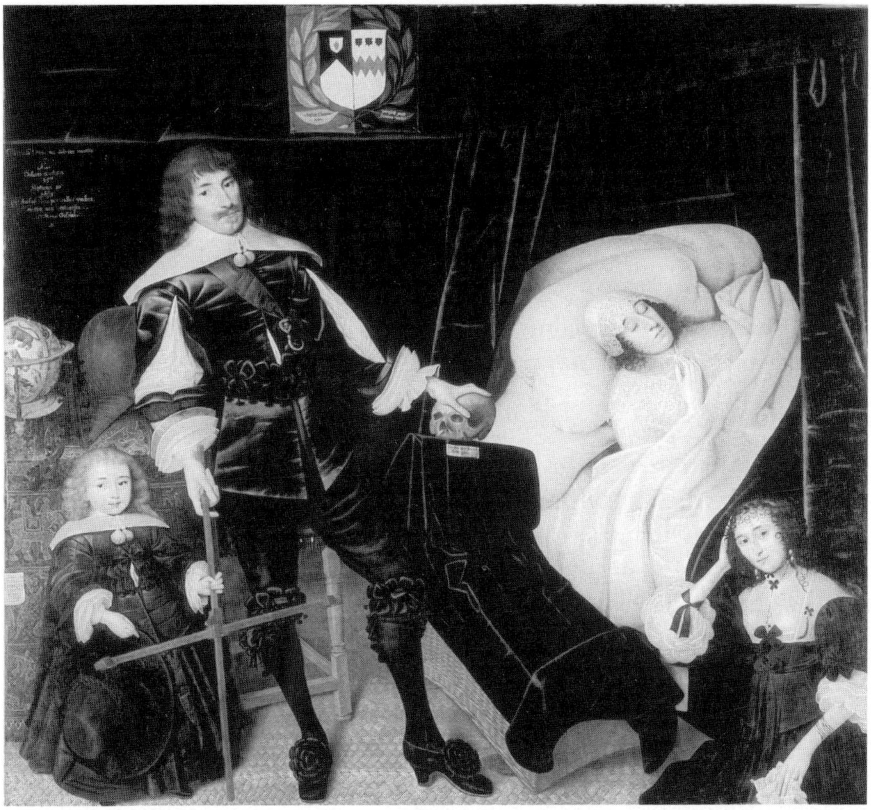

Figure 4.13: John Souch, portrait of Sir Thomas Aston and his wife Magdelene Aston who died in childbirth, 1635. Manchester City Galleries.

feeling that the institutional scaffolding of heraldry is an inadequate mediator of loss. Lady Aston's death does not constitute, therefore, a sudden cessation of her maternal influence, nor a complete transference of her son's devotion to the father. That the mysterious woman's posture mirrors that of Elizabeth Russell's monument, with which we began this chapter, as well as the touching effigies which subsequently borrowed their melancholic iconography from the commemorative programme instituted by Elizabeth Hoby Russell and her daughter Anne, is no coincidence. What all these memorial gestures point to is the subtle reconceptualisation of the processes which underpinned the institution and transmission of maternal memory.

Elizabeth Hoby Russell's ghost is not, it seems, confined to the half-lit rooms of Bisham Abbey where she is said to roam, but also haunts the maternal tombs which were erected in imitation of her daughter's monument. Young Elizabeth's death would have drawn special attention because she was in fact no less a personage than the god-daughter of Elizabeth I herself, an honour accorded her, so her father claimed, as a kind of consolation for the 'great fear and torment' in which his wife was 'delivered', when he stood in 'danger . . . of losing both' mother and child to the potential crises of childbirth.[52] As such Elizabeth's generosity in agreeing to baptise her younger namesake becomes a celebration of heroic maternity. Yet the ghost-story that has developed around the village of Bisham hints at a darker side to the maternal zeal which was one of Elizabeth Hoby Russell's most oft-noted traits. Visitors to the abbey where she once lived claim to have seen a mournful apparition of a woman engaging in a perpetual act of hand-washing in the manner of Lady Macbeth, as if trying to cleanse herself from the bloody remnants of some terrible crime. These sightings have made the abbey, reputedly, one of the most haunted houses in England, with a gruesome story to match.

A legend which has been passed down from generation to generation of Bisham's inhabitants relates that Lady Hoby Russell had another son named William who failed consistently to meet the expectations of his mother, a particularly hard task-master when it came to the education of her children. One morning as she was conducting their private instruction in the abbey, William had incensed her by blotting the copy-books in which he had been transcribing the day's lesson. Unable to tolerate sloppiness of any kind, and determined to instil in her offspring the appreciation of learning that she had imbibed as the daughter of the renowned humanist pedagogue Sir Anthony Cooke, she beat William with a heavy wooden ruler until he was dead. In 1840, when structural repairs were being carried out inside the abbey, workmen discovered a secret stash of papers which had been deliberately concealed in a hidden compartment beneath one of the windows. Some of these turned out to be blotted copy-books with, as one witness reported, the name 'William Hoby' inscribed on them.[53] Did these events really take place? Or were they merely rumours which circulated while Lady Hoby Russell was still alive? If either of these is the case is it then possible that her determination to use the ritual concomitants of memorialisation to fashion a public persona for herself as an ideal mother was a way of compensating for this? We will probably never know. It is more likely that the stories were shaped after her death, though what fires cast the smoke of these scandals into the local community is uncertain. What the legend does reveal is that there has always been an abiding interest in Lady Hoby Russell's role as a maternal figure, a role which has been continually mythologised for centuries. This testifies, in a way, to the success of her own programme of self-commemoration, since she has come today to epitomise all aspects of maternal identity as it is encoded within our culture, in all its complexity and heterogeneity. These are features which ultimately escape the narrow paradigms of femininity represented in the heraldic rites of death.

As I have attempted to show, the memorialising practices of the Russell women were both influenced by, and in turn precipitated, changes to the English death-ritual.[54] In particular writing women like Elizabeth Hoby Russell, and those who subsequently left behind their 'mothers' legacies', indulged in a range of memorialising practices which deftly circumvented the stringent laws of the heralds. Their courage in speaking out in the face of the maternal crises which threatened the integrity of the familial unit discloses the fraught nature of women's attempts at gaining some measure of control over the impact of their own inevitable separation from their kindred and children. The obstacles facing them are very much apparent in a period in which learned divines, heralds and politicians regularly joined their voices to those of men like Thomas Salter who announced, in *A Mirrhor mete for all Mothers* (1579), that 'far more convenient the Distaffe, and Spindle, Nedle, and Thimble were for them with a good and honest reputation, then the skill of well using a pen or wrightying a loftie vearse with diffame and dishonour'.[55] It was, I argue, the carefully crafted, and daringly public maternal identity of Elizabeth Hoby Russell that turned her daughter's monument into a prototype for the memorialising of motherhood. Such practices emerged at a time when the traditions of a nobility purely defined in masculine terms were coming under increased pressure from alternative forms of familial commemoration. That a feminised language of death, circulated through the unique postures of the maternal body, was also finding its way onto the public stage of the theatre during Shakespeare's age will become apparent as we turn to the performance of maternity in *Antony and Cleopatra*.

A Celerity in Dying: The Maternal Postures of Death in Shakespeare's *Antony and Cleopatra*

The Alexandrians gathered
To see the children of Cleopatra,
Caesarion, and his younger brothers,
Alexander and Ptolemy . . . there to proclaim them kings . . .
The Alexandrians, doubtless, understood
That this was nothing more than a show of words, nothing more than theatre.

C. P. Cavafy, 'Alexandrian Kings'[56]

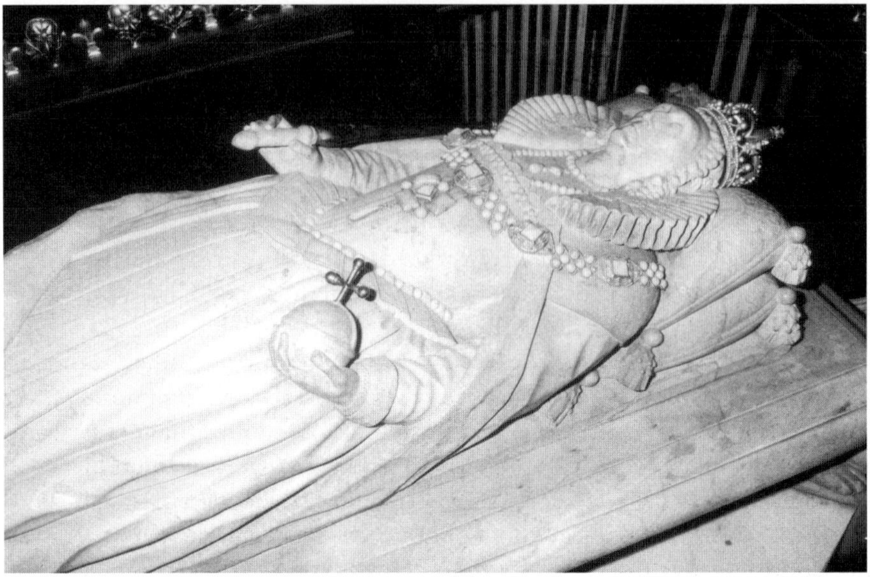

Figure 4.14: Monument of Elizabeth I, 1606, Westminster Abbey. By kind permission of the Dean and Chapter of Westminster.

Perhaps the earliest audiences of Shakespeare's *Antony and Cleopatra* would have been moved to seek parallels between Cleopatra's monumental death, in which she dons the trappings of royalty to become 'marble-constant' (V, ii, 239),[57] and the recumbent effigy of Elizabeth I in her golden finery, laid out on the splendid heraldic tomb which was completed by Maximilian Colt for Westminster Abbey around 1606, the very same year as the postulated first performance of the play (Fig. 4.14).[58] It would be all too easy to assume that the success of Cleopatra's dying postures relies on their conformity to such officially ratified modes of memory. I hope to show, however, that while the play's visual and textual vocabulary does indeed evoke traditional constructions of royal commemoration, it does so only to challenge their ideological totality, presenting instead a memorialised femininity which resists definition within a purely heraldic context.[59]

Antony and Cleopatra does not merely present us with a meditation on the universality and timelessness of man's ongoing battle with mortality, but confronts the audience with a historically delimited range of possibilities for the ritualisation of death. These possibilities manifest themselves in the varying postures of dying which find their way onto the stage, sometimes palpably embodied in the play's memorable death-scenes, at other times glimpsed more obliquely in the characters' struggle for control over the process of memorialisation itself. Indeed, the play culminates in Octavius Caesar's stage-managing of the memorial rites of the ill-fated lovers, whose imminent ceremonial apotheosis is invested with the narrative properties of chronicle history:

> No grave upon the earth shall clip in it
> A pair so famous. High events as these
> Strike those that make them, and their story is
> No less in pity than his glory which
> Brought them to be lamented. Our army shall
> In solemn show attend this funeral . . . (V, ii, 359–63)

The posthumous rites which Octavius initiates bear all the hallmarks of the heraldic funeral, with its full complement of military honours. The central place of this paraphernalia of warfare as well as the hierarchical scheme of the proceedings, suggested in his demand for '[h]igh order in this great solemnity' (V, ii, 365), indicate that the funereal 'show' will serve to authorise a concept of civic rectitude which is specifically masculine. In the *Booke of Heraldrye . . . Burialls and Enterementes*, Robert Commaundre identifies such trappings of burial as belonging exclusively to men, for 'yt is not Convenient, that a woman should have a ban[er] or Pen[n]on of Armes . . . or shield, helme and Crest, the which is not lawefull to saye a vallyante woman . . . But it very well correspondeth to saye a valliant man of armes or a good man of warre.'[60] In the formal service of lamentation Octavius has planned there is no room for a paean to female virtue.

By removing Cleopatra from the monumentalised feminine space which she shares with 'her women' (V, ii, 356), by insisting that she 'be buried by her Antony' (V, ii, 357), Octavius decentralises her body, placing it within a dynastic setting which will constitute a visible document of succession; the incorporation of her wealth, property and power into his own person. The commemorative enterprise which he seeks to implement allows him to become official chronicler, at once recorder and author, of the 'high events' whose memorial inscription will serve as a barometer of his own 'glory'. However the ritual gestures which are intended to facilitate his status as the sole contriver of Cleopatra's 'story', and hence of her memorial legacy, have already lost their potency by the time his apparent victory is realised. As we will see, Cleopatra's own dying postures pre-empt and thus diffuse the meanings which Octavius intends to impose upon her 'grave', challenging the ideological contours of such histories in stone. This process relies on the implicit recognition of Octavius as a mouthpiece for imperially-authorised protocols of death, something which Shakespeare dextrously emphasises by deliberately deviating from one of his key source-texts,

Thomas North's translation of *Plutarch's Lives of the Noble Grecians and Romanes* (1579):

> ANTONY . . . he [Octavius] hath waged
> New wars 'gainst Pompey; made his will, and read it
> To public ear;
> Spoke scantly of me; when perforce he could not
> But pay me terms of honour, cold and sickly
> He vented them; most narrow measure lent me . . . (III, iv, 3–8)

In Plutarch's history Antony is himself the author of the offending 'will' in which he asks, in defiance of Roman propriety, 'that his bodie, though he dyed at Rome, should be brought in funerall pompe . . . into Alexandria unto Cleopatra'.[61] Shakespeare, on the other hand, attributes the will to Octavius, making him a master-manipulator of Antony's public image while simultaneously weakening the latter's proficiency in the art of self-memorialisation. This is in keeping with Shakespeare's delineation of Antony as undergoing a crisis of identity in which his own 'visible shape' becomes as mutable as the 'signs' which adorn 'black vesper's pageants', perhaps an ominous allusion to the empty theatricality of funereal observance (IV, xiv, 7–14).[62] The catalyst for this crisis is an anxiety that his 'remembrance [will] suffer ill report' (II, ii, 165), something echoed by Cleopatra when she hints that Antony, while in Rome, would be desirous to conceal the fact that his 'remembrance lay/In Egypt with his joy' (I, v, 60–1). That Shakespeare deliberately presents Antony's contacts with the Egyptian queen as having a destabilising effect on his ability to govern the ritual concomitants of memory is made apparent when we compare him to his more assertive alter ego in *Julius Caesar* (c. 1599). In this play it is Antony who reads Caesar's will to the plebeians, commandeering the legacy tradition in order to incite his audience to rebellion. The context for the will is clearly a heraldic funeral, in which Caesar's body is conveyed on a 'hearse' (III, ii, 159) in a procession flanked by the public. As Antony appears in the role of chief mourner (III, ii, 38), his funeral oration makes Caesar's heroic bleeding body coterminous with the very process of legacy-giving:

> But here's a parchment with the seal of Caesar.
> I found it in his closet. 'Tis his will.
> Let but the commons hear this testament . . .
> And they would go and kiss dead Caesar's wounds,
> And dip their napkins in his sacred blood,
> Yea, beg a hair of him for memory,
> And, dying, mention it within their wills,
> Bequeathing it as a rich legacy
> Unto their issue. (III, ii, 125–34)

With its allusions to Catholic martyrdom, the 'memory' which Antony fashions, and which allows him to control the meanings of the death-ritual, is based on a Renaissance doctrine which sees the sanctity of kingship as transmissible within the primogenitural framework of the legacy tradition.[63] In *Antony and Cleopatra*, however, Antony's reaction to Octavius' will reveals the degree to which his own identity is subject to the ideologically freighted ceremonials which are a part of his enemy's representational arsenal, as he tells Octavia: 'If I lose mine honour,/I lose myself; better I were not yours/Than yours so branchless' (III, iv, 22–4). The branches referred to not only recall the offshoots of a family tree but also the victory-garland of war, a common motif in funerary decoration and heraldic custom alike, similar to that depicted in the Aston family portrait (Fig. 4.13). Antony thus locates within the image of a debased armorial body his fears that he will remain outside the very patrilineal system upon which the perpetuity of his honour among later generations depends. Significantly, Octavia's speech in this scene has, in part, been lifted from that of her Plutarchan prototype, but with one notable difference. In the earlier text she is visibly pregnant, being 'at that time . . . great with child', and is moreover a mother to 'a second daughter'.[64] By eliminating her maternal status and making her Antony's auditor as he recollects Octavius' will, Shakespeare accentuates the fact that Antony has 'Forborne the getting of a lawful race' (III, xiii, 112). This is reflected in his own self-portrait as a cuckolded husband when he muses upon the 'hotter hours,/Unregistered in vulgar fame' that Cleopatra has 'Luxuriously picked out', making him a member of the 'hornèd herd!' (III, xiii, 123–5).

Antony's language raises the spectre of an ignoble form of memorialisation, the 'vulgar fame' which Octavius, in a rhetorical sleight-of-hand, had already opposed to those more legitimate registers of memory which 'reported' how Antony had once 'borne [himself] so like a soldier' (I, iv, 68–71). Octavius undermines Antony's legendary status by presenting his attempts at reclaiming this heroic persona before the 'public eye' as a travesty of the legacy tradition:

> I'th' market-place, on a tribunal silvered,
> Cleopatra and himself in chairs of gold
> Were publicly enthroned. At the feet sat
> Caesarion, whom they call my father's son,
> And all the unlawful issue that their lust
> Since then hath made between them . . .
> His sons he there proclaimed the kings of kings:
> Great Media, Parthia and Armenia
> He gave to Alexander; to Ptolemy he assigned
> Syria, Cilicia and Phoenicia. (III, vi, 3–16)

By focusing on the illegitimacy of his 'issue', Antony's distribution of land and property in the 'common showplace' (III, vi, 12) becomes not only a breach of social and familial propriety, but a flagrant violation of the law. Octavius juxtaposes this scandalous public pageant with the lawful displays which should attend, and thus ratify, Antony's legitimate family, as he explains to Octavia: 'The wife of Antony/Should have an army for an usher, and/The neighs of horse to tell of her approach/Long ere she did appear . . . But you are come/A market maid to Rome, and have prevented/The ostentation of our love' (III, vi, 44–53). In the Renaissance these were the very trappings supplied by the College of Arms for the public processions which magnified royalty and honoured dignitaries. And it is in this context that we can better understand why Cleopatra chooses to adopt the similar stance of a 'maid that milks/And does the meanest chares' as one of her many dying postures (IV, xv, 78–9). If Octavius succeeds in partially dismantling Antony's iconic notoriety by manipulating the honorific codes enshrined in heraldic practice, his strategy is exposed and demystified by the more resilient queen after Antony's bungled suicide:

> CAESAR . . . by taking
> Antony's course, you shall bereave yourself
> Of my good purposes, and put your children
> To that destruction which I'll guard them from
> If thereon you rely. I'll take my leave.
> CLEOPATRA And may through all the world! 'Tis yours, and we,
> Your scutcheons and your signs of conquest, shall
> Hang in what place you please. (V, ii, 128–35)

Behind his assertion that he has nothing but 'good purposes' towards her children, Octavius holds out the promise of their relegitimation through the mechanisms of inheritance, a response to Cleopatra's former request to give legacies to her heirs: 'If he please/To give me conquered Egypt for my son,/He gives me so much of mine own as I/Will kneel to him with thanks' (V, ii, 18–21). But Cleopatra, in her apparent willingness to participate in a ritual of warfare which culminates in the formalised transmission of conquered property, actually questions the value of the conventions which underpin it. Demonstrating a particular sensitivity to the kinds of emblematic measures which Octavius characteristically employs throughout the play in order to exert his control over the communal memory and reputations of his enemies, she parodies his role as a heraldic choreographer, forcing it to its *reductio ad absurdum* by turning herself and her children into mere ciphers of heraldry, 'scutcheons' and 'signs of conquest'. Cleopatra discloses her awareness that her self-authored death would strike at the very heart of an ideological programme which relies so heavily on the public recognition of such symbolic rites of incorporation. Her defiant utterances rest on a recognition of the ideological commensurability between heraldic and cosmic order as it is expressed in Renaissance emblem-theory. In *The True Use of Armorie* (1592) William Wyrley presents the worldly purveyors of these rites as wielding nothing less than a Godly power:

> [T]he bearing of Armes, raising and advauncing of Standerds, Banners and Ensignes, using of obsequies, erecting of moniments, enroling and regestrings of pedegrees and descents have joyned to the auncient customes and Lawes both of this Land and all other nations, the authoritie of Gods word being very well accompanied with discretion, reason, and judgement, for God having by his sacred institution ordeined Kingdomes, Provinces, and Seignories, and that over them Kings, Princes and Magistrates, shall commaund, rule and governe his people, to the ende chiefly that his heavenly kingdom may be replenished with the blessed soules of his servants . . .[65]

It is this very impulse towards the *naturalisation* of imperialist memorialisation – which makes the heraldic scheme synonymous with the divinely-sanctioned and parthenogenically self-replicating law of nature – that Cleopatra's postures of death work to destabilise; postures which, as I hope to show, evade the contingent signs of patriarchal hegemony. She achieves this by exposing the artificiality of Octavius' commemorative project in relation to what she constructs as the most *natural* of death's affective hieroglyphs: the maternal body. How Shakespeare conceived Cleopatra's role as mother can be gleaned through a consideration of another of his possible source-texts, *The Tragedie of Antonie* (1590) by Mary Sidney, Countess of Pembroke.[66] That the play subtly interrogates the human cost of maintaining the heraldic world-view is suggested by the 'Chorus of Romaine souldiors': 'shall thick in each land/our wretched trophees stand,/to tell posteritie,/what madd Impietie/our stonie stomacks led/against the place us bred?' (IV, 378–83). The function of armorial 'trophees', to memorialise acts of valour and record the acquisition of land and property which arises from this martial success, is here overturned. Rather than extolling the vertues of the deceased for 'posteritie' they will serve as markers for a ravished maternal landscape.[67] The debate which the play stages around the validity and significance of formalised repositories of genealogy is, however, mainly centred on a small community of women in Cleopatra's court. Together they form a female circle of mourning through which the protocols of death are both implemented and contested. When Cleopatra resolves to die for Antony, Charmion labels her a 'Hardharted mother!' since her death would dissolve her children's 'royall right' and leave them 'deprive[d] of heritage' (II, 319–23). She advises her to seize command of the death-ritual for her own purposes, insisting that the implementation of the appropriate funerary customs are the only means of rehabilitating Antony's reputation and of securing her children's safety:

> builde for him a tombe
> Whose statelinesse a wonder new may make.
> Let him, let him have sumptuous funeralls:
> Let grave thereon the horror of his fights . . .
> Make all his combats, and couragious acts:
> And yearley plaies to his praise institute:
> Honor his memory: with doubled care
> Breed and bring up the children of you both
> In *Caesars* grace: who as a noble Prince
> Will leave them Lords of this most glorious realme. (II, 369–82)

Elements of this fantasy may well have appealed to the Countess of Pembroke who, like Elizabeth Hoby Russell, was actively engaged in expanding the limits of women's engagement in the public demonstration of grieving. That her literary endeavours enabled her to fashion successfully a persona for herself as Sir Philip Sidney's chief mourner is suggested by Abraham Fraunce's mythologised portrait of her in his *Ivychurch*, in which she appears as the very axis of a coterie of women who meet on an annual basis to conduct the fitting memorial rites.[68] However, in Pembroke's *Antonie*, Charmion presents such histrionic customs as ultimately serving the political interests of Octavius, becoming a propagandist vehicle for the demonstration of his 'grace'. As such Cleopatra's reproductive body is reduced to a mere vessel for dynastic legitimation.

The play does not, as we might expect, show us an alternative to this construction of maternity. Though Cleopatra refuses to perform what she sees as the fruitless ritual aggrandising of Antony's 'high estate' (II, 389), wishing instead to base her actions on 'vertue' (II, 408), this is a specifically 'wively' virtue (II, 354) which she pointedly opposes to her role as mother (II, 320). In her last moments, with her children appearing by her side, Cleopatra performs what sounds very much like an epitaphic utterance, one which equates her death with what she imagines to be the worst fate that can possibly befall them; the loss of the specifically paternal inheritance in which the family's 'remembrance' is invested: 'Adieu deare children, children deare adieu . . ./Remember not, my children, you were borne/Of such a Princely race . . ./That this great *Antony* your father was, *Hercules* bloud' (V, 55–65). Even her protestations that she is able to outdo the 'weeping *Niobe*' in 'griefe' do not serve unproblematically to align her with this most legendary of mourning mothers, whose monumental apotheosis she fails to acquire: 'Thy children thou, mine I poore soule have lost,/And lost their Father, more then them I waile,/Lost this faire realme; yet me the heavens wrath/Into a stone not yet transformed hath' (V, 95–104). She could be suggesting that she laments the fate of her children all the more, not because they will be without a mother, but because they will live bereft of a father whose lineage would have assured them the 'realm' now eternally beyond their reach; or that she mourns the loss of her husband and her kingdom 'more *th[a]n*' that of her children. Either way, her slippery and ambiguous rhetoric serves to de-emphasise the sufficiency of the fractured maternal bond as a focus for the public postures of mourning.

Though Pembroke's Cleopatra is unable finally to achieve the status of monumentalised mother within the confines of a dynastically oriented etiquette of memorialisation, this cannot be said for Shakespeare's creation. In her appropriations of the death-ritual this Cleopatra confronts the audience with an affective vocabulary of dying which cannot be entirely supplanted by the threat of paternal privation which, as we saw in the first part of this chapter, is the justificatory engine for heraldic commemoration. She does this by situating her body in an entirely different nexus of meanings, one in which it is no longer purely an instrument of primogeniture. Indeed, Cleopatra, who has 'such a celerity in dying' (I, ii, 151), proves herself to be as deft a manipulator of the rites of memory as Octavius. In the very first act she exploits the death of Fulvia in order to monopolise Antony's attention at the expense of his duties in Rome:

> ANTONY . . . At the last, best,
> See when and where she died.
> CLEOPATRA O most false love!
> Where be the sacred vials thou shouldst fill
> With sorrowful water? Now I see, I see,
> In Fulvia's death how mine received shall be . . .
> I prithee, turn aside and weep for her,
> Then bid adieu to me, and say the tears
> Belong to Egypt. Good now, play one scene
> Of excellent dissembling, and let it look
> Like perfect honour. (I, iii, 62–81)

Antony's statement is equivocal, either praising Fulvia for having *died well* or simply indicating his saving the best news (of her death) for last. Not surprisingly, Cleopatra seizes on the latter interpretation. The 'sacred vials' to which she refers are not only the tear-filled eyes of grief but the lachrymatories or ritual offerings of Roman funereal custom.[69]

Antony is accused of neglecting the proper rites of burial which belong to his wife, an imposture which Cleopatra imagines will be repeated after her own death. In an ingenious rhetorical flourish she insists that since Antony is the embodiment of the 'oblivion' to which she will eventually succumb, at a time when she will be 'all forgotten' (I, iii, 92–3), it necessarily follows that all formal protestations of sorrow are merely theatrical contrivances. Claiming to stand aloof from these debased ceremonials she locates her own feelings of love outside the shows of ritualised mourning and within the idea of a suffering maternity: ''Tis *sweating labour*/To bear such idleness so near the heart/As Cleopatra this. But, sir, forgive me,/Since *my becomings kill me* when they do not/Eye well to you. Your honour calls you hence;/. . . Upon your sword/Sit laurel victory' (I, iii, 95–102, my italics). The depth of her emotion, she maintains, results in a painful 'labour' which kills the mother during delivery. In a final oratorical twist she juxtaposes these natural signs of female honour with the empty emblems of masculine distinction after which Antony strives: the 'target', 'sword' and the 'laurel [of] victory' (I, iii, 83–102). This is not the only instance in which Cleopatra seeks to adopt the tragic role of a dying mother. Indeed, it becomes one of the play's persistent leitmotifs. When Antony accuses her of sheltering divided loyalties, she protests her devotion in an emphatic speech which draws on the deepest recesses of her maternal instincts:

> if I be so,
> From my cold heart let heaven engender hail
> And poison it in the source, and the first stone
> Drop in my neck; as it determines, so
> Dissolve my life! The next Caesarion smite,
> Till by degrees the memory of my womb,
> Together with my brave Egyptians all,
> By the discandying of the pelleted storm
> Lie graveless, till the flies and gnats of Nile
> Have buried them for prey! (III, xiii, 163–72)

This nightmare vision of Cleopatra's self-destroying generativity culminates in the ignominious abortion of the ceremonial order which will leave her people 'graveless'. While the maternal body is presented as outgrowing the familiar bounds of the death-ritual, it also provides a locus for a female sense of honour which finds its most authentic correlation within the 'memory' of Cleopatra's womb. Since in Shakespeare's day the word 'memory' could designate a memorial inscription of any kind, including that preserved on a tomb, the very act of commemoration is here redefined as a specifically feminine prerogative.[70]

Though Cleopatra is often described as the most 'theatrical' of Shakespeare's tragic figures, the structural device which actually informs her monumental end is, surprisingly, the deliberate elision of theatricality as an appropriate medium for an epistemology of death. Highlighting the visual vocabulary which Octavius intends to deploy in order to become 'eternal in . . . triumph' (V, i, 66), Cleopatra juxtaposes her own memorialisation with forms of 'imperious show' which are illusory, lubricious and debased (IV, xv, 24). Her fears that Octavius will turn her into 'an Egyptian puppet', patronising Rome's 'quick comedians' who will 'stage' her in 'th' posture of a whore' (V, ii, 207–20), are realised in Proculeius' own injunction: 'Do not abuse my master's bounty by/Th' undoing of yourself. Let the world *see*/His nobleness *well acted*, which your death/Will never let come forth' (V, ii, 42–5, my italics). The expressly masculine parthenogenic 'bounty' which Octavius seeks to flaunt as a measure of his 'nobleness' is, however, invalidated by the pathos which Cleopatra draws from the evocation of a perverted fertility, answering Proculeius with the words: 'Rather a ditch in Egypt/Be gentle grave unto me! Rather on Nilus' mud/Lay me stark naked, and let the waterflies/Blow me into abhorring' (V, ii, 56–9). Here she conjures yet another image of a maimed burial rite, one which nullifies by its extremity of 'horror' (V, ii, 62) the effectiveness of any violence which Octavius could possibly perpetrate against her memory. The epitome for this concept of posthumous virtue is the spectacle of the naked female body 'blown' as if pregnant, the very cradle of the death-boding fly. And it is the fate of the doomed maternal body, as a potent emblem of how 'all labour/Mars what it does' (IV, xiv, 48–9), that becomes the subject of the false death-bed narrative which Cleopatra asks Mardian to fashion, insisting that he 'word . . . piteously' her tragic end in the 'monument' (IV, xiii, 9–11):

> The last she spake
> Was 'Antony! Most noble Antony!'
> Then, in the midst, a tearing groan did break
> The name of Antony; it was divided
> Between her heart and lips. She rendered life,
> Thy name so buried in her. (IV, xiv, 29–34)

Mardian appropriates the rhetorical scheme of the 'good death', fashioning a tableau which evokes the anguish of a mother's childbed demise. Cleopatra's body becomes the grave or tomb of Antony's name which, like a newly-formed baby, she struggles to deliver with her 'tearing groans', recalling the sad fate of many a Renaissance mother. During the late sixteenth and early seventeenth centuries pictorial representations of this kind of tragic loss were more widely disseminated than at any other

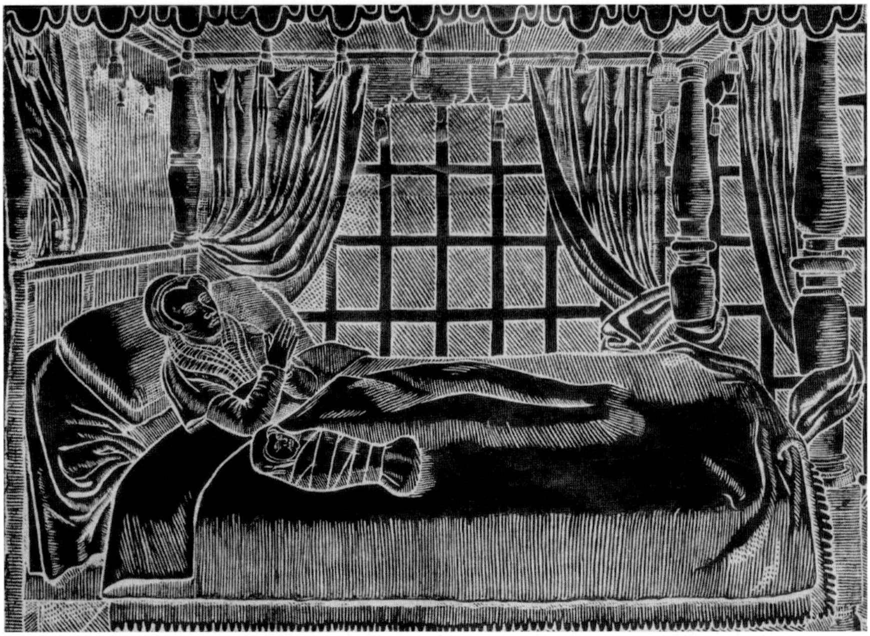

Figure 4.15: Funerary brass plaque of Anne Savage, d. 1605, Wormington, Gloucestershire. Reproduced by kind permission of English Heritage, National Monuments Record.

time in history, particularly on tomb brasses and wall monuments. When Anne Savage died in childbirth in 1605, the brass plaque erected to her memory in Wormington, Gloucestershire, described her fiery apotheosis, for 'Like another Phoenix she perished thus giving birth' (Fig. 4.15).[71] In 1639 Jane Crewe was commemorated in Westminster Abbey. Her wall plaque, attributed to Epiphanius Evesham, recaptures the drama and the trauma of her last moments (Fig. 4.16). In the centre of a stylised interior the dead mother lies on a tomb-shaped bed, one hand stretched over her womb. Her newly-born infant appears in the foreground, reclining upon a diminutive copy of his mother's sepulchral couch, while her husband and surviving children adopt the conventional attitudes of mourning. These memorials illustrate the opportunities for experimentation afforded those who designed and commissioned monuments of women. The extremity of such loss, the tragic severing of the mother-child bond in death, licensed the creation of monumental styles which resisted the formalised postures of more heraldic models.

That Cleopatra's dying postures exploit the affective and even 'theatrical' elements which inform the creation of these poignant memorials cannot be denied. When she employs the anti-theatrical discourse

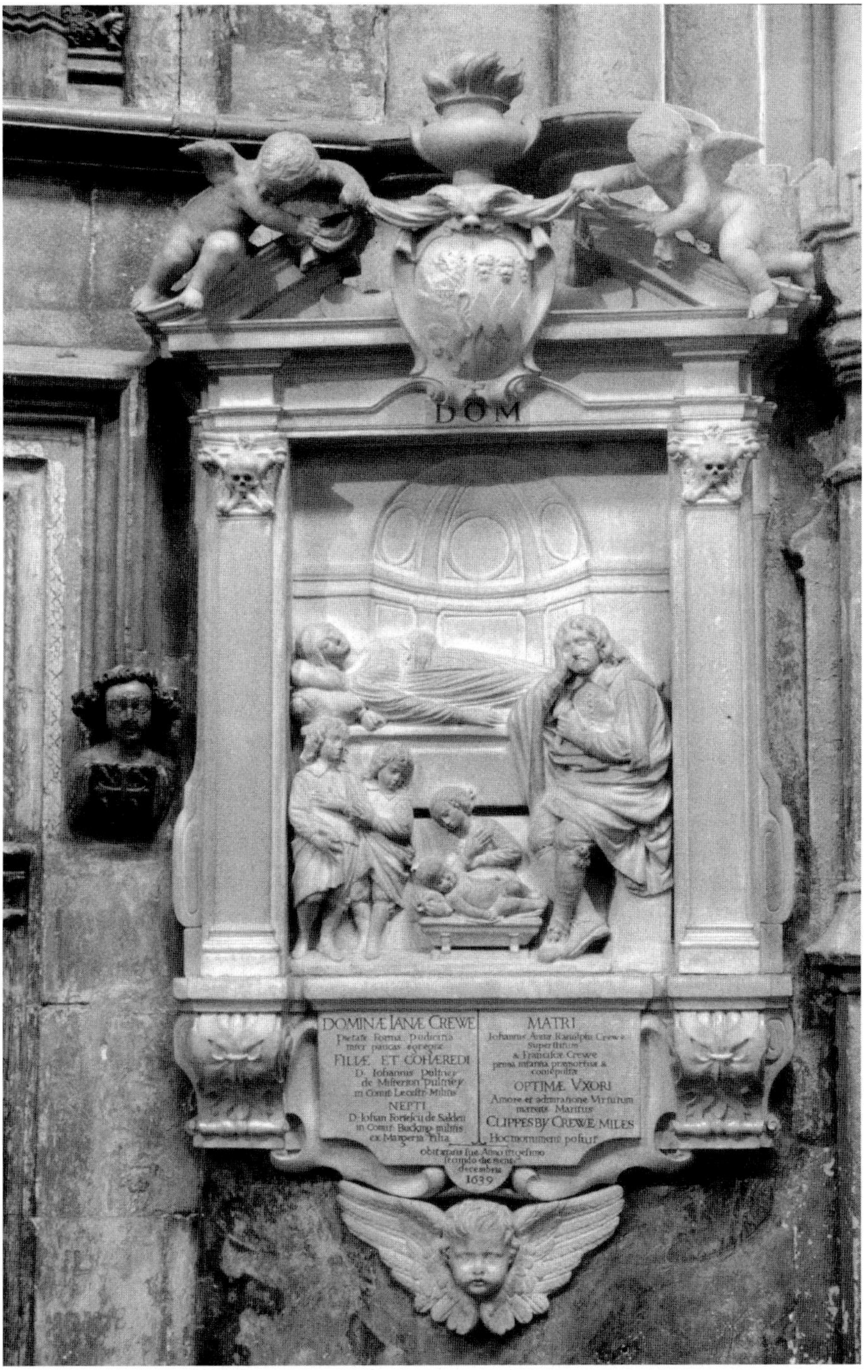

Figure 4.16: Monument of Jane Crewe, 1639, Westminster Abbey. By kind permission of the Dean and Chapter of Westminster.

against Octavius, however, she is drawing the battle-lines across a debate which surrounded the controversial use of funereal and commemorative customs in Renaissance England. From the late sixteenth century onwards, texts which dealt with the arts of remembrance increasingly expressed an anxiety regarding the validity of such rituals of display as expressions of true virtue. In *The Holy State* (1642) Thomas Fuller insisted that '*Tombes ought in some sort to be proportioned not to the wealth but deserts of the party interred.*' Churches and cathedrals should be populated only by 'monuments to mens merits' for, he observed, '[I]n some monuments . . . the red veins in the marble may seem to blush at the falshoods written on it. He was a witty man that first taught a stone to speak, but he was a wicked man that taught it first to lie'.[72] Similarly John Weever, author of a disquisition on *Ancient Funerall Monuments* (1631), insisted that 'stately monuments' should not be provided for 'every man that was of ability to erect the same' since 'by some epitaphs more honour is attributed to a rich quondam Tradesman, or griping usurer, then is given to the greatest Potentate entombed in Westminster'. Such sentiments cannot be divorced from the demands of a historiographical enquiry which sought to legitimate the claims of the ruling classes. While Weever, like many a fellow antiquarian, looked to his classical forebears to provide the template for the ideal community of the dead, this glorious necropolis was invaded by a generation of upstart crows, whose unwanted effigial lodgers turned the most hallowed mausolea into the repositories of the age's most 'monstrous' vanities. Because they were often 'veiled under . . . fantasticke habits and attires', these monumental figures became 'rather provocations to vice, then incitations to vertue', making the Temple of God 'a Schoolehouse . . . wherein Taylors may find out new fashions'.[73] This kind of imagery is remarkably similar to that deployed in the antitheatrical texts of the time. In his *Playes Confuted in Five Actions* (1582), Stephen Gosson sees the theatre as 'being but a[n] assemblie of Tailers'. These are given first billing among a range of other debased theatre-goers, including 'Tinkers, Cordwayners, [and] Saylers',[74] a roll-call reminiscent of Cleopatra's reference to the 'Saucy lictors' and 'Mechanic slaves/With greasy aprons, rules, and hammers' who will theatricalise her memory (V, ii, 208–13). These ideas find an apt corollary in John Webster's *The Duchess of Malfi* (c. 1612–13). Masquerading as a tomb-maker whose 'trade is to flatter the dead' (IV, ii, 139), Bosola asks the Duchess 'of what fashion' she will have her tomb:

DUCHESS Why, do we grow fantastical in our death-bed?
Do we affect fashion in the grave?

> BOSOLA Most ambitiously. Princes' images on their tombs do not lie,
> as they were wont, seeming to pray up to heaven: but with their
> hands under their cheeks, as if they died of the tooth-ache. They
> are not carved with their eyes fixed upon the stars, but as their minds
> were wholly bent upon the world, the selfsame way they
> seem to turn their faces. (IV, ii, 146–53)[75]

The new method of monumental representation Bosola decries is presented as a visible challenge to the purely dynastic tombs whose perpetual tenants seemed 'to pray/Up to Heaven'.[76] The former not only evokes the seated pose of the Russell monument, in which the effigy props up a languid cheek with her cupped hand (Fig. 4.1), but may also allude to another stylistic innovation. By the end of the sixteenth century stone figures began to appear resting on their sides, often 'with their hands under their cheeks'. This arrangement, with its emphasis upon the horizontal field of the statue's gaze, reflected a fundamental shift in attitudes as well as taste. Looking out at the world, rather than upwards to God, sculptures of women in particular could deal with everyday concerns, with their roles as wives and mothers. The tomb of Sir Edward Seymour, who died in 1593, and his son, who died in 1613, praises the fecundity of the latter's wife Elizabeth who, says the epitaph, 'had isshew 11 children by him' (Fig. 4.17). But the tomb, which can be seen in Berry Pomeroy, Devon, constitutes a split register of values. The portion depicting Elizabeth is very different from the effigies of her husband and father-in-law, decked in full military regalia. She is dressed in contemporary clothing and clutches a tiny bible in her hand, a symbol of her spiritual courage in the face of death, as well as of her desire to impart sacred knowledge to her children. Below her head a baby reposes in a cradle while at her feet an effigy of a child is rendered with touching realism; her cheeks puffy, her eyes attentive, seated in a chair just as she would be at home under the care of her mother. The monument of Elizabeth Williams (d. 1622), executed by Samuel Baldwin for the Lady Chapel of Gloucester Cathedral, also shows the deceased mother holding a gold-embellished bible as she leans protectively over her swaddled child (Fig. 4.18). This scriptural motif may reflect a way in which women were able to participate in the private gestures of legacy-giving. In anticipation of her death in 1619, for example, Lady Strode of Newingham bequeathed a gift to her children, one which acted as a legitimate vehicle for a textual 'mother's legacy', imparting advice as well as blessing, for she 'left certain Bibles to be delivered to her daughters, with this writ on them; *I have said, that my flesh shall perish and rot: but the word of the Lord shall endure for ever: and blessed shall you be, if you constantly, unto the end, delight to seek and follow that, with*

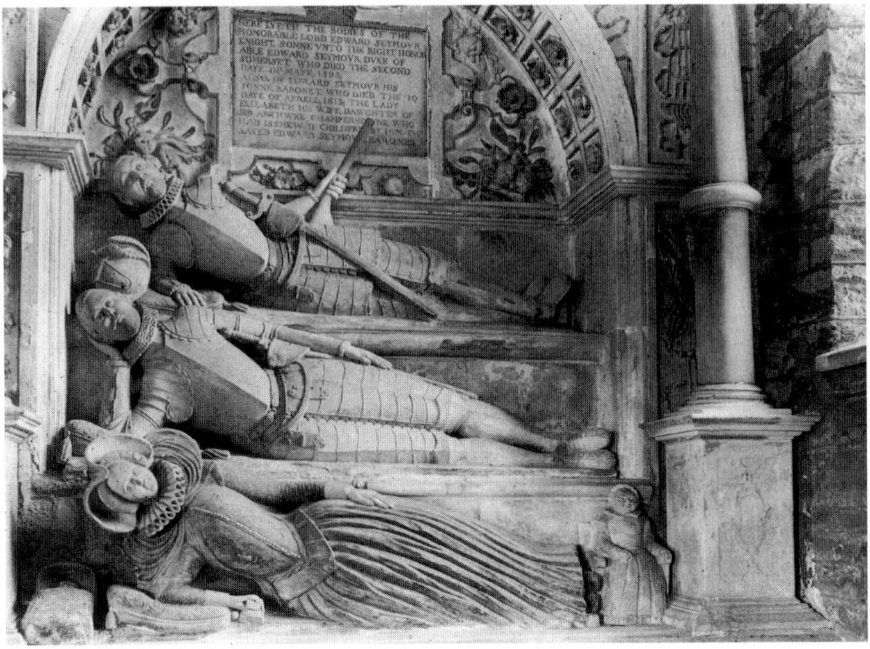

Figure 4.17: Monument of Edward Seymour, d. 1593 and his son, d. 1613, Berry Pomeroy, Devon. Conway Library, The Courtauld Institute of Art, London.

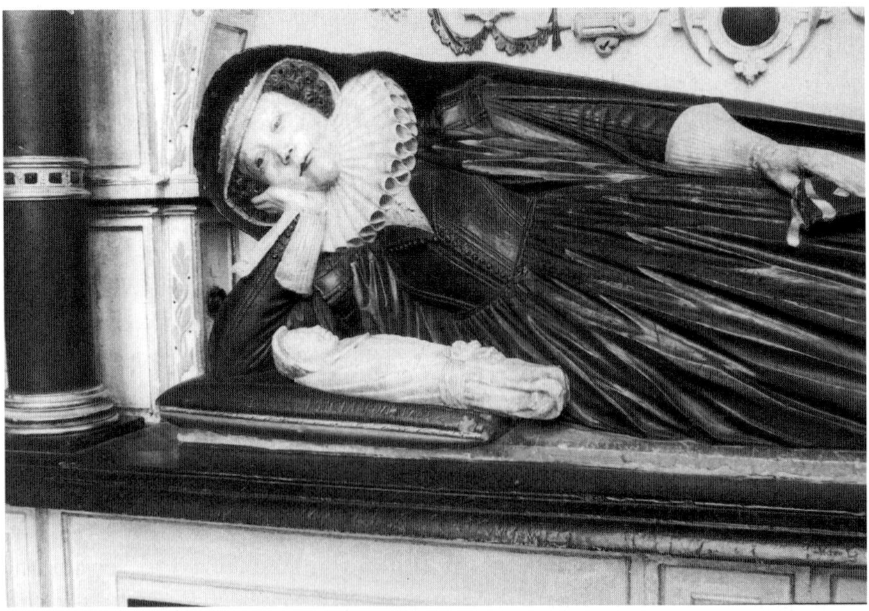

Figure 4.18: Monument of Elizabeth Williams, d. 1622, Lady Chapel, Gloucester Cathedral. Conway Library, The Courtauld Institute of Art, London.

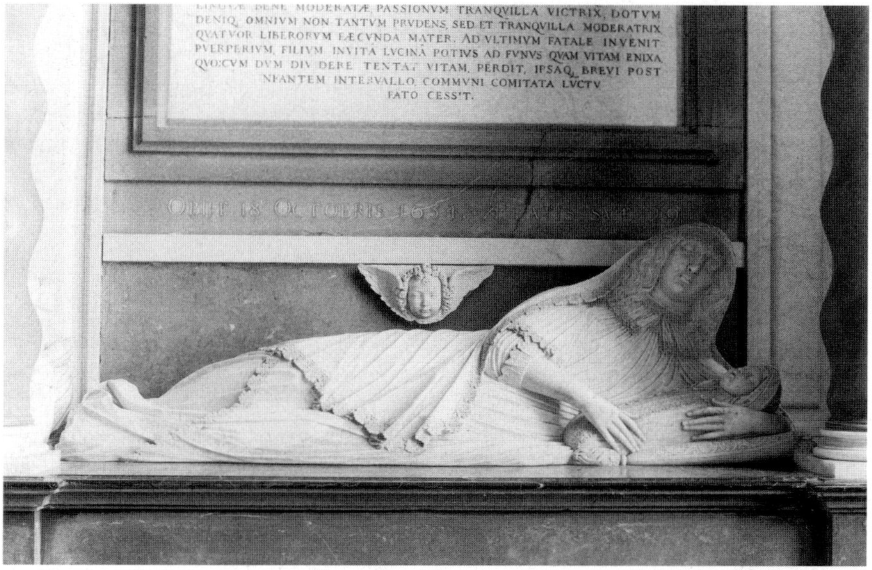
MODERATÆ PASSIONVM TRANQVILLA VICTRIX, DOTVM
DENIQ. OMNIVM NON TANTVM PRVDENS, SED ET TRANQVILLA MODERATRIX
QVATVOR LIBERORVM FÆCVNDA MATER. AD VLTIMVM FATALE INVENIT
PVERPERIVM, FILIVM INVITA LVCINA POTIVS AD FVNVS QVAM VITAM ENIXA
VITAM, PERDIT, IPSAQ. BREVI POST
COMMVNI COMITATA LVCTV
FATO

Figure 4.19: Monument of Mary Coventry, d. 1634, Croome d'Abitot, Worcestershire. Conway Library, The Courtauld Institute of Art, London.

faithfull and true hearts'. That she believed her maternal role could be most aptly enshrined in a form of memorialisation shorn of ceremonial excess is evident in her own death-bed will which expresses 'her desire . . . that there might be no blacks worne for her, at her Funerals, except by her owne house at the most', thus making the domestic sphere the centre of mourning.[77]

Just as the *mother's legacy* tradition centralised the feminine scene of death, allowing dying women to gain a voice and even, as funerary sermons of the age indicated, an audience by playing out the drama and trauma of their own fatal maternity, the maternal monument recapitulated the space in which many Renaissance mothers had met their untimely ends: the beds upon which they had given birth. In 1634 Mary Coventry died in childbirth and was commemorated in Croome d'Abitot in Worcestershire (Fig. 4.19). Her effigy is sumptuously dressed in bed-clothes and embellished with an epitaph which describes her as a 'fruitful mother' (*faecunda mater*), a phrase which may also carry oratorical connotations since the word *faecunda* is reminiscent of the Latin *facundus*, meaning 'eloquent'. Variations of this posture also emerged in the shape of the near-recumbent, though not static effigy. The tomb of Elizabeth Coke, in Bramfield, Suffolk, records that she died in childbirth in 1627 (Fig. 4.20). She is captured in stone, reclining on a deep pillow with her child, covered up to her waist with lace-trimmed

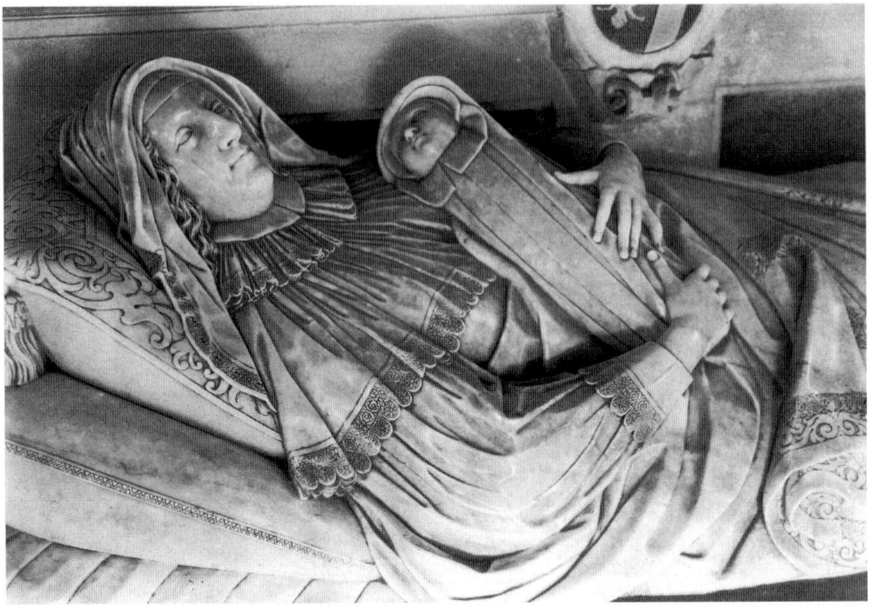

Figure 4.20: Monument of Elizabeth Coke, d. 1627, Bramfield, Suffolk. Conway Library, The Courtauld Institute of Art, London.

bed-sheets.[78] This is echoed in the posture and dress of Anne Leighton, who died during the birth of her thirteenth child (Fig. 4.21). Her monument was commissioned in 1634 by her husband, Sir John St John, in Lydiard Tregoze, Wiltshire, and is the work of Samuel Baldwin. The monuments of these nurturing women, repeating the witnessing process which takes place at the feminine death-bed, do not signify the cessation of their maternal duties, but display the imminence of loss as a pretext for an affirmation of those responsibilities.[79]

Such tombs, I would argue, embody a specifically gendered dichotomy, straddling two different traditions of monumental design. Whereas the dynastic or purely heraldic tomb usually presents the female body as a vehicle for the perpetuation of patrilineage, as an expendable vessel for the production of future heirs, tombs which begin to include women in maternal postures show mothers in the dynamic act of nurturing. No longer passive receptacles for the male parthenogenic fantasy which underpins legal constructions of inheritance and primogeniture, they are actively engaged in maternal work. Sharing the public space, these tombs visibly stake a claim for the shaping influence of maternity in the cultivation of civic virtue, re-inscribing the domestic sphere as the training-ground for public life. We must, however, exercise caution here. The visual vocabulary deployed by these memorials should not be seen as

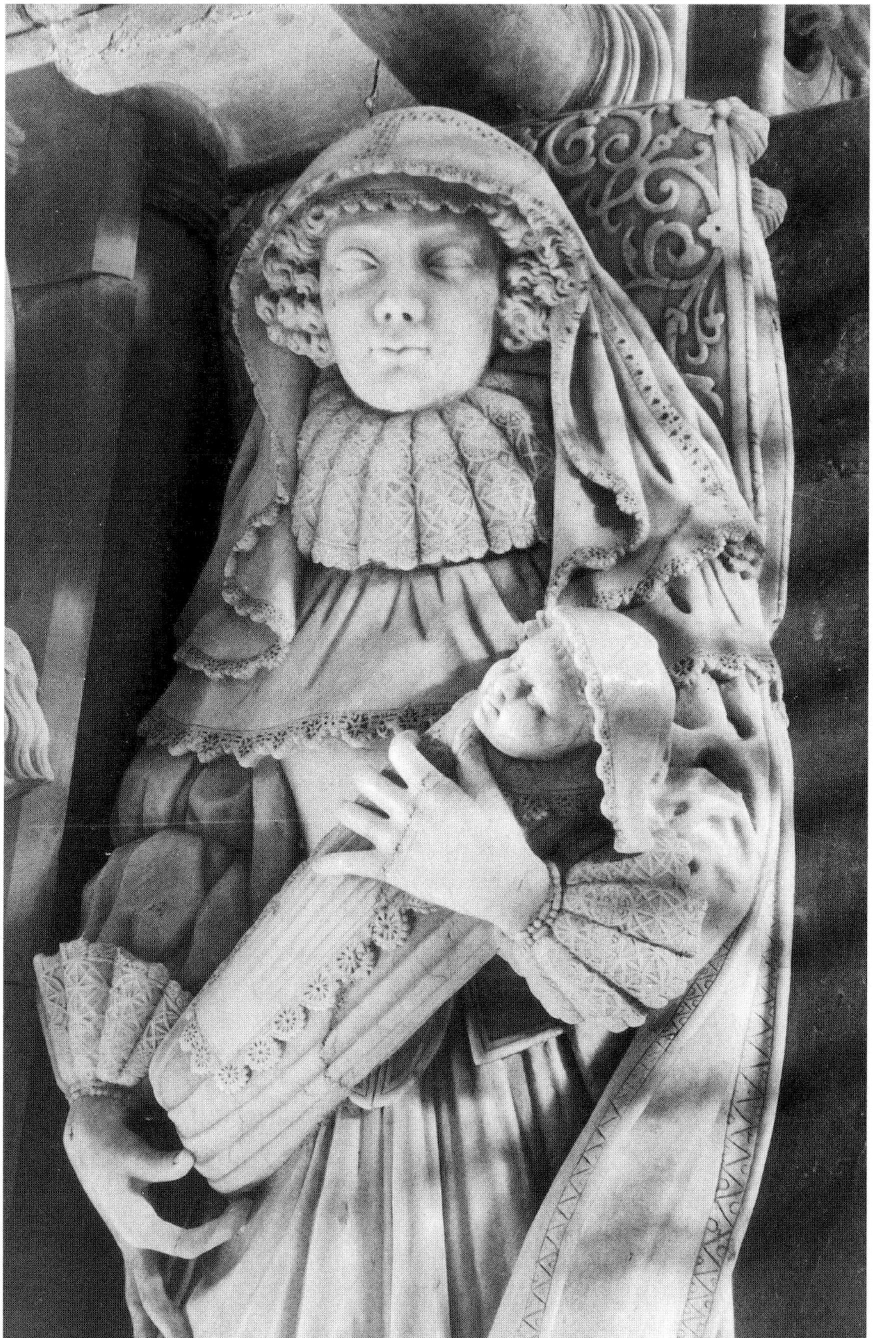

Figure 4.21: Monument of Anne Leighton, d. 1634, Lydiard Tregoze, Wiltshire. Conway Library, The Courtauld Institute of Art, London.

constituting a proto-feminist utterance. Rather it allowed the rising classes, in an age of increased social mobility, to base the honour and nobility which they claimed on more than the precarious accoutrements of heraldry.[80] In his treatise on *The Nobles or of Nobilitye* (1563) Lawrence Humfrey praised the 'Magnificence of monumentes, tombes, funeral oractions, Images, Chappelles, and Epitaphes' fashioned in classical times as paeans to 'noble actes, and praise worthy offices'. These admirable endeavours were to be contrasted with the all too often empty ostentation of his contemporaries, whose honour consisted only in 'outwarde shewe and vaunt'.[81] Placing the emphasis on 'private vertues', he urged his contemporaries to cultivate a 'domestical discipline', turning the home into the very well-spring of nobility, the only bulwark against the excessively theatricalised politic world, where one may 'as in a free schoole shape & forme him selfe: before thence he be thruste abroade as into an open stage'.[82]

There was always a danger that those who erected lavish memorials, with all their gorgeous apparel, would find themselves at the wrong end of the elite community's censuring finger, and come to epitomise what Henry Peacham most despised: 'neither must we Honour or esteeme those ennobled . . . [because they] weare the Cloath of a Noble Personage, or have purchased an ill Coat at a good rate; no more then a Player upon the Stage, for wearing a Lords cast suit'.[83] The maternal monument both engaged with, and attempted to efface, its own theatricality by displaying what its textual and visual apparatus claimed were essential qualities. If it 'spoke' of the importance of the deceased's private virtue to the quotidian world upon which it often gazed, it did so by paradoxically insisting on the insufficiency of the outward, the visual, as accurate indicators of merit. What I am not suggesting is that Shakespeare's Cleopatra fully embodies all the traits of the exemplary mother as they are conveyed in such commemorative practices. Rather the play's many references to her maternity constantly foreground a sense of dissatisfaction with the traditional conventions of the death-ritual. While Octavius manipulates heraldic codes of honour, as we have seen, in order to delegitimise Cleopatra's line of succession, referring to her children as her 'unlawful issue' (III, vi, 7), the Egyptian queen exploits an emerging language of maternal memory in order to emphasise her inherent, her *natural* nobility. This is conveyed in her own self-appointed role as Antony's memorialiser which she takes on in the guise of being 'No more but e'en a woman' (IV, xv, 77): 'O withered is the garland of the war,/The soldier's pole is fallen; young boys and girls/Are level now with men; the odds is gone' (IV, xv, 66–8). Whereas the heraldic death-ritual was instituted to preserve distinctions, to pass them on as the due inheritance of the deceased's progeny, Cleopatra presents the loss of Antony as signalling the expiration of all heraldry and its concomitant armorial codes. She shatters, in effect, the primogenitural programme by burying it with Antony. Shakespeare's Cleopatra thus differs from that of Samuel Daniel, whose *Tragedy of Cleopatra* (1599) dramatises the impossibility of escaping such ritualised badges of nobility. Her own desire to procure 'Honor' means that she will be unable 'to purchase grace/For my distressed seede after my death', leaving them without a fitting inheritance:

> That's it alas detaines me from my tombe,
> Whiles Nature brings to contradict my soule
> The argument of mine unhappy wombe . . .
> Bloud, Children, Nature, all must pardon me.
> My soule yeeldes Honor up the victory,
> And I must be a Queene, forget a mother,
> Though mother would I be, were I not I;
> And Queene would not be now, could I be other. (I, 77–98)

The roles of honoured queen and 'wofull mother' (I, 83) are presented as entirely incompatible.[84] If she is to be noble in her end then she must relinquish her parental claims. In other words, her death will be a decidedly unmaternal, that is to say *unnatural* act. Though Shakespeare's Cleopatra claims the paraphernalia of royalty for herself, in her injunction to her women to 'Show me . . . like a queen' in 'My best attires . . . crown and all' (V, ii, 226–31), this image of queenship is not permitted to become coterminous with traditional models of monumentalised nobility. That this is the case may be gleaned from a text which has long been recognised as a possible source for the play by such commentators as Walter R. Coppedge and Janet Adelman.[85] Plutarch's essay 'Of Isis and Osiris', which appears in Philemon Holland's 1603 translation of the *Moralia*, presents Isis as a universal mother whose nurturing qualities are transmissible specifically because of her 'infinite' variety:

> For Isis is the feminine part of nature, apt to receive all generation, upon which occasion called she is by Plato, the nurse and *Pandeches*, that is to say, capable of all: yea and the common sort name her *Myrionymus*, which is as much to say, as having an infinite number of names, for that she receiveth all formes and shapes . . . and is great therewith [i.e. pregnant], ready to be delivered.[86]

In the public legacy-giving scene, which we explored earlier, Cleopatra appears 'In th' habiliments of the goddess Isis' in which she 'oft before gave audience' (III, vi, 17–18). Holland also refers to 'the habilliments of Isis' which, he insists, are fashioned 'of different tinctures and colours: for her whole power consisteth and is emploied in matter which . . . becommeth all maner of things, to wit . . . fire, water, life, death, beginning and end'.[87] This may remind us of Cleopatra's own dying words in which, like Isis, she undergoes a metaphysical transmutation into 'fire and air' (V, ii, 288). Suggestively, she rejects the 'baser' (V, ii, 289) elements of earth and water, the very constituents of the marble-constancy she had previously claimed as her own, and which she had associated with the elision of her femininity (V, ii, 237–8), thus further distinguishing herself from the play's barren Octavia who 'shows a body rather than a life,/A statue than a breather' (III, iii, 20–1). Just what is at stake in her appropriation of the figure of Isis may be more clearly delineated if we consider a text, often overlooked, which Shakespeare may well have read. Mary Sidney's translation of Philippe de Mornay's *Discourse of Life and Death* (1592) was published along with her rendering of Garnier's *Tragedie of Antonie* in its first edition, and contains a telling reference to the Egyptian goddess. This is situated within a refutation of the false signs of 'honor' which embellish those weighed down by 'rich stuffes' and 'appareled in purple, in scarlet, and in cloth of gould', for

> Let but fortune turne her backe, every man turnes from them . . . [L]et them once be disroabed of their triumphall garment, no body will any more knowe them. Againe, let there be apparelled in it the most unworthie, and infamous whatsoever: even he without difficultie by vertue of his robe, shall inherit all the honours the other had done him. In the meane time they are puffed up, and growe proude, as the Asse which caried the image of *Isis* was for the honours done to the Goddesse, and regard not that it is the fortune they carry which is honored, not themselves, on whome as on Asses, many times she will be caried.[88]

The structural homology upon which this anecdote is based, and which becomes the vehicle for its opening out of the dubious nature of all protestations to legitimate inheritance, turns Isis into an embodiment of Fortuna. In the same way Cleopatra, whose motivation towards suicide is a fear that she will become yet another piece of adornment on Octavius' own 'triumphall garment', refers to her enemy as an 'ass/Unpolicied!' (V, ii, 306–7). The honour which Octavius therefore sees as his due belongs in actuality to Fortune: ''Tis paltry to be Caesar. /Not being Fortune, he's but Fortune's knave,/A minister of her will. And it is great/To do that thing that ends all other deeds . . ./Which sleeps and never palates more the dung,/The beggar's nurse, and Caesar's' (V, ii, 2–8). The process of nurturing is here a socially levelling one, replacing an artificially-imposed masculine hierarchy of rank and distinction with a gauge of value based on humanity's most *natural* inheritance: the du[n]g. As Isis/Fortuna then, Cleopatra's final apotheosis is achieved through an overturning of the cult of distinctions by making the maternal body and its productions the very fountainhead of history itself. Indeed, the play's most consistent meditation on fortune does not separate its apparently erratic machinations from the will of Isis:

> CHARMIAN . . . Prithee, how many boys and wenches must I have?
> SOOTHSAYER If every of your wishes had a womb,
> And fertile every wish, a million . . .
> CHARMIAN . . . Alexas – come, his fortune, his fortune! O, let him marry a woman that cannot go [i.e. become pregnant], sweet Isis, I beseech thee, and let her die too, and give him a worse, and let worse follow worse, till the worst of all follow him laughing to his grave, fiftyfold a cuckold! Good Isis, hear me this prayer, though thou deny me a matter of more weight; good Isis, I beseech thee! (I, ii, 38–71)

Isis is here appealed to as Queen of Fortune, and her power to destabilise the patrilineal basis of the social order is refracted through the emblem of the debased death-ritual. The barren wife who, in a parodic enactment of the funeral procession, follows her cuckolded husband's coffin to burial with laughter rather than tears, turns what should be the sacred solemnising of succession into an instance of the precariousness of traditional honorific codes when set against the wayward female body. Placing her own body before the sacrificial altar of Isis, Charmian is willing to forgo 'a matter of more weight' in exchange for the fulfilment of her prayer, a possible allusion to the 'weight' of pregnancy. This meaning also colours the virtually identical usage of the word in relation to Cleopatra. When the Egyptian queen fashions her arresting elegy for the dead Antony, she turns him once more into the embodiment of heraldry, a colossus whose 'reared arm/Crested the world' (V, ii, 81–2). However, this idol proves to be unsustainable in the quotidian realm and is iconoclastically obliterated by Cleopatra herself: 'Think you there was or might be such a man/As this I dreamt of? . . ./But if there be nor ever were one such,/It's past the size of dreaming' (V, ii, 92–6). Dolabella responds to this by providing a corporealised locus for her bereavement which evades the 'strange forms' and shadows of fancy: 'Your loss is as yourself, *great*, and you *bear* it/As answering to the *weight*' (V, ii, 97–101, my italics). Cleopatra's greatness, her honour in grief, is thus presented as deriving its impetus from a type of nobility which is inherently maternal, one which in effect turns her into the mother of loss, or rather of Death.

That *Antony and Cleopatra* encapsulates what was a new epistemological culture of memorialisation, which developed in the first half of the seventeenth century, is perhaps most clearly delineated in Ben Jonson's elegiac poetry. In his elegy 'To the Memory of . . . Lady Jane . . . Countess of Shrewsbury', who died in 1625, he imagines himself gazing mournfully at the monuments in Westminster Abbey, which provides the backdrop for the Countess' commemoration: 'No stone in any wall here, but can . . . venture one's descent to hit,/And Christian name too, with a herald's wit./But, I would have thee to know something new'.[89] This 'something new' is her wifely devotion in death, the essence of which the purely historiographical productions of heraldry fail to capture. Similarly, in 'An Elegy on the Lady Jane Pawlet, Marchion[ess] of Winton', Jonson again claims to be the mouthpiece for 'something new' (17). Rejecting what 'the heralds can tell' (20) about the lineage of the deceased, he divulges instead how Lady Pawlet's 'last act, taught the standers-by,/With admiration, and applause to die!'. This 'last act' of death constituted a ratification of her maternal status, since she 'blessed her son' with her final breath (57–62).[90] That Cleopatra abandons the elemental substances of earth and water, which, as we have seen, form the compositional constituents of stone, indicates her rejection of the static marble-constancy which proves so inadequate a memorial to her infinite variety. Indeed, it is not generally known that the theoretical underpinnings of that most heraldic of emblems, the coat of arms, are in fact *elementally* conceived. Henry Peacham enumerates the significance of the coloured backgrounds which embellish armorial standards:

> Armes or ensignes . . . [are] composed of two or moe colours, whereof one was ever white or yealow, which we now tearme Mettals . . . [F]or without the mixture of one of these, the other as too darke of themselves, could not be discerned farre, neyther of white and yealow onely, as participating too much of the light. Hence they say . . . where there is wanting colour or mettal, it is false armorie . . . The colours, to say truth, immediately proceeding from the elements, are yellow and white: yellow beeing an effect of the fire, and all heate . . . [and what] lie[s] boyled, [in] the bellies of hot venemous Serpents and the like. The white is proper to the water and earth, as we may see in all watery bodies congealed . . . Concerning the aire it selfe, it hath no colour at all.[91]

Could Cleopatra's rejection of the 'metalls' made up of earth and water be a deliberate, albeit buried reference to this heraldic tradition? Infused with the fiery poison of the serpents and the air which is 'no colour at all', she necessarily participates 'too much of the light'. She thus incorporates the armorial body only to shatter it. Since the coat of arms requires a minimum of two 'colours' in order to be a legitimate heraldic sign of honour, her unwillingness to take on the 'darke' ground which will complement and balance the 'light', means that she has created a 'false armorie'. Indeed, her disaffection for the 'baser' elements (V, ii, 289), echoed in her fear that a lack of celerity in reaching Antony before Iras will be an error which 'proves [her] base' (V, ii, 299), may carry a suggestion of the *base* 'Mettals' which make up the heraldic shield. Because she is as changeable as Fortune, as endlessly creative and fertile as Isis, Cleopatra evades the restrictive delineations of a memorialising heraldry which seeks to contain and control the *memory* of the female body. She thus refuses to put herself 'under . . . [Octavius'] shroud' (III, xiii, 75), for doing so would prevent her from being 'noble to myself' (V, ii, 191).

Unlike Elizabeth I's monumental likeness, Cleopatra is not the fixed, static icon of death which is conventionally the lot of the royal personage in the heraldic death-ritual, but adopts instead an 'infinite variety' of dying postures which are at once both tragic and self-empowering. She becomes a devoted wife to her 'Husband' (V, ii, 286), as well as a supplier of nourishment, a 'maid that milks' (IV, xv, 78), and ultimately, in her most poignant and telling of endings, a breast-feeding mother or nurse. Crying in her final throes, 'Dost thou not see my baby at my breast/That sucks the nurse asleep?' (V, ii, 308–9), her death is caught between the performance of maternal nurture and the imminence of bodily dissolution; the fatal generativity which provides the pretext for the memorialising of maternity:

CAESAR Bravest at the last,
She levelled at our purposes and, being royal,
Took her own way . . . O noble weakness!
. . . she looks like sleep,
As she would catch another Antony
In her strong toil of grace.
DOLABELLA Here on her breast
There is a vent of blood, and something blown . . . (V, ii, 334–48)

Cleopatra's fantasy of blissful maternal embrace, suggested by her breast-feeding of the serpent/baby,[92] is continued after her death in an analogous dream of 'toil' in which she struggles to catch hold of Antony in her loving arms. The 'vent of blood' at her breast is indicative of lactation, of a body escaping its own confines in its nurturing death. In her own monumental end Cleopatra 'looks like sleep', having performed that 'noble act' through which her 'courage prove[s her] . . . title' (V, ii, 284–7). It is because she dies as a mother that she will be remembered as a queen. Ending where we began, it seems pertinent to recall the monument of Elizabeth Russell (Fig. 4.1); her effigy too 'is not dead but sleepeth' and, like the maternal monuments which came after it, is intended to accentuate those virtues through which a claim to a specifically feminine nobility is vindicated beyond what is strictly accorded by heraldic rite. Even Octavius' instinctive response to the spectacle of Cleopatra's body partially encodes the feminised discourse of the death-bed, investing her with the 'grace' which is the sign of divine favour. Her ending thus recapitulates the 'good death' of the Renaissance mother as it was reconceived by those women whose legacies are ours to cherish today; legacies which were not only part of, but contributed towards, changes in the ritual and epistemological constitution of the most harrowing of all maternal crises.

Notes

1. Lawrence Durrell, *Collected Poems 1931–1974*, ed. James A. Brigham (London and Boston: Faber and Faber, 1985), p. 145.
2. This was John Boswell, who visited the abbey around 1755, and recorded his impressions of the monuments in *A description of the royal tombs in the Chapel of the Kings & the Chapel of King Henry the VII together with those of the nobility & others in . . . the Collegiate Church of St Peter Westminster*. He adds that the monument stands as a reminder of Russell's desire to die well, 'signifying the composed situation of her mind at the approach of Death, which she consider[e]d only as a profound sleep, from which she was again to wake in joyfull resurrection', BL, additional MS 33379, f. 20v.
3. I owe my knowledge of Elizabeth Russell's unmarried status to Ann Mitchell, archivist at Woburn Abbey, the Russell family seat in Bedfordshire. I would also like to thank Dr Anthony Trowles of the Westminster Abbey Library, Geoffrey Fisher of the Courtauld Institute, Robert Yorke, archivist at the College of Arms and Jerry McIntosh, for their valuable assistance with my research into all aspects of the Renaissance death-ritual.
4. This monument is described as wearing a 'widow's hood' in *Royal Commission on Historical Monuments (England)*, London West, vol. 2 (London: HM Stationery Office, 1925), p. 32 (2). However, this is not the case as such items of clothing were fashionable attire for women. Her husband, Sir Peter Legh, was clearly living at the time of her death and commissioned the monument.
5. For more on the depiction of children in monumental art, see Katharine A. Esdaile, *English Monumental Sculpture since the Renaissance* (New York and Toronto: Macmillan, 1927), pp. 79–86.
6. College of Arms, Vincent MS 151, 1568, ff. 58–9.
7. The 'offertory' was conducted before the altar of the church in which the funeral service took place and the 'hatchments' were usually taken directly from the hearse of the deceased upon which they had been displayed. For accounts of formal ceremonial procedures at heraldic funerals see BL, additional MS 14417; College of Arms, MS 151; and Westminster Abbey MSS, WAM (i.e. Westminster Abbey Muniments) 6348 and 6351, accounts for the funerals of the Countess of Lennox in 1606 and the Countess of Exeter in 1609 respectively.

8. In the funeral of Lady Deane, for example, the chief mourner, Lady Webbe, made an offering of 'a peice of gould': Nicholas Charles, *Book of Proceedyng at Funerals*, 1613, BL, additional MS 14417, f. 6.
9. College of Arms, Vincent MS 92, f. 198, dated 1570.
10. BL, additional MS 35324, f. 20.
11. See Clare Gittings, *Death, Burial and the Individual in Early Modern England* (Sydney: Croom Helm, 1984), pp. 175–8. Gittings records in particular that 'only the eldest of any sons could act as mourner to a dead father, and daughters could rarely mourn officially for their own mothers': p. 175. For more on the ceremonial procedures conducted at the funerals of women, in comparison with those of men, see *Parentalia or Funerall Rites, Ceremonies, and Solemnities . . .*, College of Arms, Vincent MS 87, ff. 83–4.
12. For a pictorial example of the differences in the mourning gestures adopted by men and women, see BL, additional MS 35324, f. 4v.
13. Nowhere was the visibility of social stratification more forcefully asserted than in the college's rigorous control over costume and mourning apparel. See the *Antiquarian Collections* of Francis Tate, Secretary to the Society of Antiquaries from 1590 to 1600, BL, Stowe MS 1045, f. 104v; and the common-place book of Francis Thynne, Lancaster Herald from 1602 to 1608, BL, Stowe MS 1047, ff. 246v-247. Allowances for the 'quantitie of cloth and other habiliments' for female mourners are also tabulated in College of Arms, Vincent MS 151, ff. 327–9.
14. WAM 6349, 'An ordre for the Funerall of the . . . lady Lenox'. WAM 6348 contains a list of 'Allowances for the church at the buriall of the countess of Lennox', including charges 'for the breaking of the ground and blackes about the church' as well as 'for composition for the hearse'.
15. WAM 6351, 'Allowances of Fees and Black[es] at the Funerall of the Countesse of Exceter. the xxth of Aprill 1609', which includes fees for 'bell-ringers' and an 'allowance for torches . . . and lights at the Buriall'.
16. College of Arms, Vincent MS 151, f. 380.
17. The College of Arms had already been feeling the effects of both public and ecclesiastical disapproval for several decades. Elaborate funerals could appear shamefully wasteful and the college's involvement in protracted legal battles with the Church over the ownership of expensive funerary paraphernalia began to corrode its credibility. The archives of Westminster Abbey afford us tantalising glimpses of the debates which raged over the funerals of Anne of Cleves, Lady Catherine Knollys, and as late as 1613, of Henry, Prince of Wales. These legal conflicts were more than mere addenda to the history of the College of Arms, rather they offered a precedent for the challenging of its authority in matters concerning the decorums of funerary procedure. For these legal disputes see Westminster Abbey manuscripts, WAM 6353, WAM 6414 and WAM 6415–7.
18. This became fashionable among James I's Scottish courtiers, whose nationality meant that they were not subject to the stringent laws of the college. See Ralph Houlbrooke, *Death, Religion and the Family in England 1480–1750* (Oxford: Clarendon Press, 1998), p. 273.
19. I am partly reacting to Clare Gittings' emphasis on 'individualism' as one of the primary catalysts for changes in the nature of the death-ritual during this period. See her *Death, Burial and the Individual*, p. 175.

20. BL, Harleian MS 1301, first half of seventeenth century, f. 12v.
21. Nigel Llewellyn, *Funeral Monuments in Post-Reformation England* (Cambridge: Cambridge University Press, 2001), p. 36.
22. College of Arms, *Book of Monuments* (1619), MS 1, p. 1.
23. To distinguish Elizabeth Russell from her mother of the same name, I will continue to refer to the latter as Elizabeth Hoby Russell.
24. Quoted in Violet A. Wilson, *Society Women of Shakespeare's Time* (London: John Lane, The Bodley Head Limited, 1924), p. 21.
25. I am deeply indebted to Patricia Burstall, Bisham church archivist, for welcoming me so warmly to Bisham and for providing me with valuable information about the Hobys, the church, and Bisham Abbey.
26. Transcriptions from the tombs of Bisham church can be found in Elias Ashmole, *The Antiquities of Berkshire* (London: 1719), vol. 2, pp. 462–76, BL, 10361.d.6. I have chosen to translate the extracts I have used in order to emphasise particular aspects of meaning which I believe to inhere in the original Latin. Full transcriptions and translations of the Cooke/Hoby cycle of epitaphs are tabulated in Louise Schleiner, *Tudor and Stuart Women Writers* (Bloomington and Indianapolis: Indiana University Press, 1994), pp. 205–12.
27. The word '*viscera*' can mean the internal organs generally, or figuratively the heart, bowels or womb. It may also designate 'child' or offspring. The phrase can thus be translated in a variety of ways; as 'alas my womb/my children', or as an expression of internal anguish, 'alas [what pain there is in] my heart'.
28. '*Sic volui mater tumulo sociarier uno,/Una quas utero laeta genensque tuli.*'
29. The marriage is recorded as having taken place on 23 December 1574: *The Register of Bisham Co. Berks*, transcribed by Edgar Powell (London: The Parish Register Society, 1898), p. 19.
30. '*O utinam mater jacuissem lumine cassa* [dead: literally devoid of light]/*Solvissetque prior justa sprema mihi!*' Transcriptions from the Russell monuments in Westminster Abbey appear in *Reges, Reginae, Nobiles, et Alij in Ecclesia Collegiata B. Petri Westmonasterij Sepulti* (London: 1606), pp. 44–6, BL, 578.b.47. Again, full translations (different from my own) are offered in Schleiner, *Tudor and Stuart Women Writers*, pp. 47–50.
31. '*Quod licuit feci, vellem mihi plura licere.*' My translation highlights the legally freighted terminology of '*licere*', which indicates an apprehension about the lawfulness or licitness of an act. It also reveals the subsidiary meaning of the word '*feci*', from *facio*, which, as a type of performance, carries ritualistic connotations, particularly as it is related to a religious practice with sacrificial or devotional significance.
32 Elizabeth Russell, Dedicatory Epistle to Anne Russell Herbert, *A Way of Reconciliation of a Good and Learned Man, Touching the ... Sacrament* (London: 1605), *The Early Modern Englishwoman: A Facsimile Library of Essential Works, Protestant Translators: Anne Lock Prowse and Elizabeth Russell*, Series I, Printed Writings, 1500–1640, Part 2, vol. 12, ed. Elaine V. Beilin (Aldershot: Ashgate, 2001).
33. Elizabeth Clinton, *The Countesse of Lincolnes Nurserie* (Oxford: 1622), p. 20, BL, C.40.d.30.

34. Elizabeth Grymeston's mother's advice-book, *Miscellanea, Prayers, Meditations, Memoratives*, was first published just one year before in 1604 (I have consulted the 1608–10(?) edition), and draws upon a specifically Catholic tradition: BL, 692.a.16. It does not identify itself in its title-page as a legacy. A later text that does, however, is M.R.'s, *The Mothers Counsell or, Live within Compasse. Being the last Will and Testament to her dearest Daughter, which may serve for a worthy Legacie to all the Women in the World which desire good report from men in this world*, possibly published around 1630: BL, Huth 128. For a reading of the 'female legacy' tradition, see Wendy Wall's insightful *The Imprint of Gender: Authorship and Publication in the English Renaissance* (Ithaca and London: Cornell University Press, 1993), pp. 283–310.
35. These figures are given in Sylvia Brown (ed.), *Women's Writing in Stuart England: The Mothers' Legacies of Dorothy Leigh, Elizabeth Joscelin and Elizabeth Richardson* (Gloucestershire: Sutton Publishing, 1999), p. vi.
36. Dorothy Leigh, *The Mothers Blessing . . .*, pp. 2–3. I am using the eighth edition (London: 1622), BL, C.107.dg.25.(2).
37. Ibid., pp. 4 and 9–10.
38. Elizabeth Joceline, *The Mothers Legacie to her unborne Childe* (London: 1624), pp. 2–3. BL, C.38.c.23.
39. Ibid., Epistle Dedicatory, 'To my truly loving and most dearly loved husband, Taurell Jocelin'.
40. Ibid. p. 11.
41. Stephen Denison, *The Monument or Tomb-Stone: Or a sermon preached . . . at the funerall of Mrs Elizabeth Juxon, the late wife of Mr John Juxon* (London: 1620), pp. 112–13 and 119, BL, 1418.i.19.
42. One contemporary legal authority defined 'Covert Baron' in these terms: 'A woman as soon as she is married is called covert, in Latine *nupta*, that is, vailed, as it were, clouded and over-shadowed . . . her new selfe is her superior, her companion, her master': T. E., *The Lawes Resolutions of Womens Rights: or the Lawes Provision for Woemen* (London: 1632), pp. 124–5, BL, 1481.b.46. For the restrictions placed upon women as disposers 'Of goods and cattelles', see Henry Swinburne, *A Brief Treatise of Testaments and Last Willes* (London: 1590), ff. 47v-48v, BL, 1609/1399. For an overview of women and laws of inheritance, see Amy Louise Erickson's *Women and Property in Early Modern England* (New York and London: Routledge, 1993) and Mary Prior, 'Wives and Wills 1558–1700', in *English Rural Society, 1500–1800: Essays in Honour of Joan Thirsk*, eds John Chartres and David Hey (Cambridge: Cambridge University Press, 1990), pp. 201–25.
43. G. Williams, *The Honour of Vertue. Or The Monument erected . . . to the immortall memory of . . . Mrs Elizabeth Crashawe. Who dyed in childbirth* (Oxford: 1620), sig. C1v, Bodleian Library, MAL.297 (12).
44. Hanniball Gamon, *The Praise of a Godly Woman. A Sermon preached at the Solemne Funeral of the Right Honourable Ladie, the Ladie Frances Roberts . . .* (London: 1627), pp. 27 and 30, BL, 1419.f.26.
45. In his *Anatomie of Mortalitie* (London: 1632), George Strode commends Jacob 'in whose last will and testament are contained many worthy and notable lessons, blessings and prophecies of the estate of his children', p. 112, BL, 875.s.12.

46. Folger MS V.a.511, in Sylvia Brown (ed.), *Women's Writing in Stuart England*, p. 254.
47. The text is also reproduced in Sylvia Brown, *Women's Writing in Stuart England*: Richardson, *Ladies Legacy to her Daughters* (1645), 'A Letter to my foure Daughters'. The *Ladies Legacy* was followed by Susanna Bell's *Legacy of a Dying Mother* in 1673.
48. *A Ladies Legacie*, presentation edition, Bodleian Library.
49. Manchester City Art Galleries.
50. For example, that of Sir Walter Ralegh with his eldest son Walter, painted around 1602 by an unknown artist, and housed in the National Portrait Gallery, London.
51. It is not known if this woman is a mourning relative or, as Nigel Llewellyn suggests, the ghostly double of Magdelene herself. See Llewellyn's *The Art of Death: Visual Culture in the English Death Ritual c. 1500-c. 1800* (London: Reaktion Books, 1991), pp. 47–8.
52. Letter from Lord Russell to Lord Burleigh: J. H. Wiffen, *Memoirs of the House of Russell from the Time of the Norman Conquest* (London: Longman et al., 1833), vol. 1, pp. 501–2.
53. The witness was the then owner of the abbey Mrs Vansittart, wife of General Vansittart. Today the copy-books are missing, or as has been claimed, stolen by the workmen who discovered them. There are no extant documents which confirm that Elizabeth Hoby Russell was ever mother to a William Hoby. It is possible that the legends refer to the young Francis Russell, the cause of whose death is not recorded, and that, over the years, the name has merely been confused. Whether or not this is actually the case must, like so much about the intriguing Russell tale, remain a mystery.
54. For more on Elizabeth Hoby Russell's interest in her lasting reputation, see Felicity Heal, 'Reputation and Honour in Court and Country: Lady Elizabeth Russell and Sir Thomas Hoby', *Transactions of the Royal Historical Society* 6 (1996), pp. 161–77.
55. T[homas] S[alter], *A Mirrhor mete for all Mothers, Matrones, and Maidens, intituled the Mirrhor of Modestie* (London: 1579), sig. C2, BL, C.40.a.20.
56. C. P. Cavafy, *Complete Poems* (Athens: K. Stroumbouki, 1984), pp. 69–70. The extract is my translation from the original Greek.
57. All quotations are taken from *Antony and Cleopatra*, ed. John Wilders (London: Arden, 1995).
58. For the dating of the play, see *The Oxford Companion to Shakespeare*, eds Michael Dobson and Stanley Wells (Oxford: Oxford University Press, 2001), p. 15.
59. There is some evidence to suggest that the tiring-house facade of outdoor theatres such as the Rose and the Globe may have been reminiscent of the architectural surrounds which were a feature of many seventeenth-century monuments, including that of England's deceased queen. The three-tiered structure flanked by classical columns is common to both. The best reconstruction of the parallels between tomb art and theatrical architecture is that of Jean Wilson, *The Shakespeare Legacy: The Material Legacy of Shakespeare's Theatre* (Surrey: Bramley Books, 1995), pp. 81–103. Wilson also mentions *Antony and Cleopatra* as an instance in which the

'tiring-house facade', before which Cleopatra may have played out her final scenes, 'can itself become a monument': p. 95. Similarly, Andrew Gurr insists that theatres like the Globe must have had 'a curtained alcove or discovery-space in the tiring-house wall, which served as a shop, tomb, cell, study or closet'. He conjectures, however, that in *Antony and Cleopatra*, the queen's death may have been performed on a 'raised platform, or even a curtained "booth" set up on stage': *The Shakespearean Stage 1574–1642* (Cambridge: Cambridge University Press, 1992), p. 149.

60. Robert Commaundre, *The Booke of Heraldrye . . . Burialls and Enterementes*, late sixteenth to early seventeenth centuries, BL, Egerton MS 2642, f. 205.
61. *Narrative and Dramatic Sources of Shakespeare*, vol. 5, ed. Geoffrey Bullough (London: Routledge and Kegan Paul, 1964), pp. 293–4.
62. Among the 'signs' Antony mentions are those which appear 'dragonish', or 'sometime like a bear or lion, [or]/A towered citadel' (IV, xiv, 2–4). Is it a coincidence that the dragon, bear, lion and citadel are all common motifs in heraldic emblemature, as well as in standards of war used in heraldic processions? In Shakespeare's *Julius Caesar*, 'the bloody sign of battle' (V, i, 14, *The Norton Shakespeare*, eds Stephen Greenblatt et al. (New York and London: W. W. Norton and Company, 1997), from which all quotations from this play are taken) refers to such heraldic standards, and as we will see later, Cleopatra identifies the 'signs of conquest' with 'scutcheons', painted shields with armorial symbols (V, ii, 134). See also David Crystal and Ben Crystal, *Shakespeare's Words: A Glossary and Language Companion* (Harmondsworth: Penguin, 2002), p. 388 ('scutcheon') and p. 400 ('sign').
63. This can be seen as a literalised manifestation of the doctrine of the king's two bodies as it is presented in such tracts of political philosophy as the manuscript version of Edmund Plowden's (1518–85) *Treatise of Succession*: '[A]ll thoughe the bodie naturall die yet the bodie pollitticke is never accounted or termed in the Lawe to die but it . . . is translated and conveyed from one bodie naturall to an other': BL, Cotton MS Caligula B. IV, '[T]reatise of the two bodies of the kinge', f. 6. With its *embodying* of the dictates of primogeniture, this kind of thinking is encapsulated in the very phrase which acts as a catalyst for the ensuing proceedings in a ruler's heraldic obsequies: 'The King is dead, long live the King.' It is this precept that Antony both appropriates and disrupts by bequeathing the 'sanctity' of kingship not to Caesar's immediate successor but to the people. It is possible that the heraldic ritual of the 'offertory' was intended to supplant the Catholic dissemination of the Eucharist (Gittings, *Death, Burial and the Individual in Early Modern England*, p. 176). Antony's language similarly presents the distribution of Caesar's 'sacred blood' within the context of specifically heraldic customs.
64. Bullough, *Narrative and Dramatic Sources*, p. 282.
65. *The True use of Armorie . . . [showing] the lawfulnes of honorable funerals and moniments . . . advancing of Banners, Ensignes, and marks of noblenesse* (London: 1592), pp. 23–4, BL, C.124.c.8 (2).
66. This is a translation of Robert Garnier's French tragedy, *Marc-Antonie*, first published in Paris in 1578. All quotations from Pembroke's translation are taken from *Three Tragedies by Renaissance Women*, ed. Diane Purkiss (Harmondsworth: Penguin, 1998).

67. The 'trophy', which could either designate a memorial itself, or the emblems of warfare which adorned it, was an important adjunct to the symbolic rites of the heraldic funeral. In *Hamlet*, Laertes commiserates over the 'obscure burial' of Polonius, executed with 'No trophy, sword, nor hatchment o'er his bones,/No noble rite nor formal ostentation' (IV, v, 213–15: *Hamlet*, ed. G. R. Hibbard (Oxford: Oxford University Press, 1987)).
68. It is the third part of *Ivychurch* which dramatises these mourning rites: BL, 80.a.28 (2). See also Schleiner, *Tudor and Stuart Women Writers*, pp. 52–5.
69. On the mistaken belief in the funereal function of these 'lachrymatories', see the note corresponding to the passage in John Wilders' Arden edition of the play.
70. *Oxford English Dictionary*, s.v. 'Memory': 'An act of commemoration, esp. of the dead . . . A memorial tomb, shrine, chapel, or the like; a monument. *Obs.*'.
71. My translation: '*Velut altera Phoenix dum partit illa perit*'. For more examples of brasses dedicated to children and mothers, see John Page-Phillips, *Children on Brasses* (London: Allen and Unwin, 1970).
72. Thomas Fuller, *The Holy State* (Cambridge: 1642), pp. 188–9, BL, 694.i.2.
73. John Weever, *Ancient Funerall Monuments* (London: 1631), pp. 10–11, BL, 209.d.1.
74. I am quoting from the 1590 edition, sig. D1, BL, C.39.a.33.
75. John Webster, *The Duchess of Malfi and Other Plays*, ed. René Weis (Oxford: Oxford University Press, 1996).
76. For examples of these dynastic tombs, see Paul Binski, *Medieval Death: Ritual and Representation* (London: The British Museum Press, 1996).
77. John Barlow, *The True Guide to Glory. A Sermon Preached at Plymptonmary in Devon, at the Funerals of the Right Worshipful, and truely Religious Lady, the Lady Strode of Newingham* (London: 1619), pp. 49–50, BL, 1417.h.1. This kind of request was particularly prevalent among women with Puritan leanings.
78. This was also produced by the workshop of Nicholas Stone, who records in his note-book that he was paid a total of £130, £60 of which was paid by her husband Arthur Coke 'in his lef tim[e]' and a further £70 by his brother Sir Robert Coke 'after the sayed After [Arthur] Cook decesed': Nicholas Stone, ed. Walter Lewis Spiers, 'The Note-Book and Account Book of Nicholas Stone', *The Walpole Society VII, 1918–1919*, ed. A. J. Finberg (Oxford: Oxford University Press, 1919), p. 73.
79. For alternative readings which deal with the relation between Shakespeare's plays and forms of sculpture, including classical, see Leonard Barkan, '"Living Sculptures": Ovid, Michelangelo, and *The Winter's Tale*', *English Literary History* 48 (1981), pp. 639–67; and Bruce R. Smith, 'Sermons in Stones: Shakespeare and Renaissance Sculpture', *Shakespeare Studies* 17 (1985), pp. 1–23. Catherine Belsey also looks at some maternal monuments, including those of Lady Margaret Legh and Catharine Savage, and their significance for the *Winter's Tale*, in *Shakespeare and the Loss of Eden: The Construction of Family Values in Early Modern Culture* (Houndmills: Palgrave, 2001), pp. 85–127. Belsey believes that in these monuments the 'affective family is shown as vulnerable' for 'the loving

nuclear family constitutes a remarkably precarious basis for a stable and well-ordered society': pp. 98–9. My reading presents the maternal monument in an antithetical light, as a vehicle for a newly emerging discourse of 'nobility' which portrays older heraldic codes as necessarily less stable markers of familial virtue and hence civic order.

80. Nigel Llewellyn explains that a large proportion of the heraldic information on tombs was inscribed 'illegally for the most part', making them 'fictions in stone': 'Honour in Life, Death and in the Memory: Funeral Monuments in Early Modern England', *Transactions of the Royal Historical Society* 6 (1996), p. 191.
81. Lawrence Humfrey, *The Nobles or of Nobilitye* (London: 1563), sigs E1 and E2v-E3, BL, 138.a.27.
82. Ibid., sigs S1v and R2.
83. Henry Peacham,*The Compleat Gentleman* (London: 1622), p. 3, BL, C.124.c.8 (1).
84. Bullough, *Narrative and Dramatic Sources of Shakespeare*, pp. 409–10.
85. Walter R. Coppedge, 'The Joy of the Worm: Dying in Antony and Cleopatra', *Renaissance Papers* (1998), pp. 41–50, and Janet Adelman, *Suffocating Mothers: Fantasies of Maternal Origin in Shakespeare's Plays, Hamlet to the Tempest* (New York and London: Routledge, 1992), pp. 183–5. Adelman sees in Cleopatra's dying body 'the memorializing site of Antony's heroic masculinity': p. 185. She goes on to add that 'Cleopatra must, in particular, die for the right reason: she can become the repository of Antony's new masculinity only insofar as she is willing to die specifically for him': p. 190. To define Cleopatra's death, however, as taking place solely for the purpose of recuperating Antony's masculinity is to undermine the power she herself derives from her remarkable dying 'postures'. Indeed, it is the peculiarly maternal nature of these postures that enable her to subvert the masculine codes of heroism and heraldry which seek both to define and contain her. Like Janet Adelman's reading, most critical assessments of maternity in the play lean heavily towards psychoanalytical interpretations. See also Constance Brown Kuriyama's reading of the maternal aspects of the play, in 'Mother of the World: A Psychoanalytic Interpretation of Shakespeare's *Antony and Cleopatra*', *English Literary Renaissance* 7 (1977), pp. 324–51.
86. Plutarch, *Moralia*, trans. Philemon Holland (London: 1603), p. 1309, BL, C.74.e.3.
87. Ibid., p. 1,318.
88. Philippe de Mornay, *Discourse of Life and Death* (London: 1592), sigs B2-B3, BL, C.57.d.16.
89. Ll. 9–12. Ben Jonson, *The Complete Poems*, ed. George Parfitt (Harmondsworth: Penguin, 1996), pp. 275–6. Line numbers are hereafter indicated in brackets.
90. Ben Jonson, *The Complete Poems*, pp. 232–4.
91. Peacham, *The Compleat Gentleman*, pp. 144–5.
92. For the epitaph written by Shakespeare's daughters for their mother Anne Hathaway (Shakespeare), which contains the affecting maternal imagery of breast-feeding, see René Weis *Shakespeare Revealed: A Biography* (London: John Murray, 2007), pp. 370–1.

Postscript: Our Maternities: The Historical Legacy

> There is no doubt that modern medicine has made astounding advances in the area of birth: infertile women become mothers, sick women deliver healthy babies, and infirm newborns grow into happy kids. But it must also be said that, for many women, over the years, this supposedly beneficial medical help has often meant isolating babies in nurseries, receiving an unnecessary episiotomy, having a breast dipped in iodine before every feeding – whatever the latest trend. If only we'd known how sceptical we should have been.[1]

The authoritative knowledge claimed by the technological and biomedical institutions which have grown up around the maternal body is founded on the prevention of the potential crises faced by conceiving women. As Tina Cassidy reveals in her engaging study, *Birth: A History*, expectant mothers are confronted with a bewildering array of professional medical opinions, childcare guidance and health advice. What should women believe? Or, to put it another way, to whose authoritative knowledge should they give credence? And when, if at all, should they introduce knowledge derived from their own personal experience into the birthing process?

The maternal body we have come to *know* – the conceptual locus for our investment as a society in the care pregnant women should receive, the nature of the pharmacological and surgical intervention applied during labour, and the level of autonomous personhood accorded the developing foetus – has a rich and complex history we are only just beginning to piece together. It is a history which reaches beyond the confines of medical and technological advancement, beyond even the environs of the home and the family, to encompass the mutually-determining and reciprocally-shaping interaction between the maternal body and the many bodies of knowledge through which it has acquired intellectual, cultural and political significance. It is hoped this study has been a first step towards recuperating a maternal body which is not historically passive – merely acted upon – but dynamic, active and challenging; not the subject but the agent of history.

Today we have come to take for granted a form of biological determinism according to which our physical health, our personalities, and even the nature of our future cognitive experiences, are in part mapped out along with the laying down of bone and soft tissue during embryological formation. The idea that the body's corporeal functions are endowed, even before birth, with an inevitability beyond both human and godly control seems to govern in so many unseen ways our knowledge of ourselves. The institutions which can commandeer, even engineer, these compelling impulses have the keys to an almost unimaginable power. In order to understand this – and to acquire the conceptual tools to manage this knowledge responsibly – we must look to the historical conditions which have given rise to this unique epistemology. It was during the age of Shakespeare that branches of learning seeking to legitimise their own professionalised status reconceived the anatomy of birth, the order of creation, the influence of the preternatural, and the inviolability of lineage and social distinction, as the adjuncts to the disciplined construction of a maternal body whose inherent properties bore the imprint of a largely autonomous nature; a nature which could be controlled and subjected to the rigours of authoritative knowledge. What the historical record has occluded, however, is the extent to which these early – loosely-defined – institutions were shaped by the maternal body they sought to control. We have for too long been prevented from seeing the truly far-reaching impact of these 'maternities' on the disciplines through which we have come to mediate our understanding not only of our origins but of our own human potential.

Note

1. Tina Cassidy, *Birth: A History* (London: Chatto and Windus, 2007), p. 257. I would like to thank Helen Hackett for drawing my attention to this marvellous book.

Selected Bibliography

Primary Manuscript Sources

Barber-Surgeons' Hall

Barber-Surgeons' accounts, *Charter Act and Ordinance Book 1461–1607*, MS A/6/1.

Barber-Surgeons' accounts, *Court Minutes 1598–1607*, MS B/1/3.

Barber-Surgeons' accounts, *Court Minutes 1607–1621*, MS B/1/4.

British Library (BL)

Basil, Simon (undated), Designs for the Theatre at Christ Church, Oxford, additional MS 15505, f. 21.

The Booke of Heraldrye . . . Burialls and Enterementes, late sixteenth to early seventeenth centuries, Egerton MS 2642.

Boswell, John (c. 1755), *A Description of the Royal Tombs in the Chapel of the Kings & the Chapel of King Henry the VII together with those of the Nobility & Others in . . . the Collegiate Church of St Peter Westminster*, additional MS 33379.

Bowker, Agnes (1568), *The Examination and Confession of Agnes Bowker*, 22 January to 18 February, Lansdowne MS 101, ff. 21–33.

Charles, Nicholas (1613), *Book of Proceedyng at Funerals*, additional MS 14417.

Chroniques de France ou de Saint Denis, second quarter of the fourteenth century, Royal MS 16 G. VI.

Circumstances to be considered in the cawse of the mayde of Hockh[a]m, for scratching of an old witch there, nowe deade . . . (undated), additional MS 28223, f. 15.

Fairfax, Edward (1621–3), *A Discourse of Witchcraft as it was Acted in the Family of M[aste]r Edward Fairfax*, additional MS 32496, ff. 1–79.

Funeral Processions, late sixteenth and early seventeenth centuries, vol. 15 (Rothschild Bequest), additional MS 35324.

Glover, Mary (1603), *Mary Glovers Late Woeful Case*, Sloane MS 831.

Johnson, Margaret (1633), *The Examinac[i]on & voluntary confession of Margret Johnson of Marsden . . .*, 9 March, additional MS 36674, f. 196.

Jones, Inigo (undated), *Inigo Jones's Original Ground Plots and Profiles of Scenes . . .*, Lansdowne MS 1171.
Magic Circle, fifteenth century, Sloane MS 3853, f. 51v.
The offenders condemned & accused for witch craft w[i]th their markes at their Attainder (1633), A list of the so-called Lancaster Witches, additional MS 36674, f. 199.
Peacham, Henry (1610), *Basilikon Doron*, Royal MS 12 A, LXVI.
A Petition from the College of Arms to the Archbishop of Canterbury, first half of seventeenth century, Harleian MS 1301, f. 12v.
Plowden, Edmund, sixteenth century, *Treatise of Succession*, Cotton MS Caligula B. IV.
Robinson, Edmund (1633), *The examinac[i]on of Edmund Robinson . . . of Pendle Forrest*, 10 February, additional MS 36674, ff. 193–3v.
Roman de la Rose (c. 1500), Harley MS 4425.
Russell, Margaret (1622), *Examinations and Confessions of Margaret Russell, Accused of Bewitching Elizabeth Jennings*, 25–7 April, additional MS 36674, ff. 134–6v. The document is signed by Henry Goodcole and includes an account of Doctor Napier's diagnosis delivered on 30 July 1622, f. 137.
Tate, Francis [Secretary to the Society of Antiquities 1590–1600], *Antiquarian Collections*, Stowe MS 1045.
Thynne, Francis [Lancaster Herald 1602–8], *Commonplace Book*, Stowe MS 1047.
Willughby, Percivall (1630–78), *Observations on Childbirth, with Descriptions of Cases in his Practice*, Sloane MS 529.

College of Arms

Antiquarian Collections including funerals, Vincent MS 92.
Book of Monuments (1619), MS 1.
Orders to be observed and kept by the Officers of Armes (1568), Vincent MS 151.
Parentalia or Funerall Rites, Ceremonies, and Solemnities . . ., Vincent MS 87.

Glasgow University Library

Master John Banister's Anatomical Tables with figures, double page showing Banister presiding over a dissection, Hunter MS 364 (V1.1), f. 1.

Guildhall Library, London

Exterior and interior of the *Domus Anatomica* in Copenhagen (1643), ref. 706.
Interior of the Barber-Surgeons' anatomy theatre, Monkwell Street, ref. 8478.
Interior of the Barber-Surgeons' Hall, ref. 705.

Hatfield House, by kind permission of the Marquess of Salisbury

A copy of a Privy Seal dealing with witchcraft (27 May 1605), MS 111.11–13.
Bills for the gardens of Hatfield House, Cecil Papers, BHH/136 (1610).

Bills for the gardens of Hatfield House, Cecil Papers, BHH/140 (1611).
Bills for the gardens of Hatfield House, Cecil Papers, BHH/267 (1611).
Bills for the gardens of Hatfield House, Cecil Papers, Bills 58, BHH/282 (1611).
Bills for the gardens of Hatfield House, Cecil Papers, Bills 58, BHH/284 (1611–12).
Bills for the gardens of Hatfield House, Cecil Papers, Bills 58, BHH/285 (1611–12).
Bills for the gardens of Hatfield House, Cecil Papers, Bills 58, BHH/286 (1611–12).
King James, letter to Viscount Cranborne (c. March 1605 [?]), MS 134.71.
Montague, James, letter to the Archbishop of Canterbury (23 February 1604–5), MS 104.39.

National Archives of Scotland, Edinburgh

Court minutes (dittays) of the examination and confession of Doctor John Fian, alias Cunningham, JC2/2, *Book of Adjournal* (26 December 1590), ff. 195–6v.
Court minutes (dittays) of the examination and confession of Barbara Napier, JC2/2, *Book of Adjournal* (8–10 May 1591), ff. 213–21.

Wellcome Institute Library

Anatomical Fugitive Sheets, *Perutilis Anatomes Interiorum Mulieris Partium*, Paris: 1539, EPB 289.5.
Anatomical Fugitive Sheets, *Tabula Foeminae Membra Demonstrans*, Wittenberg: 1573, EPB 298.17.
Anatomical Fugitive Sheets, *Tabula Exhibens Insigniora Maris Viscera*, Wittenberg: 1573, Wellcome EPB 298.17.
Anatomical and Medical Treatises (c. 1420), MS 49 [Apokalypse].
Boaistuau, Pierre (1560), *Histoires Prodigieuses*, MS 136.
Pseudo-Galen, mid-15th century, *Anathomia*, MS 290.

Westminster Abbey Library

Accounts for the funeral of the Countess of Lennox (1606), WAM 6348.
Accounts for the funeral of the Countess of Exeter (1609), WAM 6351.
'An Ordre for the Funerall of the . . . Lady Lenox' (1606), WAM, 6349.
Anne of Cleves, Disputes over the funerary paraphernalia of Anne of Cleves, WAM 6353.
Henry, Prince of Wales, Disputes over the funerary paraphernalia of Henry, Prince of Wales, WAM 6415–17.
Knollys, Catherine, Disputes over the funerary paraphernalia of Lady Catherine Knollys, WAM 6414.

Windsor Castle Royal Library

Natural historical drawings of the Lincean Academy, Vincenzo Leonardi, 'Pregnant' citrus-fruit, RL19328.

Natural historical drawings of the Lincean Academy, Vincenzo Leonardi, Orange or tangerine with a tumescent outgrowth, RL19329/RL19330.
Natural historical drawings of the Lincean Academy, Deformed chick foetus, RL19341.
Natural historical drawings of the Lincean Academy, Vincenzo Leonardi, 'Siamese' melon, RL19365.
Natural historical drawings of the Lincean Academy, Vincenzo Leonardi, Malformed citrus-fruit, RL19324, RL19340, RL19355, RL19367.
Natural historical drawings of the Lincean Academy, Vincenzo Leonardi, 'Fingered' lemon, RL19379.

Worcester College Library, Oxford

Inigo Jones' designs for the Cockpit Theatre, Drury Lane, Jones/Webb, I/7B and 7C.

Primary Printed Sources

Acosta, Joseph de [1604] (1880), *The Natural and Moral History of the Indies*, ed. Clements R. Markham, London: Hakluyt Society, BL, AC.6172/54.
Agricola, Georgius (1566), *De Re Metallica Libri XII*, Basileae, BL, 32.g.13.
Albertus Magnus (1992), *Womens' Secrets: A Translation of Pseudo-Albertus Magnus's De Secretis Mulierum with Commentaries*, trans. Helen Rodnite Lemay, New York: State University of New York Press.
—(1999), *Albertus Magnus on Animals: A Medieval Summa Zoologica*, trans. Kenneth F. Kitchell Jr and Irven Michael Resnick, vol. 2, Baltimore: The John Hopkins University Press.
Aldrovandi, Ulisse (1642), *Monstrorum Historia*, vol. 1, Bononiae, BL, 38.g.11.
Allen, Robert (1603), *The Odifferous Garden of Charitie*, London, BL, Huth 53. STC 367.5.
The Apprehension and confession of three notorious Witches. Arreigned and by Justice condemned and executed at Chelmes-forde, in the Countye of Essex, the 5. day of Julye, last past. 1589 . . . (1589), Lambeth Palace Library, (zz)1597.15.03. STC 5114.
Aquinas, Thomas (1998), *Thomas Aquinas: Selected Writings*, trans. Ralph McInerny, Harmondsworth: Penguin.
Aretino, Pietro (1976), *Aretino: Selected Letters*, trans. George Bull, Harmondsworth: Penguin.
Aristotle (1991), *History of Animals [Historia Animalium]*, trans. D. M. Balme, Loeb Classical Library, Cambridge: Harvard University Press.
Ashmole, Elias (1719), *The Antiquities of Berkshire*, vol. 2, London, BL, 10361.d.6.
Augustine (1972), *City of God*, trans. Henry Bettenson, London: Penguin.
—(1991), *Confessions*, trans. Henry Chadwick, Oxford: Oxford University Press.
Bacon, Francis (1875), *The Works of Francis Bacon*, ed. James Spedding, vol. 4, London: Longmans and Co.
—(1996), *Francis Bacon: A Critical Edition of the Major Works*, ed. Brian Vickers, Oxford: Oxford University Press.

Barlow, John (1619), *The True Guide to Glory. A Sermon Preached at Plympton-mary in Devon, at the Funerals of the Right Worshipful, and truely Religious Lady, the Lady Strode of Newingham*, London, BL, 1417.h.1. STC 1440.

Basset, Robert (1637), *Curiosities: or The Cabinet of Nature*, London, BL, CUP.407.f.43. STC 1557.

Bedel, Henry (1572), *A Sermon Exhortyng to Pitie the Poore. Preached the 25 of November anno. 1571 at Christes Church in London . . . Which treasure maye well be called the mouth of the poore*, London, BL, C.142.cc.4. STC 1783.

Berengario da Carpi, Jacopo (1521), *Carpi Commentaria . . . Anatomia Mu[n]dini*, Bologna, BL, 548.f.1.

—(1523), *Isagogae Breves*, Venice, BL, C.107.bb.5.

—(1959), *A Short Introduction to Anatomy (Isagogae Breves)*, trans. L. R. Lind, Chicago and London: University of Chicago Press.

Bernard of Clairvaux (1976), *On the Song of Songs II*, trans. Kilian Walsh, Michigan: Cistercian Fathers Series, no. 7.

Bernard, Richard (1627), *A Guide to Grand-Jury Men*, London, BL, 518.a.4. STC 1943.

Besson, Jacques (1579), *Theatre des instrumens mathematiques et mechaniques*, Lyons, BL, C.97.f.1.

Blagrave, Joseph (1671), *Blagraves Astrological Practice of Physick*, London, BL, 1034.b.23. WING B3112.

Boethius (1969), *The Consolation of Philosophy*, trans. V. E. Watts, Harmondsworth: Penguin.

Bolton, Edmund (1624), *Nero Caesar, or Monarchie Depraved; an Historical Worke*, London, BL, 196.e.15. STC 3221.

Breton, Nicholas (1607), *A Murmurer*, London, BL, C.27.d.7. STC 3671.

Bright, Timothie (1586), *A Treatise of Melancholy, Contayning the causes thereof and reasons of the straunge effects it worketh in our minds and bodies*, London, BL, C.95.b.30. STC 3747.

Brooks-Davies, Douglas (1992), *Silver Poets of the Sixteenth Century*, London: Everyman.

Brown, Sylvia (ed.) (1999), *Women's Writing in Stuart England: The Mothers' Legacies of Dorothy Leigh, Elizabeth Joscelin, and Elizabeth Richardson*, Gloucestershire: Sutton Publishing.

Browne, Thomas (1928), *The Works of Sir Thomas Browne*, ed. Geoffrey Keynes, vol. 1, London: Faber and Faber.

—(1995), *Thomas Browne: Selected Writings*, ed. Claire Preston, Manchester: Carcanet.

Bullough, Geoffrey (ed.) (1964), *Narrative and Dramatic Sources of Shakespeare*, vol. 5, London: Routledge and Kegan Paul.

—(1973), *Narrative and Dramatic Sources of Shakespeare*, vol. 7, London: Routledge and Kegan Paul.

Burton, Robert (2001), *The Anatomy of Melancholy*, ed. Holbrook Jackson, New York: New York Review Books.

A catalogue of all the chiefest rarities in the publick theater and anatomie-hall of the university of Leyden (1591), Leyden, BL, 7421.b.19.

Caus, Salomon de (1615), *Les Raisons des forces mouvantes avec diverses machines . . . grotes et fonteines*, Frankfurt, BL, L.40/65.

Chaucer, Geoffrey (1987), *The Riverside Chaucer*, ed. Anthony Burgess, Oxford: Oxford University Press.

Clinton, Elizabeth (1622), *The Countesse of Lincolnes Nurserie*, Oxford, BL, C.40.d.30. STC 5432.

Colombo, Realdo (1559), *De re anatomica libri XV*, Venice, Wellcome Library, 1546.

Colonna, Francesco (1999), *Hypnerotomachia Poliphili: The Strife of Love in a Dream*, trans. Joscelyn Godwin, London: Thames and Hudson.

Corbin, Peter and Douglas Sedge (eds) (1986), *Three Jacobean Witchcraft Plays: The Tragedy of Sophonisba; The Witch; The Witch of Edmonton*, Manchester and New York: Manchester University Press.

Corner, George W. (trans.) (1927), *Anatomical Texts of the Earlier Middle Ages: A Study in the Transmission of Culture*, Washington: Carnegie Institution of Washington.

Cotta, John (1616), *The triall of witch-craft, shewing the true and right methode of the discovery with a confutation of erroneous wayes*, London, BL, 1608/727. STC 5836.

Crompton, William (1630), *A Lasting Jewell for Religious Women. In the summe of a sermon preached at the funerall of Mistris Mary Crosse, late wife of Mr Henry Crosse of Barnestaple . . . Nov. 11 1628*, London, BL, 4903.cc.46. STC 6058.

Crooke, Helkiah (1615), *Microcosmographia: A Description of the Body of Man*, London, BL, 781.k.1. STC 6062.

Dalton, Michael [1618] (1635), *The Countrey Justice*, London, BL, 1602/355. STC 6211 [First edition of 1618, STC 6210].

Davies, John [1599] (1602), *Nosce Teipsum*, London, BL, C.117.b.53. STC 6356.

A Declaration of the State of the Colony and Affaires in Virginia [1620] (1622), London, BL, C.32.g.28. STC 24844.

Dekker, Thomas (1980), *The Whore of Babylon: A Critical Edition*, ed. Marianne Gateson Riely, New York and London: Garland Publishing.

Denison, Stephen (1620), *The Monument or Tomb-Stone: or a sermon preached . . . in London, Novemb. 21 1619 at the funerall of Mrs Elizabeth Juxon, the late wife of Mr John Juxon*, London, BL, 1418.i.19. STC 6603.5.

A Detection of Damnable Driftes, practized by three Witches arraigned at Chelmisforde in Essex, at the laste Assises there holden, whiche were executed in Aprill 1579 (1579), London, BL, C.27.a.8. STC 5115.

Donne, John (1990), *John Donne: A Critical Edition of the Major Works*, ed. John Carey, Oxford: Oxford University Press.

—[1971] (1996), *John Donne: The Complete English Poems*, ed. A. J. Smith, Harmondsworth: Penguin.

Downame, John (1600), *Spiritual Phisicke to Cure the Diseases of the Soule*, London, BL, 4406.df.28. STC 7147.

—(1616), *The Plea of the Poore. Or a Treatise of Beneficence and Almes-Deeds*, London, BL, 873.h.3. STC 7146.

Durrell, Lawrence (1985), *Collected Poems 1931–1974*, ed. James A. Brigham, London and Boston: Faber and Faber.

The Earle of Gowries Conspiracie Against the Kings Majestie of Scotland (1600), London, BL, G.5126. STC 21466.

Estienne, Charles (1545), *De Dissectione Partium Corporis Humani*, Paris, Wellcome Library, 6706.
Evelyn, John (1955), *The Diary*, ed. E. S. de Beer, Oxford: Clarendon press.
Ewen, C. L'Estrange (1929), *Witch Hunting and Witch Trials*, London: Kegan Paul, Trench, Trubner.
—(1933), *Witchcraft and Demonianism*, London: Heath Cranton.
The Examination and Confession of certaine Wytches at Chensforde in the Countie of Essex (1566), London, Lambeth Palace Library, (zz)1587.12.03. STC 19869.5.
Fabricius, Hieronymus (1624), *De Formato Foetu*, Francofurti, BL, 549.1.20.(1).
—(1625), *Opera Anatomica . . . De Formato Foetu, Formatione Ovi et Pulli*, Patavii, BL, 781.1.1.
—(1942), *The Embryological Treatises of Hieronymus Fabricius of Aquapendente: The Formation of the Egg and of the Chick; The Formed Fetus*, trans. Howard B. Adelmann, New York: Cornell University Press.
Fenton, Edward (1569), *Certaine Secrete Wonders of Nature, containing a descriptio[n] of sundry strange things, seming Monstrous in our eyes and judgement, bicause we are not privie to the reasons of them*, London, BL, C.31.d.8. STC 3164.5.
Ferrari, Giovanni Battista (1646), *Hesperides, Sive de Malorum Aureorum Cultura et Usu Libri Quartuor*, Rome, BL, 35.g.2.
Fludd, Robert (1617), *Utriusque Cosmi*, Francofurti, BL, 30.g.9.
Fonte, Moderata (1997), *The Worth of Women: Wherein is Clearly Revealed their Nobility and their Superiority to Men*, trans. Virginia Cox, Chicago and London: University of Chicago Press.
Ford, John (1968), *'Tis Pity She's a Whore*, ed. Brian Morris, London: A. and C. Black.
The forme and shape of a Monstrous Child, borne at Maydstone in Kent, the xxiiii. of October 1568 (1568), London, BL, Huth 50.38. STC 17194.
Fuller, Thomas (1642), *The Holy State*, Cambridge, BL, 694.i.2.
Gamon, Hanniball (1627), *The Praise of a Godly Woman. A sermon preached at the solemne Funerall of the Right Honourable Ladie, the Ladie Frances Roberts . . . the tenth of August, 1626*, London, BL, 1419.f.26. STC 11548.
Geminus, Thomas (1553), *Compendiosa totius anatomie delineatio*, trans. N. Udall, London, BL, C.43.h.2. STC 11716.
Gifford, George (1587), *A Discourse of the subtill Practises of Devills by Witches and Sorcerers*, London, BL, 8630.e.19. STC 11852.
—[1593] (1603), *A Dialogue concerning Witches and Witchcrafts*, London, BL, 1395.b.5. STC 11851.
Gouge, William (1622), *Of Domesticall Duties: Eight Treatises*, London, BL, 722.i.23. STC 12119.
Griffith, Matthew (1633), *Bethel: Or, a Forme for Families*, London, BL, 4409.ddd.1. STC 12368.
Grimeston, Edward (1607), *Admirable and Memorable Histories containing the Wonders of our Time*, London, BL, 12356.b.35.
Grymeston, Elizabeth (c. 1608–10?), *Miscellanea, Prayers, Meditations, Memoratives*, London, BL, 692.a.16. STC 12408.

Guerric of Igny (1971), *Liturgical Sermons*, trans. the monks of Mount Saint Bernard Abbey, vol. 1, Ireland: Cistercian Fathers Series, no. 8.

Guillemeau, Jacques (1612), *Childbirth, or the Happy Deliverie of Women*, London, BL, 1177.d.40. STC 12496.

Hakluyt, Richard (1598), *The Principal Navigations, Voiages, Traffiques and Discoveries of the English Nation*, vol. 1, London, BL, 683.h.5. STC 12626.

Harrington, John (1596), *A New Discourse of a Stale Subject, Called the Metamorphosis of Ajax*, London, BL, C.21.a.5. STC 12773.

Hartmanus, Schopperus (1568), *Omnium illiberalium mechanicarum*, Francfurti, BL, C.27.a.40.

Hatton, Edward (1708), *A New View of London*, London, BL, 577.d.1–2.

Heseler, Baldasar (1959), *Andreas Vesalius' First Public Anatomy At Bologna 1540: An Eyewitness Report*, trans. Ruben Eriksson, Uppsala and Stockholm: Almqvist and Wiksells.

Holland, Henry (1590), *A Treatise against Witchcraft*, Cambridge, BL, 1608/2297. STC 13590.

Howell, T. B. (ed.) (1809), *Cobbett's Complete Collection of State Trials and Proceedings for High Treason and other Crimes 1603–1627*, vol. 2, London.

Humfrey, Lawrence (1563), *The Nobles or of Nobilitye*, London, BL, 138.a.27. STC 13964.

Joceline, Elizabeth [1624] (1632), *The Mothers Legacie, To her unborne Childe*, London, BL, C.38.c.23. STC 14625.5.

Jonson, Ben (1969), *The Complete Masques*, ed. Stephen Orgel, New Haven and London: Yale University Press.

—(1998), *Five Plays*, ed. G. A. Wilkes, Oxford: Oxford University Press.

—(1996), *The Complete Poems*, ed. George Parfitt, Harmondsworth: Penguin.

Jorden, Edward (1603), *A Briefe discourse of a Disease called the Suffocation of the Mother*, London, BL, 1177.c.1.(1). STC 14790.

Ketham, Johannes de (1495), *Fasciculus Medicinae*, Wellcome Library, 3544.3E.13.

Leigh, Dorothy (1622), *The Mothers Blessing: or, the godly counsaile of a Gentle-woman not long since deceased, left behind her for her children*, 8th edn, London, BL, C.107.dg.25 (2). STC 15404.3 [First edition of 1616, STC 15402].

Lindley, David (ed.) (1995), *Court Masques: Jacobean and Caroline Entertainments 1605–1640*, Oxford: Oxford University Press.

Lorris, Guillaume de, Jean de Meun (1995), *The Romance of the Rose*, trans. Charles Dahlberg, 3rd edn, New Jersey: Princeton University Press.

Lyly, John (1606), *Euphues: The Anatomie of Wit*, London, BL, C.190.a.2. STC 17061.

Markham, Gervase [1615] (1623), *Countrey Contentments, or the English Huswife. Containing the inward and outward vertues which ought to be in a compleate woman*, London, BL, 7074.c.31. STC 17343.

Marston, John (1598), *The Metamorphosis of Pigmalions Image and Certaine Satyres*, London, BL, 238.b.54. STC 17482.

—(1925), *The Scourge of Villainie*, ed. G. B. Harrison, New York: E. P. Dutton and Company.

Martins Months Minde (1589), London, BL, C.37.d.39. STC 17452.

Martin, Randall (ed.) (1997), *Women Writers in Renaissance England*, London and New York: Longman.

Melanchthon, Philip (1988), *A Melanchthon Reader*, trans. Ralph Keen, American University Studies, Series 7: Theology and Religion, New York: Peter Lang.

—(1999), *Orations on Philosophy and Education*, ed. Sachiko Kusukawa and trans. Christine F. Salazar, Cambridge: Cambridge University Press.

Middleton, Thomas and William Rowely (1990), *The Changeling*, ed. Joost Daalder, London: A. and C. Black.

Milwarde, John (1610), *Jacobs Day of Trouble, and Deliverance. A Sermon preached at Pauls Crosse, the fifth of August 1607. upon his Majesties Deliverance from the Earle of Gowries Treason and Conspiracie*, London, BL, 4479.bb.33. STC 17942.

Montaigne, Michel de (1991), *The Complete Essays*, trans. M. A. Screech, Harmondsworth: Penguin.

More, John (1596), *A Lively Anatomie of Death*, London, BL, 1418.c.44. STC 18073.

Mornay, Philippe de (1592), *Discourse of Life and Death*, trans. Mary Sidney, London, BL, C.57.d.16.

Moryson, Fynes (1907), *The Itinerary of Fynes Moryson*, vol. 1, Glasgow: James MacLehose and Sons Ltd.

A Most certain report of a monster borne at Oteringham in Holdernesse, the 9. of Aprill last past. 1595. Also of a most strange and huge fish, which was driven on the sand at outhorn in holdernesse in February not passing two months before this monster was brought into the world, and within 4 miles distance . . . (1595), London, BL, 1476.b.3. STC 18895.5.

The most cruell and bloody murther committed by an Inkeepers Wife, called Annis Dell . . . With the severall Witchcrafts, and most damnable practises of one Johane Harrison and her Daughter . . . (1606), London, BL, C.27.c.28. STC 6553.

The most strange and admirable discourse of the three Witches of Warboys, arraigned, convicted, and executed at the last Assies at Huntington, for the bewitching of the five daughters of Robert Throckmorton Esquire . . . (1593), London, BL, G.2393. STC 25018.5.

The most wonderfull and true storie, of a certaine Witch named Al[i]se Gooderige of Stapen hill, who was arrainged and convicted at Darbie at the Assises there. As also a true report of the strange torments of Thomas Darling, a boy of thirteene yeres of age, that was possessed by the Devill . . . (1597), London, Lambeth Palace Library, (zz)1597.15. STC 6170.7.

M. R. (c. 1630), *The Mothers Counsell or, Live within Compasse. Being the last Will and Testament to her dearest Daughter, which may serve for a worthy Legacie to all the Women in the World which desire good report from men in this world*, London, BL, Huth 128. STC 20583.

Nashe, Thomas [1589] (1590), *The Anatomie of Absurditie,* London, BL, 96.b.15.(10). STC 20583.

—[1594] (1987), *The Unfortunate Traveler*, in *An Anthology of Elizabethan Prose Fiction*, ed. Paul Salzman, Oxford: Oxford University Press.

Newes from Scotland, Declaring the damnable life and death of Doctor Fian . . . With the true examinations of the saide Doctor and Witches, as they uttered them in the presence of the Scottish King . . . (1591–2), London, Lambeth Palace Library, (zz)1597.15.04. STC 10842.

Normand, Lawrence and Gareth Roberts (2000), *Witchcraft in Early Modern Scotland: James VI's Demonology and the North Berwick Witches*, Exeter: University of Exeter Press.

Palissy, Bernard (1580), *Discours Admirables, de la Nature des Eaux et Fonteines*, Paris, BL, 1171.d.3.

—[1557] (1876), *Resources: A Treatise on 'Water and Springs' Written by Bernard Palissy in 1557*, trans. E. E. Willett, Brighton: W. J. Smith.

Paré, Ambroise (1982), *On Monsters and Marvels*, trans. Janis L. Pallister, Chicago: University of Chicago Press.

Peacham, Henry (1622), *The Compleat Gentleman*, London, BL, C.124.c.8 (1). STC 19052.

Perkins, William (1608), *A Discourse of the Damned Art of Witchcraft, so farre forth as it is revealed in the Scriptures, and manifest by true experience*, Cambridge, BL, 1607/788.(1). STC 19697.

Petronius (1997), *The Satyricon*, trans. P. G. Walsh, Oxford: Oxford University Press.

Pico della Mirandola (1965), *On the Dignity of Man, On Being and the One, Heptaplus*, trans. Charles Glenn Wallis, Paul J. W. Miller and Douglas Carmichael, Indianapolis: Hackett Publishing Company.

Pizan, Christine de (1999), *The Book of the City of Ladies*, trans. Rosalind Brown-Grant, Harmondsworth: Penguin.

A Plaine Description of the Auncient Petigree of Dame Slaunder, togither with hir Coheires and fellow members, Lying, Flattering, Backebyting (1573), London, BL, 245.d.4. STC 22630.

Plato (1921), *Theaetetus*, trans. Harold North Fowler, Loeb Classical Library, Cambridge: Harvard University Press.

—(1993), *Republic*, trans. Robin Waterfield, Oxford: Oxford University Press.

Platter, Thomas (1937), *Thomas Platter's Travels in England 1599*, trans. Clare Williams, London: Jonathan Cape.

Pliny (1942), *Natural History*, trans. H. Rackham, Loeb Classical Library, Cambridge: Harvard University Press.

Plutarch (1603), *Moralia*, trans. Philemon Holland, London, BL, C.74.e.3. STC 200663.

Potts, Thomas (1613), *The Wonderfull Discoverie of Witches in the Countie of Lancaster*, London, BL, C.27.b.37. STC 20138.

Powell, Edgar (1898), *The Register of Bisham Co. Berks.*, London: The Parish Register Society.

Purchas, Samuel (1619), *Purchas his Pilgrim: Microcosmus or the Historie of Man*, London, BL, 1113.b.2. STC 20503.

Purkiss, Diane (ed.) (1998), *Three Tragedies by Renaissance Women*, Harmondsworth: Penguin.

Quintilian (1921), *Institutio Oratoria*, trans. H. E. Butler, Books VII–IX, Loeb Classical Library, Cambridge: Harvard University Press.

Ramelli, Agostino (1588), *Le diverse et artificiose machine*, Paris, BL, G.60.55.

Raynalde, Thomas (1564), *The Birth of Mankynde, otherwyse named the Womans Booke*, London, BL, 1177.h.1. STC 21157 [First edition of 1545, STC 21154].

Reges, Reginae, Nobiles, et Alij in Ecclesia Collegiata B. Petri Westmonasterij Sepulti (1606), London, BL, 578.b.47. STC 4518.

A Rehearsall both straung and true, of hainous and horrible actes committed by Elizabeth Stile, Alias Rockingham, Mother Dutten, Mother Devell, Mother Margaret, Fower notorious Witches, apprehended at Winsore . . . executed, on the 26 daye of Februarie laste Anno. 1579 (1579), London, BL, C.27.a.11. STC 23267.

Returne from Parnassus: or the Scourge of Simony, Part 2 (1949), *The Three Parnassus Plays (1598–1601)*, ed. J. B. Leishman, London: Ivor Nicholson and Watson Ltd.

Richardson, Elizabeth (1645), *A Ladies Legacy to her Daughters*. Presentation edition, Bodleian Library.

Rogers, Thomas (1576), *A Philosophical Discourse, Entituled, The Anatomie of the minde*, London, BL, 1387.a.10. STC 21239.

Rueff, Jacob (1637), *The Expert Midwife, or An Excellent and most necessary treatise of the Generation and Birth of Man*, London, BL, C.112.c.1. STC 21442.

Sadler, John (1636), *The Sicke Womans Private Looking-Glasse*, London, BL, 1175.a.7. STC 21544.

S[alter], T[homas] (1579), *A Mirrhor mete for all Mothers, Matrones, and Maidens, intituled the Mirrhor of Modestie*, London, BL, C.40.a.20. STC 21634.

Scot, Reginald (1584), *The Discoverie of Witchcraft*, London, BL, G.19129. STC 21864.

Serlio, Sebastiano [1619] (1964), *Tutte L'Opere d'Architettura*, ed. Ludovico Roncone, A photographic re-print of the edition published in Venice in 1619, from a copy once in the possession of Inigo Jones . . . Annotations by John Webb, BL, X.423/159.

—[1611] (1982), *The Five Books of Architecture: An Unabridged Reprint of the English Edition of 1611*, New York: Dover Publications.

—(1996), *On Architecture, vol. 1, Books I–V of 'Tutte L'Opere D'Architettura et Prospetiva' by Sebastiano Serlio*, trans. Sebastiano Serlio, Vaughan Hart and Peter Hicks, New Haven: Yale University Press.

Shakespeare, William (1623), *Mr William Shakespeare's Comedies, Histories, and Tragedies: A Facsimile of the First Folio, 1623*, New York and London: Routledge.

—(1962), *The Comedy of Errors*, ed. R. A. Foakes, London: Arden.

—(1987), *Hamlet*, ed. G. R. Hibbard, Oxford: Oxford University Press.

—(1987), *The Tempest*, ed. Stephen Orgel, Oxford: Oxford University Press.

—(1990), *Macbeth*, ed. Nicholas Brooke, Oxford: Oxford University Press.

—(1993), *As You Like It*, ed. Alan Brissenden, Oxford: Oxford University Press.

—(1994), *Twelfth Night*, eds Roger Warren and Stanley Wells, Oxford: Oxford University Press.

—(1995), *Antony and Cleopatra*, ed. John Wilders, London: Arden.

—(1996), *Othello*, ed. E. A. J. Honigmann, Surrey: Arden.

—(1997), *The Norton Shakespeare*, eds Stephen Greenblatt et al., New York and London: W.W. Norton and Company.

—(1997), *King Lear*, ed. R. A. Foakes, Surrey: Arden.

—(1997), *Shakespeare's Sonnets*, ed. Katherine Duncan-Jones, London: Arden.

Sharp, Jane (1999), *The Midwives Book, Or the Whole Art of Midwifry Discovered*, ed. Elaine Hobby, Oxford: Oxford University Press.

Spenser, Edmund (1970), *Complete Poetical Works*, eds J. C. Smith and E. de Selincourt, Oxford: Oxford University Press.

—(1977), *The Faerie Queene*, ed. A. C. Hamilton, London and New York: Longman.

Stone, Nicholas (1919), ed. Walter Lewis Spiers, 'The Note-Book and Account Book of Nicholas Stone', *The Walpole Society VII, 1918–1919*, Oxford: Oxford University Press.

Strachey, William [1610] (1624), *A true repertory of the wracke, and redemption of Sir Thomas Gates . . . from the Ilands of the Bermudas: his coming to Virginia . . . July 15 1610*, included in *Purchas his Pilgrimes*, Part 4, London, BL, 679.h.14. STC 20508.

Strode, George (1632), *The Anatomie of Mortalitie*, London, BL, 875.s.12. STC 23365 [First edition of 1618, STC 23364].

Stuart, Arabella (1994), *The Letters of Lady Arabella Stuart*, ed. Sara Jayne Steen, Oxford: Oxford University Press.

Stubbes, Philip (1583), *The Anatomie of Abuses*, London, BL, G.10369. STC 23376.

Suetonius (1989), *The Twelve Caesars*, trans. Robert Graves, Harmondsworth: Penguin.

Swinburne, Henry (1590), *A Brief Treatise of Testaments and Last Willes*, London, BL, 1609/1399. STC 23547.

T. E. (1632), *The Lawes Resolutions of Womens Rights: or the Lawes Provision for Woemen*, London, BL, 1481.b.46. STC 7437.

Three Sermons or Homelies, To Move Compassion towards the Poor and Needie in these Times (1596), London, BL, 4479.bb.37. STC 13681.

Tradescant, John, the younger (1656), *Musaeum Tradescantianum: or, a Collection of Rarities*, London, BL, 957.d.34. WING T2005.

Traveller, C. (1596), *An Anatomie of the Metamorphosed Ajax*, London, BL, G.10364.(3). STC 12771.5.

A True and Sincere Declaration of the Purpose and Ends of the Plantation Begun in Virginia (1610), London, BL, C.32.d.13. STC 24832a.

Tusser, Thomas (1571), *A Hundreth Good Points of Husbandrie, Lately Maried unto a Hundrethe Good Points of Huswifry . . . with Dyvers Proper Lessons for Housholders*, London, BL, G.11233. STC 24374.

Vaughan, William (1611), *The Spirit of Detraction Conjured and Convicted in Seven Circles*, London, BL, C.122.bb.26. STC 24622.

Vasari, Giorgio (1965), *Lives of the Artists*, vol. 1, trans. George Bull, Harmondsworth: Penguin.

Vesalius, Andreas (1543), *De Humani Corporis Fabrica*, Basel, Wellcome Library, DA.CA.AA5.

—(1949), *The Epitome*, trans. L. R. Lind, New York: Macmillan.

Vicary, Thomas (1577), *A Profitable Treatise of the Anatomie of Mans Body*, London, BL, C.31.b.20. STC 24713.

—(1586), *The Englishe Mans Treasure, or Tresor for Englishmen: With the True Anatomye of Mans Body*, London, Wellcome Library, 6580. STC 24707.

Wagenaer, Lucas [1588] (1590), *The Mariner's Mirrour*, London, BL, MAPS C.8.b.4. STC 24931.

Webster, John (1996), *The Duchess of Malfi and Other Plays*, ed. René Weis, Oxford: Oxford University Press.

Weever, John (1631), *Ancient Funerall Monuments*, London, BL, 209.d.1. STC 25223.

Whyte, Rowland (undated), *The Correspondence of Rowland Whyte and Robert Sidney, first Earl of Leicester*, eds. Michael G. Brennan, Noel J. Kinnamon and Margaret P. Hannay, unpublished version.

Wiffen, J. H. (1833), *Memoirs of the House of Russell from the Time of the Norman Conquest*, vol. 1, London: Longman et al.

Williams, G. (1620), *The Honour of Vertue. Or The Monument erected . . . to the immortall memory of . . . Mrs Elizabeth Crashawe. Who dyed in child-birth*, Oxford, Bodleian Library, MAL.297 (12). STC 6030.

The wonderful discoverie of the Witchcrafts of Margaret and Phillip Flower, daughters of Joan Flower neere Bever Castle: Executed at Lincolne, March 11 1618 (1619), BL, C.27.b.35. STC 11107.

Woolton, John (1576), *A Newe Anatomie of Whole Man, Aswell of his Body, as of his Soule*, London, BL, C.130.a.3.

Wright, Edward (1599), *Hydrographiae Descriptio*, London, BL, MAPS 920.(290.).

Wyrley, William (1592), *The True use of Armorie . . . [showing] the lawfulnes of honorable funerals and moniments . . . advancing of Banners, Ensignes, and marks of noblenesse*, London, BL, C.124.c.8 (2). STC 26062.

W. W. (1582), *A true and just Recorde of the Information, Examination and Confession of all the Witches, taken at S. Oses in the countie of Essex . . .*, London, BL, C.27.a.2. STC 24922.

Young, Sidney (ed.) (1890), *Annals of the Barber-Surgeons of London*, 2 vols, London: East and Blades.

Secondary Sources

Adams, Alice E. (1994), *Reproducing the Womb: Images of Childbirth in Science, Feminist Theory, and Literature*, Ithaca and London: Cornell University Press.

Adams, John Crawford (1989), *Shakespeare's Physic*, London: The Royal Society of Medicine Press.

Janet Adelman, (1992), *Suffocating Mothers: Fantasies of Maternal Origin in Shakespeare's Plays, Hamlet to The Tempest*, New York and London: Routledge.

—(1996), '"Born of Woman": Fantasies of Maternal Power in Macbeth', in Shirley Nelson Garner and Madelon Sprengnether (eds), *Shakespearean Tragedy and Gender*, Bloomington and Indianapolis: Indiana University Press, pp. 105–31.

Alexandratos, Rea (2007), '"With the True Eye of the Lynx": The Paper Museum of Cassiano dal Pozzo', in David Attenborough (ed.), *Amazing Rare Things: The Art of Natural History in the Age of Discovery*, London: Royal Collection Publications, pp. 74–105.

Amico, Leonard N. (1996), *Bernard Palissy: In Search of Earthly Paradise*, Paris and New York: Flammarion.

Anderson, Christy (2000), 'Wild Waters: Hydraulics and the Forces of Nature', in Peter Hulme and William H. Sherman (eds), *The Tempest and Its Travels*, London: Reaktion Books, pp. 41–7.

Anthony, John (1991), *The Renaissance Garden in Britain*, Buckinghamshire: Shire Garden History.

(2006) *Art Classics: Titian*, New York: Rizzoli.

Banks, Amanda Carson (1999), *Birth Chairs, Midwives, and Medicine*, Jackson: University Press of Mississippi.

Barber, Peter, Oliver Cox and Michael Curwen (1993), *Lauderdale Revealed: A History of Lauderdale House, Highgate. The Building, its Owners and Occupiers: 1582–1993*, London: The Lauderdale House Society.

Barkan, Leonard (1981), '"Living Sculptures": Ovid, Michelangelo, and *The Winter's Tale*', *English Literary History* 48: 639–67.

—(1999), *Unearthing the Past: Archaeology and Aesthetics in the Making of Renaissance Culture*, New Haven and London: Yale University Press.

Bell, Millicent (2002), *Shakespeare's Tragic Skepticism*, New Haven and London: Yale University Press.

Belsey, Catherine (2001), *Shakespeare and the Loss of Eden: The Construction of Family Values in Early Modern Culture*, Houndmills: Palgrave.

Bicks, Caroline (2003), *Midwiving Subjects in Shakespeare's England*, Aldershot: Ashgage.

Binski, Paul (1996), *Medieval Death: Ritual and Representation*, London: The British Museum Press.

Bishop, T. G. (1996), *Shakespeare and the Theatre of Wonder*, Cambridge: Cambridge University Press.

Blakiston, Georgiana (1980), *Woburn and the Russells*, London: Constable.

Blanchard, W. Scott (1995), *Scholar's Bedlam: Menippean Satire in the Renaissance*, London and Toronto: Associated University Presses.

Blumenfeld-Kosinski, Renate (1990), *Not of Woman Born: Representations of Caesarean Birth in Medieval and Renaissance Culture*, Ithaca and London: Cornell University Press.

Boose, Lynda E. (1994), 'The 1599 Bishops' Ban, Elizabethan Pornography, and the Sexualization of the Jacobean Stage', in Richard Burt and John Michael Archer (eds), *Enclosure Acts: Sexuality, Property, and Culture in Early Modern England*, Ithaca and London: Cornell University Press, pp. 185–200.

—(2003), '"Let it be hid": The Pornographic Aesthetic of Shakespeare's *Othello*', in Lena Cowen Orlin (ed.), *Othello*, New Casebook Series, London: Palgrave Macmillan, pp. 22–48.

Brockbank, William (1968), 'Old Anatomical Theatres and What Took Place Therein', *Medical History* 12: 371–84.

Brook, Alan and David Brandon (2004), *Tyburn: London's Fatal Tree*, London: Sutton Publishing.

Bunn, I. A. W. (1982), '"A Devil's Shield": Notes on Suffolk Witch-Bottles', *Lantern* 39 (Autumn): 3–7.

Burnett, Mark Thornton (2002), *Constructing 'Monsters' in Shakespearean Drama and Early Modern Culture*, Houndmills: Palgrave.

Bynum, Caroline Walker (1982), *Jesus as Mother: Studies in the Spirituality of the High Middle Ages*, Berkeley: University of California Press.

—(1992), *Fragmentation and Redemption: Essays on Gender and the Human Body in Medieval Religion*, New York: Zone Books.
Calbi, Maurizio (1995), *Approximate Bodies: Gender and Power in Early Modern Drama and Anatomy*, New York and London: Routledge.
Campbell, Oscar James (1959), *Comicall Satyre and Shakespeare's Troilus and Cressida*, San Marino: Huntingdon Library.
Carlino, Andrea (1994), *Books of the Body: Anatomical Ritual and Renaissance Learning*, trans. John Tedeschi and Anne C. Tedeschi, Chicago and London: University of Chicago Press.
—(1999), *Paper Bodies: A Catalogue of Anatomical Fugitive Sheets 1538–1687*, trans. Noga Arikha, Medical History, Supplement 19, London: The Wellcome Institute for the History of Medicine.
Cassidy, Tina (2007), *Birth: A History*, London: Chatto and Windus.
Castiglioni, Arturo (1941), 'The Origin and Development of the Anatomical Theater to the End of the Renaissance', *Ciba Symposia* 3: 841–2.
Charney, Maurice (1988), *Hamlet's Fictions*, New York and London: Routledge.
Clark, Stuart (2001), *Languages of Witchcraft: Narrative, Ideology and Meaning in Early Modern Culture*, London: Macmillan Press.
Cleugh, James (1965), *The Divine Aretino: Pietro of Arezzo, 1492–1556: A Biography*, London: Anthony Blond.
Cohen, Nathalie (1997), 'The Hall of the Barber Surgeons', *London Archaeologist* 8 (6) (Autumn): 162–7.
Coppedge, Walter R. (1998), 'The Joy of the Worm: Dying in Antony and Cleopatra', *Renaissance Papers*: 41–50.
Corbin, Peter and Douglas Sedge (eds) (1986), *Three Jacobean Witchcraft Plays: The Tragedy of Sophonisba, The Witch, The Witch of Edmonton*, Manchester: Manchester University Press.
Cressy, David (1993), 'Purification, Thanksgiving and the Churching of Women in Post-Reformation England', *Past and Present* 141: 106–46.
—(1999), *Birth, Marriage and Death: Ritual, Religion, and the Life-Cycle in Tudor and Stuart England*, Oxford: Oxford University Press.
—(2000), *Travesties and Transgressions in Tudor and Stuart England*, Oxford: Oxford University Press.
Croft, Pauline and Karen Hearn (2003), ' "Only matrimony maketh children to be certain . . ." Two Elizabethan Pregnancy Portraits', *The British Art Journal* 3 (3) (Autumn): 19–24.
Crystal, David and Ben Crystal (2002), *Shakespeare's Words: A Glossary and Language Companion*, London: Penguin.
Cunningham, Andrew (2000), 'Luther and Vesalius', in Keith Whitlock (ed.), *The Renaissance in Europe: A Reader*, New Haven and London: Yale University Press, pp. 275–87.
Daston, Lorraine and Katharine Park (1998), *Wonders and the Order of Nature 1150–1750*, New York: Zone Books.
Daston, Lorraine (1999), 'Marvelous Facts and Miraculous Evidence in Early Modern Europe', in Peter G. Platt (ed.), *Wonders, Marvels, and Monsters in Early Modern Culture*, Newark: University of Delaware Press, pp. 76–104.
Davidson, Jane P. (1987), *The Witch in Northern European Art, 1470–1750*, Science and Research, vol. 2, Freren: Luca Verlag.

Davies-Floyed, E. and Carolyn F. Sargent (1997), *Childbirth and Authoritative Knowledge: Cross-Cultural Perspectives*, Berkeley, Los Angeles and London: University of California Press.

Demand, Nancy (1994), *Birth, Death and Motherhood in Classical Greece*, Baltimore and London: Johns Hopkins University Press.

Dewhurst, John (1980), 'The Alleged Miscarriages of Catherine of Aragon and Anne Boleyn', *Medical History* 28: 49–56.

(1994), *Dictionary of Mythology*, London: Chancellor Press.

Dobson, Jessie and R. Milnes Walker (1979), *Barbers and Barber-Surgeons of London*, Oxford: Alden Press.

Dobson, Michael and Stanley Wells (2001), *The Oxford Companion to Shakespeare*, Oxford: Oxford University Press.

Dolan, Frances E. (1994), *Dangerous Familiars: Representations of Domestic Crime in England 1550–1700*, Ithaca and London: Cornell University Press.

Donnison, Jean (1988), *Midwives and Medical Men: A History of the Struggle for the Control of Childbirth*, New Barnet: Historical Publications.

Dubrow, Heather (1999), *Shakespeare and Domestic Loss: Forms of Deprivation, Mourning and Recuperation*, Cambridge: Cambridge University Press.

Duden, Barbara (1993), *Disembodying Women: Perspectives on Pregnancy and the Unborn*, trans. Lee Hoinacki, Cambridge: Harvard University Press.

Duffy, Eamon (1992), *The Stripping of the Altars: Traditional Religion in England 1400–1580*, New Haven: Yale University Press.

Duncan-Jones, Katherine (2001), *Ungentle Shakespeare: Scenes from his Life*, London: Arden.

Dunstan, G. R. (ed.) (1990), *The Human Embryo: Aristotle and the Arabic and European Traditions*, Exeter: University of Exeter Press.

Eccles, Audrey (1982), *Obstetrics and Gynaecology in Tudor and Stuart England*, London: Croom Helm.

Egmond, Florike (2003), 'Execution, Dissection, Pain and Infamy – A Morphological Investigation', in Florike Egmond and Robert Zwijnenberg (eds), *Bodily Extremities: Preoccupations with the Human Body in Early Modern European Culture*, Aldershot: Ashgate, pp. 92–128.

Erickson, Amy Louise (1993), *Women and Property in Early Modern England*, New York and London: Routledge.

Esdaile, Katharine A. (1927), *English Monumental Sculpture since the Renaissance*, New York and Toronto: Macmillan.

Ferrari, Giovanna (1987), 'Public Anatomy Lessons and the Carnival: The Anatomy Theatre of Bologna', *Past and Present* 117: 50–106.

Fildes, Valerie (ed.) (1990), *Women as Mothers in Pre-Industrial England*, New York and London: Routledge.

Findlen, Paula (1989), 'The Museum: Its Classical Etymology and Renaissance Genealogy', *Journal of the History of Collections* 1 (1): 59–78.

Finucci, Valeria and Kevin Brownlee (eds) (2001), *Generation and Degeneration: Tropes of Reproduction in Literature and History from Antiquity to Early Modern Europe*, Durham and London: Duke University Press.

Fissell, Mary E. (2004), *Vernacular Bodies: The Politics of Reproduction in Early Modern England*, Oxford: Oxford University Press.

Forbes, Thomas R. (1962), 'Midwifery and Witchcraft', *Journal of the History of Medicine* 17: 264–83.

Fox, Alice (1979), 'Obstetrics and Gynecology in *Macbeth*', *Shakespeare Studies* 12: 127–41.

Fraser, Antonia (1984), *The Weaker Vessel: A Woman's Lot in Seventeenth-Century England*, London: Phoenix Press.

Freedberg, David (2002), *The Eye of the Lynx: Galileo, his Friends, and the Beginnings of Modern Natural History*, Chicago and London: University of Chicago Press.

French, Roger (1999), *Dissection and Vivisection in the European Renaissance*, Aldershot: Ashgate.

Frye, Roland Mushat (1984), *The Renaissance Hamlet: Issues and Responses in 1600*, Princeton: Princeton University Press.

Gaimster, David (1997), *German Stoneware 1200–1900*, London: British Museum Press.

Gaskill, Malcolm (2005), *Witchfinders: A Seventeenth-Century English Tragedy*, London: John Murray.

Gelis, Jacques (1991), *History of Childbirth: Fertility, Pregnancy and Birth in Early Modern Europe*, Cambridge: Polity Press.

Gittings, Clare (1984), *Death, Burial and the Individual in Early Modern England*, Sydney: Croom Helm.

Goodare, Julian (ed.) (2002), *The Scottish Witch-Hunt in Context*, Manchester: Manchester University Press.

Gowing, Laura (2003), *Common Bodies: Women, Touch and Power in Seventeenth-Century England*, New Haven and London: Yale University Press.

Gray, Lisa (undated), *Assessment of Bottle Contents from a Pit, High Street, Guildford, TVAS, HSG 01/08 TS, SU 99600 49490*, unpublished.

Grazia, Margreta de (1996), 'Imprints: Shakespeare, Gutenberg and Descartes', in Terence Hawkes (ed.), *Alternative Shakespeares*, vol. 2, New York and London: Routledge, pp. 63–94.

Greenfield, Susan C. and Carol Barash (eds) (1999), *Inventing Maternity: Politics, Science, and Literature, 1650–1865*, Kentucky: The University Press of Kentucky.

Gurr, Andrew (1992), *The Shakespearean Stage 1574–1642*, Cambridge: Cambridge University Press.

Hackett, Helen (1995), *Virgin Mother, Maiden Queen: Elizabeth I and the Cult of the Virgin Mary*, London: Macmillan.

—(1999), ' "Gracious be the Issue": Maternity and Narrative in Shakespeare's Late Plays', in Jennifer Richards and James Knowles (eds), *Shakespeare's Late Plays: New Readings*, Edinburgh: Edinburgh University Press, pp. 25–39.

Harcourt, Glenn (1987), 'Andreas Vesalius and the Anatomy of Antique Sculpture', *Representations* 17: 28–61.

Harley, David (1990), 'Historians as Demonologists: The Myth of the Midwife-Witch', *Social History of Medicine* 3: 1–26.

Harris, John and A. A. Tait (1979), *Catalogue of the Drawings by Inigo Jones, John Webb and Isaac de Caus at Worchester College Oxford*, Oxford: Clarendon Press, Warburg Institute, CML 230.

Hart-Davis, Adam (2002), *What the Tudors and Stuarts Did for Us*, London: Macmillan.

Hawkes, Nigel (1997), 'Grisly Surgery Site Discovered', *The Times*, 3 September, Guildhall Library, A.45/9.

Headley, Gwyn and Wim Meulenkamp (1986), *Follies, Grottoes, and Garden Buildings*, London: Aurum Press.

Heal, Felicity (1984), 'The Idea of Hospitality in Early Modern England', *Past and Present* 102 (February): 66–93.

—(1996), 'Reputation and Honour in Court and Country: Lady Elizabeth Russell and Sir Thomas Hoby', *Transactions of the Royal Historical Society* 6: 161–77.

Hearn, Karen (2000), 'A Fatal Fertility? Elizabethan and Jacobean Pregnancy Portraits', *Costume: The Journal of the Costume Society* 34: 39–43.

—(2002), *Marcus Gheeraerts II, Elizabethan Artist: In Focus*, London: Tate Publishing.

Held, Julius S. (1982), 'Rubens and Titian', in David Rosand (ed.), *Titian: His World and His Legacy*, New York: Columbia University Press, pp. 312–20.

Hellegers, Desiree (2000), *Handmaid to Divinity: Natural Philosophy, Poetry, and Gender in Seventeenth-Century England*, Norman: University of Oklahoma Press.

Henderson, Paula (2005), *The Tudor House and Garden: Architecture and Landscape in the Sixteenth and Seventeenth Centuries*, New Haven and London: Yale University Press.

Herrlinger, Robert and Edith Feiner (1964), 'Why did Vesalius not Discover the Fallopian Tubes?', *Medical History* 8: 335–41.

Highet, Gilbert (1962), *The Anatomy of Satire*, Princeton: Princeton University Press.

Hodges, Devon L. (1985), *Renaissance Fictions of Anatomy*, Amherst: University of Massachusetts Press.

Holmes, Clive (1993), 'Women: Witnesses and Witches', *Past and Present* 140 (August): 45–78.

Houlbrooke, Ralph (1998), *Death, Religion and the Family in England 1480–1750*, Oxford: Clarendon Press.

Hulme, Peter and William H. Sherman (eds) (2000), *The Tempest and its Travels*, London: Reaktion Books.

Hunt, John Dixon (1996), *Garden and Grove: The Italian Renaissance Garden in the English Imagination 1600–1750*, Philadelphia: University of Pennsylvania Press.

Jackson, Hazelle (2001), *Shell Houses and Grottoes*, Buckinghamshire: Shire Publications.

Janson, H.W. (1946), 'Titian's Laocoön Caricature and the Vesalian-Galenist Controversy', *Art Bulletin* 28: 49–56.

Jardine, Lisa (1993), *Erasmus, Man of Letters: The Construction of Charisma in Print*, Princeton: Princeton University Press.

—(1996), *Worldly Goods: A New History of the Renaissance*, London: Macmillan.

Kahn, Coppélia (1986), 'The Absent Mother in *King Lear*', in Margaret W. Ferguson, Maureen Quilligan and Nancy J. Vickers (eds), *Rewriting the*

Renaissance: The Discourses of Sexual Difference in Early Modern Europe, Chicago: University of Chicago Press, pp. 33–49.
Kaplan, E. Ann (1994), 'Sex, Work, and Motherhood: Maternal Subjectivity in Recent Visual Culture', in Donna Bassin, Margaret Honey and Meryle Mahrer Kaplan (eds), *Representations of Motherhood*, New Haven and London: Yale University Press, pp. 256–71.
Kay, Dennis (1999), 'Who says "Miracles Are Past?": Some Jacobean Marvels and the Margins of the Known', in Peter G. Platt (ed.), *Wonders, Marvels, and Monsters in Early Modern Culture*, Newark: University of Delaware Press, pp. 164–86.
Keele, Kenneth D. (1964), 'Leonado da Vinci's Influence on Renaissance Anatomy', *Medical History* 8: 360–70.
Kellett, C. E. (1964), 'Two Anatomies', *Medical History* 8: 342–53.
Kemp, Martin (2000), *Visualizations: The Nature Book of Art and Science*, Oxford: Oxford University Press.
—(2006), *Seen/Unseen: Art, Science, and Intuition from Leonardo to the Hubble Telescope*, Oxford: Oxford University Press.
Kennedy, Ian G. (2006), *Titian*, Köln and London: Taschen.
Kieckhefer, Richard (1989), *Magic in the Middle Ages*, Cambridge: Cambridge University Press.
Korda, Natasha (2002), *Shakespeare's Domestic Economies: Gender and Property in Early Modern England*, Philadelphia: University of Pennsylvania Press.
Kozikowski, Stanley J. (1980), 'The Gowrie Conspiracy against James VI: A New Source for Shakespeare's *Macbeth*', *Shakespeare Studies* 13: 197–212.
Krier, Theresa M. (2001), *Birth Passages: Maternity and Nostalgia, Antiquity to Shakespeare*, Ithaca and London: Cornell University Press.
Kuriyama, Constance Brown (1977), 'Mother of the World: A Psychoanalytic Interpretation of Shakespeare's *Antony and Cleopatra*', *English Literary Renaissance* 7: 324–51.
Kusukawa, Sachiko (1995), *The Transformation of Natural Philosophy: The Case of Philip Melanchthon*, Cambridge: Cambridge University Press.
La Belle, Jenijoy (1980), ' "A Strange Infirmity": Lady Macbeth's Amenorrhea', *Shakespeare Quarterly* 31: 381–6.
Laoutaris, Chris (2007), 'Speaking Stones: Memory and Maternity in Shakespeare's *Antony and Cleopatra*', in Kathryn M. Moncrief and Kathryn R. McPherson (eds), *Performing Maternity in Early Modern England*, Aldershot: Ashgate, pp. 143–69.
Larner, Christina (1981), *Enemies of God: The Witch-Hunt in Scotland*, Edinburgh: John Donald.
Lind, Levi Robert (1975), *Studies in Pre-Vesalian Anatomy: Biography, Translations, Documents*, Philadelphia: The American Philosophical Society.
Llewellyn, Nigel (1991), *The Art of Death: Visual Culture in the English Death Ritual c. 1500–c. 1800*, London: Reaktion Books.
—(1996), 'Honour in Life, Death and in the Memory: Funeral Monuments in Early Modern England', *Transactions of the Royal Historical Society* 6: 179–200.
—(2001), *Funeral Monuments in Post-Reformation England*, Cambridge: Cambridge University Press.

Lupton, Julia Reinhard (2000), 'Creature Caliban', *Shakespeare Quarterly* 51 (1): 1–23.

MacDonald, Michael (1981), *Mystical Bedlam: Madness, Anxiety, and Healing in Seventeenth-Century England*, Cambridge: Cambridge University Press.

—(ed.) (1991), *Witchcraft and Hysteria in Elizabethan London: Edward Jorden and the Mary Glover Case*, New York and London: Tavistock/Routledge.

MacFarlane, Alan (1970), *Witchcraft in Tudor and Stuart England: A Regional and Comparative Study*, New York and London: Routledge.

Maloney, Catherine (1980), 'A Witch-Bottle from Dukes Place, Aldgate', *Transactions of the London & Middlesex Archaeological Society* 31: 157–8.

Marchitello, Howard (1997), 'Shakespeare's *Othello* and Vesalius's *Fabrica*: Anatomy, Gender, and the Narrative Production of Meaning', in *Narrative and Meaning in Early Modern England: Browne's Skull and Other Histories*, Cambridge: Cambridge University Press, pp. 10–38.

Massey, Alan (2003), 'Spooky or What?', *Period House Magazine* (November): 92–5.

—(undated), *The Bedfordshire Witch Bottle: A Preliminary Report*, unpublished.

—Brian Hoggard, Patrick Stone and Andrew Wilson (2004), 'The Felmersham Witch Bottle', *Bedfordshire County Magazine*: 7–8.

Massey, Alan, Roger M. Smith, Tim A. D. Smith (2003), 'A Witch Bottle from Dorset', *Education in Chemistry* (July): 97–100.

Mauries, Patrick (2002), *Cabinets of Curiosities*, London: Thames and Hudson.

McLaren, Angus (1984), *Reproductive Rituals: The Perception of Fertility in England from the Sixteenth to the Nineteenth Century*, London and New York: Methuen.

Medine, Peter E. (1976), 'Isaac Casaubon's *Prolegomena* to the *Satires* of Persius: An Introduction, Text and Translation', *English Literary Renaissance* 6 (3) (Autumn): 271–98.

Mendelson, Sara and Patricia Crawford (1998), *Women in Early Modern England 1550–1720*, Oxford: Clarendon press.

Merchant, Carolyn (1980), *The Death of Nature: Women, Ecology and the Scientific Revolution*, San Francisco: Harper Collins.

Merrifield, Ralph (1969), 'Folk-Lore in London Archaeology, Part 2: The Post-Roman Period', *London Archaeologist* 2: 99–104.

—(1987), *The Archaeology of Ritual and Magic*, London: B. T. Batsford.

—and Norman Smedley (1958–60), 'Two Witch-Bottles from Suffolk', *Proceedings of the Suffolk Institute of Archaeology* 28: 97–101.

Miller, Naomi (1982), *Heavenly Caves: Reflections on the Garden Grotto*, Boston, London and Sydney: George Allen and Unwin.

Miller, Naomi J. and Naomi Yavneh (eds) (2000), *Maternal Measures: Figuring Caregiving in the Early Modern Period*, Aldershot: Ashgate.

Moncrief, Kathryn M. and Kathryn R. McPherson (eds) (2007), *Performing Maternity in Early Modern England*, Aldershot: Ashgate.

Moncrief, Moncrief M. (2007), ' "Show me a child begotten of thy body that I am father to": Pregnancy, Paternity and the Problem of Evidence in *All's Well That Ends Well*', in Kathryn M. Moncrief and Kathryn R. McPherson (eds), *Performing Maternity in Early Modern England*, Aldershot: Ashgate, pp. 29–43.

Morley, Henry (1855), *Palissy the Potter*, London: Chapman and Hall.

Mullaney, Steven (1980), 'Lying like Truth: Riddle, Representation and Treason in Renaissance England', *English Literary History* 47: 32–47.

Mussachio, Jacqueline Marie (1999), *The Art and Ritual of Childbirth in Renaissance Italy*, New Haven and London: Yale University Press.

Needham, Joseph (1959), *A History of Embryology*, Cambridge: Cambridge University Press.

Neill, Michael (1997), 'Opening the Moor: Death and Discovery in *Othello*', in *Issues of Death: Mortality and Identity in English Renaissance Tragedy*, Oxford: Clarendon Press, pp. 141–67.

Newman, Karen (1996), *Fetal Positions: Individualism, Science, Visuality*, Stanford: Stanford University Press.

Newman, William (1999), 'The Homunculus and his Forebears: Wonders of Art and Nature', in Anthony Grafton and Nancy Siraisi (eds), *Natural Particulars: Nature and the Disciplines in Renaissance Europe*, Cambridge and London: MIT Press, pp. 321–45.

Nilsson, Lennart (1990), *A Child Is Born*, London and New York: Doubleday.

Nunn, Hillary M. (2005), *Staging Anatomies: Dissection and Spectacle in Early Stuart Tragedy*, Aldershot: Ashgate.

Nutton, Vivian (2000), 'Wittenberg Anatomy', in Keith Whitlock (ed.), *The Renaissance in Europe: A Reader*, New Haven and London: Yale University Press, pp. 290–300.

O'Malley, C. D. (1964), *Andreas Vesalius of Brussels 1514–1564*, Berkeley: University of California Press.

Orrell, John (1988), *The Human Stage: English Theatre Design 1567–1640*, Cambridge: Cambridge University Press.

Page-Phillips, John (1970), *Children on Brasses*, London: Allen and Unwin.

Paige, Karen Ericksen and Jeffery M. Paige (1981), *The Politics of Reproductive Ritual*, Berkeley, Los Angeles and London: University of California Press.

Park, Katherine (1994), 'The Criminal and the Saintly Body: Autopsy and Dissection in Renaissance Italy', *Renaissance Quarterly* 47: 1–33.

—(1999), 'Natural Particulars: Medical Epistemology, Practice, and the Literature of Healing Springs', in Anthony Grafton and Nancy Siraisi (eds), *Natural Particulars: Nature and the Disciplines in Renaissance Europe*, Cambridge: MIT Press, pp. 347–67.

—(2006), *Secrets of Women: Gender, Generation, and the Origins of Human Dissection*, New York: Zone Books.

Parker, Patricia (1996), *Othello* and *Hamlet*: Spying, Discovery, Secret Faults', in *Shakespeare from the Margins: Language, Culture, Context*, Chicago: University of Chicago Press.

Paster, Gail Kern (1993), *The Body Embarassed: Drama and the Disciplines of Shame in Early Modern England*, Ithaca and London: Cornell University Press.

Platt, Peter G. (1997), *Reason Diminished: Shakespeare and the Marvelous*, Lincoln and London: University of Nebraska Press.

—(ed.) (1999), *Wonders, Marvels, and Monsters in Early Modern Culture*, Newark: University of Delaware Press.

Plumwood, Val (1993), *Feminism and the Mastery of Nature*, New York and London: Routledge.

Pomata, Gianna (2001), 'Menstruating Men: Similarity and Difference of the Sexes in Early Modern Medicine', in Valeria Finucci and Kevin Brownlee (eds), *Generation and Degeneration: Tropes of Reproduction in Literature and History from Antiquity through Early Modern Europe*, Durham and London: Duke University Press, pp. 109–52.

Potter, Jennifer (2006), *Strange Blooms: The Curious Lives and Adventures of the John Tradescants*, London: Atlantic Books.

Power, D'Arcy K. B. E. (1912), *Notes on the Early Portraits of John Banister, of William Harvey, and the Barber-Surgeon's Visceral Lecture in 1581 . . . Reprinted from the Proceedings of the Royal Society of Medicine*, BL, 10.804.h.19(2).

Preus, Anthony (1970), 'Science and Philosophy in Aristotle's *Generation of Animals*', *Journal of the History of Biology* 3: 1–52.

—(1977), 'Galen's Criticism of Aristotle's Conception Theory', *Journal of the History of Biology* 10: 65–85.

Prior, Mary (1990), 'Wives and Wills 1558–1700', in John Chartres and David Hey (eds), *English Rural Society, 1500–1800: Essays in Honour of Joan Thirsk*, Cambridge: Cambridge University Press, pp. 201–25.

Pryor, Felix (1992), *The Mirror and the Globe: William Shakespeare, John Marston and the Writing of Hamlet*, London: Handsaw.

Purkiss, Diane (1996), *The Witch in History: Early Modern and Twentieth-Century Representations*, New York and London: Routledge.

Pye, Christopher (2000), *The Vanishing: Shakespeare, the Subject, and Early Modern Culture*, Durham and London: Duke University Press.

Randolph, Mary Claire (1941), 'The Medical Concept in English Renaissance Satiric Theory: Its Possible Relationships and Implications', *Studies in Philology* 38 (2) (April): 125–57.

Rath, Gernot (1964), 'Charles Estienne: Contemporary of Vesalius', *Medical History* 8: 354–9.

Rhodes, Neil (2006), 'Hamlet and Humanism', in *Early Modern English Drama: A Critical Companion*, Oxford: Oxford University Press, 2006, pp. 120–9.

Rich, Adrienne (1986), *Of Woman Born: Motherhood as Experience and Institution*, New York and London: W. W. Norton and Company.

Rifkin, Benjamin A., Michael J. Ackerman and Judith Folkenberg (2006), *Human Anatomy: Depicting the Body from the Renaissance to Today*, London: Thames and Hudson.

Roberts, K. B. and J. D. W. Tomlinson (1992), *The Fabric of the Body: European Traditions of Anatomical Illustration*, Oxford: Oxford University Press.

Rose, Jacqueline (1986), *Sexuality in the Field of Vision*, London and New York: Verso.

Rose, Mary Beth (1991), 'Where are the Mothers in Shakespeare? Options for Gender Representation in the English Renaissance', *Shakespeare Quarterly* 42 (fall): 291–314.

(1925) *Royal Commission on Historical Monuments (England)*, London West, vol. 2, London: HM Stationery Office.

Russell, Elizabeth (Hoby) [1605] (2001), *A Way of Reconciliation of a Good and Learned Man, Touching the . . . Sacrament*, London, *The Early Modern*

Englishwoman: A Facsimile Library of Essential Works, Protestant Translators: Anne Lock Prowse and Elizabeth Russell, Series I, Printed Writings, 1500–1640, Part 2, vol. 12, ed. Elaine V. Beilin, Aldershot: Ashgate.

Sacks, Elizabeth (1980), *Shakespeare's Images of Pregnancy*, London: Macmillan.

Saunders, J. B. de C. M. and Charles D. O'Malley (1950), *The Illustrations from the Works of Andreas Vesalius of Brussels*, New York: Dover Publications.

Sawday, Jonathan (1990), 'The Fate of Marsyas: Dissecting the Renaissance Body', in Lucy Gent and Nigel Llewellyn (eds), *Renaissance Bodies: The Human Figure in English Culture c.1540–1660*, London: Reaktion Books, pp. 111–35.

—(1995), *The Body Emblazoned: Dissection and the Human Body in Renaissance Culture*, New York and London: Routledge.

Saxl, F. (1939), 'Pagan Sacrifice in the Italian Renaissance', *Journal of the Warburg and Courtauld Institutes* 2: 346–67.

Schleiner, Louise (1994), *Tudor and Stuart Women Writers*, Bloomington and Indianapolis: Indiana University Press.

Schoenbaum, S. (1977), *William Shakespeare: A Compact Documentary Life*, Oxford: Oxford University Press.

Schoenfeldt, Michael C. (1999), *Bodies and Selves in Early Modern England: Physiology and Inwardness in Spenser, Shakespeare, Herbert and Milton*, Cambridge: Cambridge University Press.

Schofield, J. R. Lear (forthcoming), *Holy Trinity Priory, Aldgate, City of London: An Archaeological Reconstruction and History*, MoLAS Monogr Ser.

Schulz, Eva (1990), 'Notes on the History of Collecting and of Museums: In the Light of Selected Literature of the Sixteenth to the Eighteenth Century', *Journal of the History of Collections* 2 (2): 205–18.

Sharpe, J. A. (1991), 'Witchcraft and Women in Seventeenth-Century England: Some Northern Evidence', *Continuity and Change* 6 (2): 179–99.

—(2001), *Witchcraft in Early Modern England*, London: Longman.

Slater, Miriam (1984), *Family Life in the Seventeenth Century: The Verneys of Claydon House*, London: Routledge and Kegan Paul.

Smedley, Norman and Elizabeth Owles (1964–6), 'More Suffolk Witch-Bottles', *Proceedings of the Suffolk Institute of Archaeology* 30: 84–93.

Smith, Bruce R. (1985), 'Sermons in Stones: Shakespeare and Renaissance Sculpture', *Shakespeare Studies* 17: 1–23.

Sparti, Donatella L. (1990), 'Carlo Antonio Dal Pozzo (1606–1689): An Unknown Collector', *Journal of the History of Collections* 2 (1): 7–19.

Stonehouse, Julia (1994), *Idols to Incubators: Reproduction Theory through the Ages*, London: Scarlet Press.

Strong, Roy (1979), *The Renaissance Garden in England*, London: Thames and Hudson.

—(1987), *Gloriana: Portraits of Queen Elizabeth I*, London: Pimlico.

Swann, June (1996), 'Shoes Concealed in Buildings', *Costume* 30: 56–9, at www.apotropaios.co.uk.

Talvacchia, Bette (1999), *Taking Positions: On the Erotic in Renaissance Culture*, Princeton: Princeton University Press.

Tanner, James M. and Gordon Rattray Taylor (eds) (1968), *Life Science Library: Growth*, London and Holland: Time-Life International.

Thomas, Keith (1971), *Religion and the Decline of Magic: Studies in Popular Beliefs in Sixteenth- and Seventeenth-Century England*, Harmondsworth: Penguin.

Twyman, Mick (2006), 'The Mystery of Margate's Shell Temple', *Bygone Kent* (September/October), at www.shellgrotto.co.uk

Waddington, Raymond B. (2004), *Aretino's Satyr: Sexuality, Satire and Self-Projection in Sixteenth-Century Literature and Art*, Toronto: University of Toronto Press.

Wall, Wendy (1993), *The Imprint of Gender: Authorship and Publication in the English Renaissance*, Ithaca and London: Cornell University Press.

Warner, Marina (2000), '"The foul witch" and Her "freckled whelp": Circean Mutations in the New World', in Peter Hulme and William H. Sherman (eds), *The Tempest and Its Travels*, London: Reaktion Books, pp. 97–113.

Weis, René (2007), *Shakespeare Revealed: A Biography*, London: John Murray.

Whitfield, Peter (1998), *New Found Lands: Maps in the History of Exploration*, London: The British Library.

Willis, Deborah (1994), 'Shakespeare and the English Witch-Hunts: Enclosing the Maternal Body', in Richard Burt and John Michael Archer (eds), *Enclosure Acts: Sexuality, Property, and Culture in Early Modern England*, Ithaca and London: Cornell University Press, pp. 96–120.

—(1995), *Malevolent Nurture: Witch-Hunting and Maternal Power in Early Modern England*, Ithaca and London: Cornell University Press.

Willis, Gary (1995), *Witches and Jesuits: Shakespeare's Macbeth*, Oxford: Oxford University Press.

Wilson, Adrian (1985), 'Participant or Patient? Seventeenth-Century Childbirth from the Mother's Point of View', in Roy Porter (ed.), *Patients and Practitioners: Lay Perceptions of Medicine in Pre-Industrial Society*, Cambridge: Cambridge University Press, pp. 129–144.

—(1990), 'The Ceremony of Childbirth and its Interpretation', in Valerie Fildes (ed.), *Women as Mothers in Pre-Industrial England: Essays in Memory of Dorothy McLaren*, New York and London: Routledge, pp. 68–107.

Wilson, Jean (1995), *The Shakespeare Legacy: The Material Legacy of Shakespeare's Theatre*, Surrey: Bramley Books.

Wilson, Richard (1994), 'Observations on English Bodies: Licensing Maternity in Shakespeare's Late Plays', in Richard Burt and John Michael Archer (eds), *Enclosure Acts: Sexuality, Property, and Culture in Early Modern England*, Ithaca and London: Cornell University Press, pp. 121–50.

—(2004), *Secret Shakespeare: Studies in Theatre, Religion and Resistance*, Manchester: Manchester University Press.

Wilson, Violet A. (1924), *Society Women of Shakespeare's Time*, London: John Lane, The Bodley Head Limited.

(2000), *Woburn Abbey*, Norwich: Woburn Abbey and Jarrold Publishing.

Wood, Michael (2003), *In Search of Shakespeare*, London: BBC.

Wroe-Brown, Robin (1998), *Barber-Surgeons Hall Garden: An Archaeological Research Evaluation* (May), Museum of London Archaeology Service: unpublished.

Zimmerman, Susan (2005), *The Early Modern Corpse and Shakespeare's Theatre*, Edinburgh: Edinburgh University Press.

Index

Entries in *italic* refer to illustrations.